The
Other Side
of
Psychotherapy

Edited by Jairo N. Fuertes

The Other Side of Psychotherapy

Understanding Clients' Experiences
and Contributions in Treatment

 AMERICAN PSYCHOLOGICAL ASSOCIATION

Published by
American Psychological Association
750 First Street, NE
Washington, DC 20002
https://www.apa.org

Order Department
https://www.apa.org/pubs/books
order@apa.org

In the U.K., Europe, Africa, and the Middle East, copies may be ordered from Eurospan
https://www.eurospanbookstore.com/apa
info@eurospangroup.com

Typeset in Meridien and Ortodoxa by Circle Graphics, Inc., Reisterstown, MD

Printer: Gasch Printing, Odenton, MD
Cover Designer: Anthony Paular Design, Newbury Park, CA

Library of Congress Cataloging-in-Publication Data

Names: Fuertes, Jairo, editor.
Title: The other side of psychotherapy : understanding clients' experiences
  and contributions in treatment / Jairo N Fuertes.
Description: Washington, DC : American Psychological Association, [2022] |
  Includes bibliographical references and index.
Identifiers: LCCN 2022003021 (print) | LCCN 2022003022 (ebook) |
  ISBN 9781433835858 (paperback) | ISBN 9781433835841 (ebook)
Subjects: LCSH: Client-centered psychotherapy. | Experiential
  psychotherapy. | Mental health counseling--Methodology. | BISAC:
  PSYCHOLOGY / Clinical Psychology | PSYCHOLOGY / Psychotherapy /
  Counseling
Classification: LCC RC481 .O84 2022 (print) | LCC RC481 (ebook) |
  DDC 616.89/14--dc23/eng/20220224
LC record available at https://lccn.loc.gov/2022003021
LC ebook record available at https://lccn.loc.gov/2022003022

https://doi.org/10.1037/0000303-000

Printed in the United States of America

10 9 8 7 6 5 4 3 2 1

I would like to dedicate my portion of the work in this book to my wife, Hnin, and my daughters, Sofia and Isabella. I also dedicate my work to my loving big brother, Pedro H. Fuertes, and to Mr. James Coyle, who taught me English as a second language the summer after I arrived in the United States. Finally, in the spirit of this book, I dedicate my work to my wonderful clients, who have taught me so much about the process and outcome of psychotherapy.
—JAIRO N. FUERTES

CONTENTS

CONTRIBUTORS

Timothy Anderson, PhD, Department of Psychology, Ohio University, Athens, OH, United States

Arthur C. Bohart, PhD, California State University, Dominguez Hills, Carson, CA, and Counseling Psychology Department, Santa Clara University, Santa Clara, CA, United States

James F. Boswell, PhD, Department of Psychology, University at Albany, State University of New York, Albany, NY, United States

Kathleen M. Collins, MA, Department of Psychology, University of Massachusetts Boston, Boston, MA, United States

Michael J. Constantino, PhD, Department of Psychological and Brain Sciences, University of Massachusetts Amherst, Amherst, MA, United States

Danielle M. Cook, BS, Department of Psychology, University of Scranton, Scranton, PA, United States

Alice E. Coyne, PhD, Department of Psychological Sciences, Case Western Reserve University, Cleveland, OH, United States

Jairo N. Fuertes, PhD, ABPP, LMHC, Gordon F. Derner School of Psychology, Adelphi University, Garden City, NY, United States

Averi N. Gaines, MA, Department of Psychological and Brain Sciences, University of Massachusetts Amherst, Amherst, MA, United States

Charles J. Gelso, PhD, Department of Psychology, University of Maryland, College Park, MD, United States

Juan Martín Gómez-Penedo, PhD, Facultad de Psicología, Universidad de Buenos Aires (CONICET), Buenos Aires, Argentina

Rodney K. Goodyear, PhD, School of Education, University of Southern California, Los Angeles, CA, and Department of Counseling and Human Services, University of Redlands, Redlands, CA, United States

Amy Greaves, PhD, private practice, San Diego, CA, United States

Martin grosse Holtforth, PhD, Department of Psychology, University of Bern; Psychosomatic Medicine, Department of Neurology, Inselspital, Bern University Hospital, University of Bern, Bern, Switzerland

Ally B. Hand, BA, Department of Psychology, University of Massachusetts Boston, Boston, MA, United States

Kathryn V. Kline, PhD, private practice, Washington, DC, United States

Heidi M. Levitt, PhD, Department of Psychology, University of Massachusetts Boston, Boston, MA, United States

Brent Mallinckrodt, PhD, Department of Psychology, Western Washington University, Bellingham, WA, United States

Cheri Marmarosh, PhD, Professional Psychology Program, The George Washington University, Washington, DC, United States

John C. Norcross, PhD, Department of Psychology, University of Scranton, Scranton, PA, United States

João Tiago Oliveira, PhD, CIPsi—Psychology Research Center, School of Psychology, University of Minho, Braga, Portugal

Matthew R. Perlman, PhD, Department of Psychology, Ohio University, Athens, OH, United States

Javier L. Rizo, BA, Department of Psychology, University of Massachusetts Boston, Boston, MA, United States

Adela Scharff, MA, Department of Psychology, University at Albany, State University of New York, Albany, NY, United States

Hideko Sera, PsyD, Office of Equity, Inclusion and Belonging, Morehouse College, Atlanta, GA, United States

Karen Tallman, PhD, Tallman Research, El Cerrito, CA, and Bay Area Rescue Mission, Richmond, CA, United States

The
Other Side
of
Psychotherapy

An Introduction to *The Other Side of Psychotherapy*

Jairo N. Fuertes

A recent clinical practicum supervisee, while reviewing the progress one of her clients had made, told me, "I can't believe how much my client has changed this semester. It's so disproportionate to what I did!" This reaction from my supervisee captures a thought that I had experienced many times as a therapist but had never been able to express, especially so succinctly. My supervisee was reviewing her work at the end of a semester and uttered what I thought was the perfect quote for this book. Mona marveled at the magnitude and pace of change that her client had achieved in 15 sessions of psychotherapy. She was pleased, of course, but uttered in wonder what she had "done" to make the changes possible and how it could be that a depressed client with a history of family abuse and isolation could have initiated so many positive changes in such a short time. We had a fruitful supervision session in which we discussed the client's courage and hard work, but we also discussed many of the therapeutic conditions and interventions that Mona had offered. It was evident to us that the client had made significant progress over the course of a semester and that it probably would not have happened without Mona being her therapist. Mona was clearly devoted and had done her job, but so had the client.

There are many books and chapters in the literature on what it takes to be a good therapist. This book focuses more on the client's side of the equation.

I thank Charles J. Gelso, Jennifer Sawicki, and Kimberly Kissoon for their comments on previous drafts of this chapter.

https://doi.org/10.1037/0000303-001
The Other Side of Psychotherapy: Understanding Clients' Experiences and Contributions in Treatment, J. N. Fuertes (Editor)

Without devaluing the important role of the therapist or therapy, the book presents ways that clients contribute to, experience, and work in psychotherapy. The authors describe, based on the available literature and their clinical experience, how clients help to make psychotherapy so effective and efficient.

A recent exchange with a colleague is also worth highlighting. He is now an accomplished therapist and psychotherapy researcher. He shared what he called one of the most surprising and memorable experiences that he had with a client when he was still in training years ago. He remarked that he remembered making a "mistake" in therapy when he was a graduate student. He disclosed his frustration with a client who had engaged over and over in self-defeating behavior. These behaviors were previously discussed and processed in earlier sessions. After sharing his frustration with the client, he pondered his reaction and disclosure, discussed it with his supervisor, and agreed that he would apologize to the client at their next session. He subsequently apologized to the client and elaborated why he had shared his feelings with her, but, surprisingly, the client found that disclosure to have been helpful and powerful.

You may have had similar experiences with clients, in which your perception of an event with a client was different from the client's perception. The purpose of mentioning my colleague's story is to highlight that clients and therapists can often agree on what has taken place in their sessions, but they can have different interpretations or associations of the same event. The literature has discussed how clients and their therapists differ in their perception of the same events in therapy (Bohart & Wade, 2013; Eugster & Wampold, 1996; Levitt & Rennie, 2004).

An extension of this phenomenon is that therapists tend to see and understand therapy primarily from their own perspective. Our profession has been, to a great extent, therapist-centric. While we readily acknowledge that psychotherapy is a collaborative process involving the client, in our hearts, we believe that our interventions are the force behind the change: the reason why the client got better. It is understandable why we do so. We care about our clients, we spend years training, and we are devoted to our work. And undoubtedly, we do help. However, we tend to view therapy from our side, from our point of view. In this volume, the authors take a more client-centric approach. I call it the "other side." While our presence and interventions are crucial to the process and outcome of psychotherapy, it seems important to get a better understanding of how clients work in psychotherapy. What strengths, capacities, behaviors, and cognitions do clients experience or use in psychotherapy? How do clients experience the therapist, the therapy relationship, and therapists' interventions? What influence do clients have on their therapists, and how do they experience outcome and termination? These are some of the questions that are discussed in this book. While I refer to the client as the "other side," this is not a prevailing mindset that I bring into therapy. Like most therapists, I see myself on the same side as the client; I see us as a team, a collaboration. However, I chose the title to highlight the fact that clients have their own views and experiences in psychotherapy and that, in some ways, their perspective remains largely unknown to us.

You may know by now that the evidence is in, from hundreds of carefully conducted studies: Psychotherapy is highly effective (American Psychological Association [APA], 2013; Cooper, 2008; Lambert, 2013). Psychotherapy is beneficial to clients who come into our offices with problems and concerns that range in severity from mild to moderate to severe (Wampold & Imel, 2015). While individuals are capable of adapting, growing, and transcending hurtful and traumatic experiences on their own, the evidence from the outcome literature shows that individuals who receive psychotherapy make greater gains, make them faster, and are able to maintain these gains longer than people who do not receive treatment (Wampold & Imel, 2015). Because research findings consistently show that client factors explain the largest proportion of outcome variance (Bohart & Wade, 2013; Cooper, 2008; Wampold & Imel, 2015), this book is dedicated to examining how clients contribute to such considerable outcomes.

The audiences that may benefit most from this book are psychologists and counselors. The book will also be of interest and benefit to faculty and graduate students in master's and doctoral programs in counseling and clinical psychology. It will also be relevant to professionals in related areas, such as social workers and counselor educators. My overall hope is that the book will be valuable in clinical practice and clinical training and may be a source of ideas for researchers interested in further advancing psychotherapy.

WHY DEVOTE AN ENTIRE BOOK TO THE CLIENT?

Despite a great deal of research that has examined client factors, there is a limit on what can be inferred about clients in psychotherapy. After reading the research about clients, it is difficult to understand what they experience in treatment or how they work and contribute to process and outcome. As Fuertes and Williams (2017) noted, studies on clients have generally isolated one or two client variables and correlated them with outcome, which is, of course, valuable, but when the literature on client factors is read in aggregate, the results are often mixed or inconclusive. Client factors are often presented as a single chapter in a book and are usually not discussed within the broader scope of psychotherapy. And yet, most clinicians and researchers would agree that the client is incredibly important to the process and outcome of psychotherapy. The client can be called the primary stakeholder in therapy—the person who holds the keys to the success of treatment—the client is a contributor, strategist, and decision maker in treatment. Clients are ultimately responsible for change and growth in treatment (Cooper, 2008); it is clients—not therapists—who make psychotherapy work (Duncan et al., 2004). In this book, we present a more complete and in-depth narrative about the client in psychotherapy. By focusing on their perspectives, we present a more complex and integrated set of story lines about their experiences and work in treatment. Moreover, we hope that by accounting for more of the work clients do, a more complete understanding can emerge of the collaboration between them and their therapists.

Fuertes and Williams (2017) noted that attending to the experiences of our clients matters because they tend to do a great deal of the work in treatment. Bohart and Tallman (2010) and Levitt et al. (2016) noted that clients contribute so much to the work in therapy that perhaps this may explain the "dodo bird hypothesis," where therapies tend to generate about the same level of effectiveness vis-à-vis outcome (Luborsky et al., 1975; Wampold & Imel, 2015). While many have discussed the role of common factors in explaining outcomes in therapy, Bohart and Tallman (2010) noted that the client is the ultimate common factor in treatment. Fuertes and Williams discussed the client as the main protagonist in treatment because clients know their lives best and are the ultimate arbiters of what is helpful, useful, or useless in therapy. They are the only ones who experience the benefits and difficulties of therapy and can implement the changes and deal with the resulting consequences.

Bergin and Garfield (1994) noted that the question is not whether the therapy works but whether the client works. And clients do work and are remarkably effective in their labor. As the outcome literature has shown repeatedly, clients make substantial gains after only 8 to 14 weeks in treatment and make clinically significant differences in about 16 to 20 hourly sessions. How does this happen? What happens in that span of time that clients can make such rapid improvements in such a brief period? The short answer is that they have the capacity to change. Clients, as human beings, have tremendous capacities for adapting, resilience, and growth. Clients change because they can change. Clients are human beings who are wired to adapt, endure, and grow—they are members of a species that has tremendous capacities for withstanding and thriving under difficult circumstances, and they have been at it for thousands of years, long, long before psychotherapy was created.

Informing my emphasis on the experiences and work of the client is the client-centered perspective of Carl Rogers. However, my perspective on the work of the client is also informed by many traditions in psychotherapy, from Freud to Klein to Rogers to Ellis. The authors of the chapters that follow also represent a diverse set of schools of thought that span the history of psychotherapy. While I believe that all of them would acknowledge the influence of Carl Rogers in their training, they would also add a list of many prominent thinkers and researchers who shaped their clinical and academic views of therapy. Thus, the emphasis in this volume on the client is informed by Rogers, but it also includes many diverse voices who came before him and since. And as mentioned earlier, the volume is also informed by the vast amount of empirical evidence pointing to the importance of the client in therapy.

Fuertes and Williams (2017) described therapy as a psychological gym and compared it to a physical gym. The therapist in this analogy is the personal trainer. While in the traditional gym, the person learns from the trainer and is encouraged to practice physical exercises to develop qualities such as physical strength, flexibility, and stamina, the client in therapy also learns and repeats exercises to develop psychological strength, flexibility, and greater tolerance and stamina in introspection. The exercises for the client in therapy are reflection, exploration of difficult experiences and emotions, and honest communication. Fuertes and Williams noted that both gyms generate similar results in that in both situations, the client or person begins to feel better about themselves and others. In both gyms, the client does a great deal of the work, in the sessions and between them. Therapists and personal trainers are present, they model and teach many of the skills that their clients have to learn and practice, and they constantly encourage and push their clients to an optimal level. But the client is key; if the client does not get with the program, they will make an experienced therapist or personal trainer ineffective, or conversely, they can make a relatively new therapist look accomplished.

There is an interesting conundrum in trying to understand the client in psychotherapy. In this volume, we are interested in understanding clients, "the other side." However, there is obviously no singular client perspective. Every client is different; every client–therapist dyad is unique; no one psychotherapy session is ever replicated. The developmental, social, and cultural influences that clients experience generate tremendous individual human diversity. However, there is also no singular therapist perspective either, and we have been fascinated with the therapist's experience, work, and activities in psychotherapy for many decades. But having studied therapists has given us a good understanding of what makes them effective and how the range of interventions they employ allows them to help their clients. My hope is that with greater study and emphasis on the client, we will be able to also understand what makes them effective in therapy and also come to appreciate the type of interventions and strategies they employ to collaborate with their therapists, to overcome their difficulties, and help heal themselves. While this volume does not delve directly into the issue of human diversity, I encourage you to learn about it, particularly as it applies to therapy. The APA (2018) has published guidelines for professionals to study and use in working with human diversity.

THIS VOLUME

Each chapter in the book reviews the empirical base in its respective area, including quantitative and qualitative research and case studies. The authors present what we can infer about clients from the literature and discuss what we do not know or what seems to be missing in the knowledge base. They also discuss implications for practice, teaching, and training new professionals, and they identify areas for future research. Chapters also include case examples demonstrating key concepts.[1]

The book is organized into three parts. Six chapters fall within Part I, Client Factors in Therapy Processes and Outcomes, and six chapters fall within Part II, Client–Therapist Interactions. The final part, Integration and Discussion, contains one chapter that looks back on the whole book.

---

[1]The identities of the individuals in the case examples throughout this book have been properly disguised to protect client confidentiality.

Part I begins with Chapter 1, "Client Expertise: The Active Client in Psychotherapy," in which Arthur C. Bohart and Karen Tallman discuss the strengths and qualities of the client that make them an expert and authority in their life and therefore another expert in the room. The authors also discuss how the expertise of the client manifests itself in therapy, how therapists can work with clients' self-expertise, and how the client's expertise can contribute to the process and outcome of treatment work. In Chapter 2, "Understanding and Enhancing Client Motivation," João Tiago Oliveira and his colleagues review the literature on what motivates clients in therapy and how therapists can promote client involvement and engagement in treatment. Chapter 3 is titled "Patient Readiness to Change: What We Know About Their Stages and Processes of Change." John C. Norcross, Danielle M. Cook, and I discuss how clients experience, negotiate, and engage in the process of change and growth in psychotherapy and the importance of therapists assessing client stage of change so that interventions can be matched and tailored to facilitate progress and outcome. In Chapter 4, "Therapist and Client Facilitative Interpersonal Skills in Psychotherapy," Timothy Anderson and Matthew R. Perlman discuss how clients experience therapists' facilitative skills and how they use these skills and their therapists' facilitative interpersonal skills to advance their progress in therapy. Chapter 5 is titled "Clients' Experiences of Attachment in the Psychotherapy Relationship," and in it, Brent Mallinckrodt discusses client attachment and its role in psychotherapy, including how clients experience attachment and achieve "earned attachment" in psychotherapy. The last chapter in Part I is titled "Clients' Agentic and Self-Healing Activities in Psychotherapy." Amy Greaves provides an innovative perspective on how clients progress through self-healing with the help of their therapist; her model is based on her research and is informed by the broader literature.

Part II begins with Chapter 7, "The Client's Function in the Psychotherapy Relationship: What Clients Experience and Contribute," in which Charles J. Gelso and Kathryn V. Kline discuss how clients experience the relationship and how they contribute to its formation and to sustaining it, including the real relationship, the working alliance, and the transference and countertransference configuration. In Chapter 8, "Client-Focused Assessment and Intervention: Tailoring the Work to the Client," James F. Boswell and Adela Scharff discuss ways of incorporating client feedback in assessment and intervention through routine outcome monitoring to better tailor and personalize therapy to the needs and perspective of the client. In Chapter 9, "Rethinking Therapists' Responsiveness to Center Clients' Experiences of Psychotherapy," Heidi M. Levitt and colleagues discuss clients' experiences of therapists' helping skills and the implications of their accounts in how therapists are prepared to maximally respond to the unique circumstances of each client. Chapter 10 is titled "Clients' Influence on Psychotherapists and the Treatment They Provide." Rodney K. Goodyear and Hideko Sera discuss the process of mutual influence in the clinical dyad and present how clients influence therapists' experiences, their ratings of therapy, and their behavior in session. The chapter also discusses how therapists and supervisors can intervene to identify and work with clients' contributions and influence. In Chapter 11, "Clients' Own Perspectives on Psychotherapy Outcomes and Their Mechanisms," Michael J. Constantino and his colleagues review the empirical literature and identify factors in treatment most closely associated with clients' perceptions of progress and outcome. In the final chapter of Part II, "Clients' Experiences of Therapy Ending," Cheri Marmarosh discusses how clients experience the end of therapy, including when a transfer to a new therapist is involved.

In the last chapter, I provide an integration and discussion based on my reading of the chapters and outline three broad themes that I identified from them about what clients experience and contribute to psychotherapy. They are (a) the role of client agency in therapy, (b) client collaboration in adapting and tailoring therapy, and (c) the role that clients play in nurturing a collaborative and therapeutic relationship. I also present ideas for future research on clients' experiences and contributions in therapy.

In closing, I want to reiterate that this book does not intend to undermine the valuable work of psychotherapists in helping their clients. Clients do a great deal of the work in therapy, but they do it with our help; before entering therapy, clients realized that they would not be able to change and grow on their own, which is why they enlisted the help of therapists. And we do help them. The psychotherapy we provide is highly effective and essential in tapping and galvanizing the client's resources and energies needed to overcome their problems. Thus, while we play an important role in psychotherapy, ours is not the only important role in the process. After having many exchanges with all the authors included in this volume, it is clear that while we acknowledge our hard work and expertise as professionals, we also acknowledge the amazing, resilient, creative, and hardworking psychotherapy client. And for our clients' courage, work, and important role in treatment, we are in awe, proud, and grateful.

REFERENCES

American Psychological Association. (2013). Recognition of psychotherapy effectiveness. *Psychotherapy, 50*(1), 102–109. https://doi.org/10.1037/a0030276

American Psychological Association. (2018, January). APA adopts new multicultural guidelines. *Monitor on Psychology, 48*(1), 47. https://www.apa.org/monitor/2018/01/multicultural-guidelines

Bergin, A. E., & Garfield, S. L. (1994). Overview, trends, and future issues. In A. E. Bergin & S. L. Garfield (Eds.), *Handbook of psychotherapy and behavior change* (4th ed., pp. 821–830). Wiley. https://doi.org/10.1176/ajp.152.5.804-a

Bohart, A. C., & Tallman, K. (2010). Clients as active self-healers: Implications for the person-centered approach. In M. Cooper, J. C. Watson, & D. Holldampf (Eds.), *Person-centered and experiential therapies work* (pp. 91–131). PCCS Books.

Bohart, A. C., & Wade, A. G. (2013). The client in psychotherapy. In M. J. Lambert (Ed.), *Bergin and Garfield's handbook of psychotherapy and behavior change* (6th ed., pp. 219–257). Wiley.

Cooper, M. (2008). *Essential research findings in counselling and psychotherapy*. SAGE.

Duncan, B. L., Miller, S. D., & Sparks, J. A. (2004). *The heroic client: A revolutionary way to improve effectiveness through client-directed, outcome-informed therapy*. Jossey-Bass.

Eugster, S. L., & Wampold, B. E. (1996). Systematic effects of participant role on evaluation of the psychotherapy session. *Journal of Consulting and Clinical Psychology, 64*(5), 1020–1028. https://doi.org/10.1037/0022-006X.64.5.1020

Fuertes, J. N., & Williams, E. N. (2017). Client-focused psychotherapy research. *Journal of Counseling Psychology, 64*(4), 369–375. https://doi.org/10.1037/cou0000214

Lambert, M. J. (2013). The efficacy and effectiveness of psychotherapy. In M. J. Lambert (Ed.), *Bergin and Garfield's handbook of psychotherapy and behavior change* (6th ed., pp. 169–218). Wiley.

Levitt, H. M., Pomerville, A., & Surace, F. I. (2016). A qualitative meta-analysis examining clients' experiences of psychotherapy: A new agenda. *Psychological Bulletin, 142*(8), 801–830. https://doi.org/10.1037/bul0000057

Levitt, H. M., & Rennie, D. L. (2004). Narrative activity: Clients' and therapists' intentions in the process of narration. In L. E. Angus & J. McLeod (Eds.), *The handbook of narrative and psychotherapy* (pp. 298–313). SAGE. https://doi.org/10.4135/9781412973496.d23

Luborsky, L., Singer, B., & Luborsky, L. (1975). Comparative studies of psychotherapies. Is it true that "everyone has won and all must have prizes"? *Archives of General Psychiatry, 32*(8), 995–1008. https://doi.org/10.1001/archpsyc.1975.01760260059004

Wampold, B. E., & Imel, Z. E. (2015). *The great psychotherapy debate: The evidence for what makes psychotherapy work* (2nd ed.). Routledge. https://doi.org/10.4324/9780203582015

I

CLIENT FACTORS IN THERAPY PROCESSES AND OUTCOMES

1

Client Expertise

The Active Client in Psychotherapy

Arthur C. Bohart and Karen Tallman

Recently, there has been increased interest in the client's experience of and contribution to the therapy process (e.g., Fuertes & Williams, 2017). In 1999, we proposed a modification to the way most of the field views psychotherapy. On the basis of the evidence we reviewed, we concluded that it is clients who ultimately make therapy work (Bohart & Tallman, 1999). This may not seem unusual; most therapists probably agree that clients make therapy work. If clients do not participate and invest in the therapeutic process and interventions offered, nothing will work.

However, we were proposing something beyond client participation. In contrast to the dominant "interventionist" model of therapy, we proposed that it is clients' creativity, agency, initiative, and inventiveness that ultimately make therapy work. Therefore, looking at therapy by focusing on therapists' interventions is like listening to half of a conversation.

The interventionist model of therapy is patterned after the medical model of practice (Wampold & Imel, 2015). Therapists choose appropriate interventions that "operate on" clients' dysfunctional ways of being (e.g., dysfunctional schemas, attachment styles, internal working models, emotion schemes, defense mechanisms) to create change. This can be diagrammed as follows:

Therapist assesses client dysfunction $\longrightarrow$ Chooses appropriate interventions that operate on client dysfunction $\longrightarrow$ To produce client change

https://doi.org/10.1037/0000303-002
The Other Side of Psychotherapy: Understanding Clients' Experiences and Contributions in Treatment, J. N. Fuertes (Editor)

The role of the therapeutic relationship in this model is twofold. It either supports the therapist implementing interventions (as in cognitive behavior therapy), or it itself is an intervention (as in the idea that the therapist is providing a corrective relational experience to modify attachment styles, internal working models of people and relationships, and the like).

It is crucial that clients "collaborate" in the interventionist model. This is similar to medical practice: If the patient does not disclose their symptoms to the doctor, and if they do not follow the doctor's prescriptions, then medicine will not "work." Client "collaboration" means compliance: willingness to do what the therapist wants them to do. If clients do not do this, they are typically viewed as resisting. The therapist then needs to find a way of "treating" the client's resistance.

By contrast, we hold that it is largely clients who make therapy work. In particular, clients are the ones who make interventions work. Clients are able to use interventions from different therapy approaches to fashion change. They actively integrate whatever the therapy is offering into their life experiences. They can use exploring the past in psychoanalysis, empathically supported self-exploration in person-centered therapy, exposure and cognitive restructuring in cognition therapy, the miracle question in solution-focused therapy, and so on. Therapists' interventions are "affordances" (Bohart, 2007) that clients can use in different ways to promote change (we go into the idea of an affordance later).

Furthermore, clients work on therapists' interventions. They creatively interpret them in their own ways to achieve what they need, as well as integrate them into their lives and life structures. In addition, they create their own interventions. They blend what they gain from therapy with their own ideas, their own aims, and the ideas of friends, ministers, culture, social media, television talk show hosts, and so on. They also actively gain their own insights that they do not necessarily share with therapists. They notice things in the therapy encounter that are of value to them—things that may not be what therapists thought were the useful things to attend to. They also manage therapists to get what they want. Clients are active agents who "operate on" therapy. We have diagrammed this thusly:

Clients ⟶ Operate on therapists' interventions ⟶ To create change

Clients are, therefore, as much interventionists as are therapists. We agreed with Prochaska et al. (1994), who suggested that therapy is professionally guided self-change. To quote Bohart (2015),

> What I continued to experience [with my clients] was interactions with intelligent others who would take my interventions, treat them as useful or not so useful tools, and use them in their own ways to get whatever they could out of them if anything. And if clients did not actively engage with them, find them useful, and utilize them, my magical interventions lost all their power. . . . Clients were active agents and I was a consultant who listened to them and, in dialogue with their own agency, offered them ideas and dialogue. I was not an interventionist . . . I did not "treat" my clients. In fact, I stood in awe of their creative capacities. I had seen far too many of my clients take my "interventions" and totally transform them in ways I never had intended. (pp. 1063–1065)

On the basis of this view of the client, we proposed an alternative model of how therapy works. We called it the "meeting of minds meta-model" (Bohart & Tallman, 1999). Contrary to the interventionist model in which the therapist is primary and "prescribes" what is best, the meeting of minds model is more genuinely collaborative, even if the therapist takes the lead. Therapists and clients work together in a coconstructive fashion to jointly share and shape clients' changes. Dialogue between therapist and client becomes the primary "intervention." The most important therapist skill is to be sensitively responsive and open to the client's creative contributions. The outcome of therapy is a joint product of two minds meeting, in which the therapists' interventions blend with the active client's creativity and expertise in terms of knowledge of their life structure, goals, theories of change, and so on. The idea of "applying" therapy "to" clients is misguided from our point of view.

We briefly summarize and give examples of research findings that led us to develop our point of view. We are unable to fully review the research base in this chapter. We refer interested readers to earlier publications (Bohart & Tallman, 1999, 2010; Bohart & Wade, 2013). In addition, we have included recent findings. We have broken up the topics into two sections: client expertise and activity and therapy as a meeting of minds. Many research findings are relevant to both sections.

CLIENT EXPERTISE: CLIENT ACTIVITY IN PSYCHOTHERAPY

For many therapists, client expertise refers to the fact that clients are experts on their own lives. We go further to emphasize clients' own active and generative activity in making therapy work.

Two concepts from Gibson's (1979) theory of perception help to understand client activity in psychotherapy. The first is the concept of an *invariant*: People extract from the flux of experience underlying constancies. Clients do this in therapy. Clients ask, "What am I supposed to be doing here? What am I supposed to be learning (i.e., what are the constancies, the meanings that I am supposed to be extracting from my experiences here)? What is the therapist up to? What am I learning about myself? Does this therapist value me and empathically understand me? If so, what does that mean about me and my experience?" and so on.

We suggest that clients are continuously extracting invariants (meaning and patterns) from what they are experiencing. For instance, with empathy, it is not necessary that therapists always be accurate with their empathy responses. As important is if clients detect an underlying constancy that therapists are trying to understand them (e.g., Bohart & Byock, 2005), even if any given response is not accurate.

The second Gibsonian concept is that of affordance. An *affordance*, as we interpret it, is something whose structure "affords" an action. Things in the environment can afford more than one use. If you are out in the woods, a long stick may afford walking—becoming a cane. If you have a string and a hook, it may become a fishing pole. If you run into a coyote, it may become a weapon of defense, and so on.

The research suggests that clients use their experiences in therapy and the interventions provided by the therapist as affordances (Bohart, 2007). A therapeutic technique, or a therapist's response, can "afford" different client interpretations and actions. For instance, as we note later, a client may use the two-chair technique in emotion-focused therapy for the purpose of assertion training, although its theoretical purpose is to help clients access and work through emotional conflicts.

Evidence Supporting the Idea That Client Activity Contributes to Therapy

In 1994, we first started thinking about the generative contribution of the client in regard to the "dodo bird" finding that all bona fide therapies work about equally well for most disorders (American Psychological Association, 2013; Wampold & Imel, 2015). We conducted a small therapy analog research study (Tallman et al., 1994) that found that clients presented with poor empathy responses worked with them to keep therapy on track while simultaneously protecting the ego of the therapist. This finding that clients may be active and creative seemed to provide an explanation for the dodo bird verdict.

The dodo bird finding that widely different approaches, using different theories and strategies, work about equally well for most disorders suggests that specific interventions are not typically needed to "treat" specific disorders. Bergin and Garfield (1994) concluded from their review of the evidence, that "With some exceptions . . . there is massive evidence that psychotherapeutic techniques do not have specific effects; yet there is tremendous resistance to accepting this finding as a legitimate one" (p. 822). Wampold and Imel (2015) estimated that techniques account for at most about 8% of the 13% of outcome variance accounted for by psychotherapy, which equates to 1% of the total outcome variance. In contrast to techniques, Norcross and Lambert (2011) estimated that the therapist and the therapeutic relationship account for about 19% of the variance accounted for by psychotherapy. Beutler et al. (2004) reported correlations between specific techniques and outcomes ranging from 0 to .11.

The interventionist model of therapy attributes the primary "force" of change to the expert therapist's interventions. The previous set of findings suggest that the interventionist model has shortcomings. Furthermore, there is ample evidence that self-help frequently works as well as, or almost as well as, professionally provided psychotherapy (e.g., Norcross, 2006). These findings suggest that even the presence of therapists and the therapeutic relationship is not always necessary for a person to make significant changes (see Bohart & Tallman, 2010, for a more thorough analysis). As Bohart and Tallman (2010) suggested, the reason widely different approaches to therapy work about the same is that clients take interventions and experiences from different approaches and are able to utilize them to resolve their problems. This does not mean that the interventions from different approaches may not be effective in their own ways. Challenging dysfunctional cognitions may indeed change dysfunctional thinking. Exploring childhood may indeed help alleviate splitting and transference. But it is the whole person who is the client that integrates changing dysfunctional cognitions or exploring early relationships and defense mechanisms into their whole life (i.e., into everyday functioning, setting goals, coping with life's frustrations, enjoying things, and so on). The client is the "common factor" across therapies.

The idea that clients make the single most important contribution to therapy outcome is supported by expert estimates. Asay and Lambert (1999) said that "extra-therapeutic factors," which consist of the client as well as factors in the client's life, accounted for about 40% of the outcome in therapy. Placebo effects accounted for 15%. Given that placebo effects are primarily due to clients' self-healing capabilities, this suggests that the client and factors in the client's life account for 55% of outcome variance. This is more than therapist factors (techniques and relationship—45%). Wampold and Imel (2015) estimated that therapy factors accounted for only about 14% of outcome variance. Of the remaining 86%, most was likely due to the client (Wampold, 2010). Finally, Norcross and Lambert (2011) suggested that 40% of the outcome variance is unexplained. Half of the remaining 60% is due to the client and a half due to all other factors combined.

These percentages do not mean that all client variance is accounted for by clients' active efforts to make therapy work. Percentages due to the client also include percentages due to client variables such as personality characteristics, level of distress, level of pathology, and so on (Bohart & Wade, 2013). Nonetheless, these findings indicate that we need to look more at the client and the client's role in therapy and not focus just on therapists and their interventions (Norcross, 2020).

Following on these percentages, the active engagement, involvement, and participation of the client in the therapeutic process have been found to be the most important factors in determining whether therapy works (Orlinsky et al., 1994). Orlinsky et al. (2004) named 11 variables that were associated with client outcome. Eight are client factors. They include the client's cooperation, the client's experience of the therapeutic relationship, the client's contribution to the relationship, the client's affirmation of the therapist, the client's interactive collaboration, the client's openness and nondefensiveness, the client's suitability for treatment, and the client's expressiveness.

More recent research examples support this. Lilliengren et al. (2019) found that patients' engagement was important for making therapy work with patients with Cluster C personality disorders. Studies of "personal growth initiative" (PGI; Robitschek et al., 2019; Weigold et al., 2013) have found that it predicts a positive outcome in the treatment of psychological distress. PGI is defined as an active and intentional engagement in the growth process (Weigold et al., 2013).

Compatible with the role of client engagement, there is evidence that client agency and empowerment are important. Client agency is a complex topic. We take it as a presupposition that clients, like all humans, are active agents.

Our view of the client (and the human being) is that the person is an entity who is always striving to make their way in the world to achieve their ends or, in the case of clients struggling with problems, to metaphorically "find a way to stay on the planet." When clients come to therapy, they carry this kind of agency into therapy. The very act of coming is agentic (even if they are court referred or dragged in by their spouse). Perhaps a good way of saying it is that we see the human as an intentional being. In this sense, all clients are agentic, and they are operating agentically, even when they are resisting therapy or lapsing into passive hopelessness. This is different from what many therapists and researchers mean by agency. For them, agency is *proactive agency*, that is, actively playing a positive and productive role in therapy. *Low agency*, from their point of view, therefore, would be feeling helpless or passive or not taking an active role.

We also distinguish between clients acting agentically versus clients feeling or seeing themselves as agentic. Clients may act agentically even if they do not feel agentic (Hanna & Ritchie, 1995). Therefore, we have focused on clients' activity more so than on their perceived agency. Nonetheless, clients' perceived agency has been found to relate to outcomes. Hoener et al. (2012) conducted a qualitative study of 11 clients. They defined clients' agency as referring to clients' dispositions to "actively make and enact choices regarding their therapy" (p. 66). Most clients reported that change resulted from their agentic efforts. They also reported that they highly valued their own contributions to therapy. An interesting finding was that different clients saw different approaches as facilitating their agency in different ways. Some reported that exploratory approaches facilitated agency. Others reported that directive therapies facilitated their agency by placing responsibility on them to do homework. Huber, Born, et al. (2019) found that changes in agency over the course of therapy correlated with outcome. Huber, Nikendei, et al. (2019) found that clients higher in agency had stronger therapeutic alliances and participated more actively in therapy. Adler et al. (2008) rated clients' narratives for a sense of empowerment to overcome circumstances rather than be at their mercy. They correlated this with a composite score of subjective well-being measures and found a significant relationship ($r = .55$). Khattra et al. (2017) found that clients attributed change to their agency in a combined motivational interviewing–cognitive-behavioral treatment, although not in a pure cognitive-behavioral treatment.

There are also studies on how therapy fosters client agency and feelings of empowerment. Von der Lippe et al. (2019) studied how therapists foster agency in low agency clients. A previous study found a pattern of low agency in poor outcome clients. This study found that therapist behaviors in the poor outcome cases tended to discourage client agency, while therapist behaviors in the good outcome cases tended to encourage it. Therapists in the good outcome cases were sensitive to clients' perspectives and invited mutual cooperation. Therapists in the poor outcome or low agency cases dominated the dialogue and were out of tune with clients' accounts. Other things that foster client agency and empowerment include client reflexive inquiry into emotionally salient personal stories (Angus & Kagan, 2013), therapist respect (Noyce & Simpson, 2018), and therapist empathy (Angus & Kagan, 2007; Timulak & Elliott, 2003).

Evidence Supporting the Role of Clients as Generative Contributors

Clients do not contribute merely by participating or even by "absorbing" or "metabolizing" therapist interventions. They go beyond their active participation to, in some sense, being therapists themselves—actively working with and creating interventions and actively integrating what they are learning into their lives. We next consider how clients work to shape, influence, and create meaning out of the therapy interaction.

In one striking study, Garfinkel (1967) had participants interact with a therapist who was behind a screen. The participants asked the therapist questions about their problems. The questions had to be framed in a "yes/no" fashion, and the therapist responded only with a "yes" or a "no." The participants did not know this, but the therapist responded randomly with yes or no. Nonetheless, the participants were able to create coherent accounts out of the therapist's answers and derive solutions for their problems.

Rennie (1990, 1992, 1994, 2000) conducted a series of seminal research studies on clients' experiences. He had clients go over tapes of their therapy sessions soon after the sessions took place and comment on what was going on with them. Rennie found that clients engaged in a great deal of covert mental activity during therapy sessions. They thought about what was happening in the session while overtly they listened to their therapists. They achieved insights that they kept to themselves and did not communicate to their therapists. They deferred to therapists overtly, but they then thought about the things they were talking about in the way they wanted. They sometimes resisted therapists' influence, particularly when they thought the therapist was misunderstanding them or what the therapist was proposing did not fit with them. They acted on therapists' directives while interpreting the meaning of techniques or relationship factors in their own unique ways. Finally, they actively managed the therapy session (see also Chapter 6, this volume). If the therapist went off course, they tried to redirect the therapist in the direction they needed while also trying to protect the therapist's feelings. They would not overtly contradict the therapist or disagree with them. Instead, they would overtly defer but then find ways of going off in the direction they needed to go in.

We share one example reported by Rennie (1994). The client begins the session by telling the therapist about a humiliating experience at work. She knows there is more to the story than she has shared but isn't ready to delve into all of it yet. She decides to go into it more thoroughly after the therapist exhibits understanding. Through telling the therapist about her experience, she privately achieves several insights but does not yet feel comfortable sharing them with the therapist. Telling the therapist about the humiliating event helps her get rid of distressing feelings the event evoked.

Levitt (2004) conducted a qualitative analysis based on interviews with clients. One finding was that clients responded to interventions differently at different times. Another finding was that clients reported managing their therapists to get what they needed. Levitt concluded that it was not sensitive to clients' experience to use blanket "manualized" interventions.

Other studies support the idea that clients are active. Elliott (1984) found in a study of interpretation and insight events in therapy that the errors therapists made in their interpretations were ignored by clients. Clients used what they found to be useful. Gold (1994) reported case studies in which clients initiated and carried out their own versions of psychotherapy integration. In a qualitative study, McKenna and Todd (1997) found that clients got different things out of therapy at different points in their lives. Greaves (2006; see also Chapter 6, this volume) used a qualitative analysis to examine the experiences of 13 clients. The pattern of results that emerged supports many of the findings that we cite, consistent with the view of clients acting as agentic self-healers.

Bohart and Boyd (1997) explored 12 clients' responses to three sessions of therapy. One client, who believed she needed support, perceived empathic responses as offering support. A client who believed she needed insight perceived empathic responses as offering insight. Similarly, a client whose goal was to become more assertive reported that the two-chair exercise in emotion-focused therapy helped her learn to be more assertive, even though the purpose of the therapist using it was to help access and process emotional conflict. Similarly, Talmon (1990) did an interview study of ex-clients. He reported,

> I had taken my interventions and my words much too seriously. Patients reported following suggestions that I could not remember having made. They created their own interpretations, which were sometimes quite different from what I recollected and sometimes more creative and suitable versions of my suggestions. (p. 60)

A group of graduate students and I (ACB) did a series of studies (Bekele et al., 2004; Bohart & Byock, 2005; Bohart et al., 2007) to explore how clients actively process their experiences in therapy. The hypothesis was that clients would perceive and "use" therapist responses in their own ways. Identical therapist responses would be reacted to differently by different clients. We were not able to directly test this in therapy. Instead, we used a "vicarious ethnographic" method. We had coresearchers (both me and graduate students) vicariously participate in published therapy videos (e.g., of Carl Rogers, Aaron Beck, and Leslie Greenberg) by going through them and imagining themselves into the role of the client in the video step by step. They would then try to imagine how they would be receiving and interpreting what the therapist was doing.

In one of these studies, Bekele et al. (2004) watched videos of a psychodynamic therapist, a Gestalt therapist, and a cognitive-behavioral therapist. They found that different vicarious clients experienced the interactions quite differently. Different meanings were extracted by different clients from the same therapist responses, and they perceived the "tools" used by the therapists—

the interventions—differently. The cultural backgrounds of the vicarious clients made a difference (we give an example later).

Bohart and Byock (2005) studied three different videos and transcripts of Carl Rogers working with three different clients. One was the famous case of Gloria. One vicarious client, imagining herself into the Gloria role and going step by step, experienced Rogers as more empathically on target than the other vicarious client did. In particular, the female researcher, imagining herself into the role of a female client, found Rogers significantly less empathic and missing more than did the male researcher. The female researcher also experienced Rogers as following an agenda more than did the male researcher.

Finally, in one study (Bohart et al., 2007), a female vicarious client from a sociocentric culture imagined herself in the role of a male client who appeared in a video working with Aaron Beck (Ratner, 1986). This was a particularly interesting example and illustrates how the client's culture plays a role in how they process what the therapist is doing. The vicarious client heard Beck as suggesting that one should not depend on people for one's happiness. She found herself privately arguing with him because relationships were fundamental in her culture. Later in the session, Beck suggested that the client handle his depression by naming names of friends. At that point, she (as the client) saw Beck as coming around to her way of thinking! Next, we give a brief excerpt of the therapy dialogue, with her private responses (as the client) to what Beck said to the actual male client, to give a flavor of this finding and of this research. "VC" stands for "vicarious client." Remember, in terms of pronouns, that the client in the video is actually a male. However, the vicarious client is a woman.

> In one response, Beck instructed the client that the client's role is to answer questions and give information and stated that the client is not responsible for how the interaction goes.
>
> The VC privately thought, "What does he mean I am not responsible? Yes, I am because what happens to me is my responsibility if my thinking causes my stomach to be upset and so on."
>
> Beck said, "Honesty has got nothing to do with performing, performing well, carrying on a good conversation, being a polished speaker, and so on. Now that we've gone through that and restructured your role, how are you feeling?"
>
> The VC said (to herself), "Therapist is teaching me the difference between 'self' and behavior and my role and checks with me where I am."
>
> Beck was trying to convince the client that he should be a whole person by himself and not rely on others for happiness.
>
> The VC thought to herself, "I understand what you are saying and feel that you are teaching me to be independent, but I am not sure if I agree with you or if it feels right to me to accept what you are saying. I am balanced when my life is interconnected with others, families, friends, community. So much to learn, share, understand, celebrate together."
>
> Beck encouraged the client to overcome the belief that he needs a woman.
>
> The VC responded, "If you think so, but it's not a belief. I see myself in relation with others therefore I can't see life, growth without others in my life."

Core to Carl Rogers's view of psychotherapy is that it is client creativity and generativity that make therapy work. Most theories of psychotherapy do not include the capacity of the client for creative thinking as an integral part of the change process. If you look up "client thinking" in the index of most books on psychotherapy, you won't find it, except perhaps for "dysfunctional thinking." You also won't find "creative thinking." It is as if the client as a generative, creative agent disappears in books on therapy.

Yet, a variety of writers have argued that creativity is a fundamental part of human life (e.g., Richards, 2007). Cantor (2003), a personality psychologist, spotlighted the human capacity for adaptive creativity:

> One of the signature features of individuals' proclivity for constructive cognition is its creativity, as contrasted with two attributes—accuracy and straightforwardness—that one might instead expect to characterize the strengths of social cognition. In fact, a great deal of what people think about themselves and others is adaptive precisely to the extent that it plays creatively with "reality." (p. 53)

Thus, it would be no surprise that clients bring their capacity for creativity into therapy. This is particularly true because many of the things therapists do promote the conditions for clients to use their creativity. These include empathic listening, providing a safe space, reducing stress, promoting openness versus defensiveness, promoting clients adopting a preaffirmative or nonjudgmental position to their experience, promoting curiosity, and providing structures (techniques, interactions) that encourage exploration.

Various aspects of the evidence we have already reviewed supports clients' creative capacity. One example is Garfinkel's (1967) study in which clients pieced together a coherent account from a therapist's random yes or no answers to their questions. Another is Talmon's (1990) interview study in which clients reported making creative modifications on suggestions that he had given. Studies that suggest that clients modify therapist responses to fit with what they need also support the idea of client creativity. Greaves (2006; see also Chapter 6, this volume) also found evidence of clients' creativity in her studies.

In addition, Selby (2004) conducted a qualitative analysis of the experiences of 20 clients in therapy. The analysis was based on 97 tape-recorded sessions. Both clients and therapists were interviewed. Ten of the 20 demonstrated creativity. Creativity was an emergent from the combined contributions of therapist and client. Selby also looked at the cases of the noncreative clients. Lack of creativity could sometimes be attributed to clients' reluctance to engage in the therapy process, and some was due to therapists' lack of receptivity to engaging with clients who were ready to be creative.

Mackrill (2008) did a qualitative multicase history study. He had clients keep diaries on their experiences both inside and outside of therapy. He also tape-recorded sessions. The case of Jane provides an example of client creativity. Jane is an adult child of an alcoholic. She comes to therapy because she is afraid that she is "going to the rats," which in Denmark, where the study takes place, means that she fears she is going crazy. She also has trouble with men, feeling that they exploit her. The existential-psychodynamic therapist she sees primarily responds to her in a supportive, empathic way in the first session. This reduces her fears that she is losing her mind. She then proceeds to generate her own creative interventions. First, she contacts her brother, who she has never talked with about their alcoholic parent and, in effect, creates her own support group. Second, she decides to deliberately experiment with saying no to men. Again, neither of these strategies was suggested by the therapist. They were creative emergents out of the therapy process.

Other evidence is indirect. Eugene Gendlin's (1980) focusing technique involves teaching clients how to listen to their internal experience and unfold it. The most basic form of this procedure has the therapist sit silently with the client while the client engages in the process. Focusing leads to clients generating their own insights and creative emergents in their experiencing. There is evidence that focusing correlates with a positive change in psychotherapy (Hendricks, 2002) as well as with indicators of creativity and health (Gendlin, 1980).

We also mention the "inner guide" exercise (Zilbergeld & Lazarus, 1987). This technique is commonly used by therapists who practice hypnosis and guided imagery. The client is taught to relax and then awaits a visit from a figure in their imagination who will be their "inner guide." They then can ask the inner guide for guidance. Clients frequently report gaining wise advice about, or insight into, their problems. Zilbergeld and Lazarus (1987) quoted a client as saying, "I ran into someone—the strongest, wisest person I've ever met" (p. 149). Thus, clients are capable of making creative variations on therapists' interventions, creatively using them in the ways they need, as well as generating their own creative interventions.

Clients also creatively utilize the therapy experience outside of therapy. Traditional theoretical models assume that therapy largely happens inside the therapy session. Researchers focus on "significant events" in therapy as if that is where change happens. The implicit model is that therapy corrects dysfunctional aspects of the patient, such as a weak ego or dysfunctional cognitions. This leads to being able to function more effectively in everyday life. However, research supports the idea that clients actively work with therapy material outside of the session. They do not merely "absorb" it in therapy and then go home and, like a drug, wait for it to make changes occur. Dreier (2000) studied the experiences of families in therapy. He found that client development extends beyond the therapy office, and in fact, most development occurs outside of therapy. Clients transform what they have learned and creatively apply it to their lives. "Clients configure the meaning of therapy within the structure of their ongoing social practice" (Dreier, 2000, p. 253).

Mackrill's (2008) qualitative study found that clients knew what would be helpful for them and proceeded to use their ideas in their everyday lives. In other words, clients translated therapy into their lived environments. Clients also compared what therapists said with what friends, family, and other people in their everyday lives had said. They were more likely to use what the therapist said if it was aligned with the opinions of others.

Clients in therapy also increase their utilization of other people to talk to about their problems (Cross et al., 1980). Some clients read self-help books, review their dialogues with their therapists, and engage in their own self-questioning activities (Levitt et al., 2006).

Mörtl and Von Wietersheim (2008) studied clients in a day clinic and found that they discussed clinic experiences with people in their everyday life and reflected on these clinic experiences while at home. They enlisted people at home to help them confront everyday problems. Similarly, Mörtl and Von Wietersheim noted that clients compared experiences at home with the feedback received at the clinic. They also learned from comparing their home and clinic relationships.

Finally, there is evidence that many clients think about their experiences with the therapist outside of the session. In psychodynamic language, they "internalize" the therapist. Hartmann et al. (2010) concluded, "It appears that differences in the way patients 'absorb' and 'metabolize' their therapy may emerge more clearly *between* sessions, when patients are not actually in contact with their therapists, than in the therapeutic process observed *during* therapy sessions" (p. 357). The research findings are complex—not all clients think about their therapists outside of session, and how they think is important to whether it is useful. Nonetheless, the fact that many do shows how clients actively work with their experiences in therapy outside of the sessions.

In summary, evidence supports the hypothesis that clients are active contributors to the psychotherapy change process. Clients monitor what is happening in therapy. They reflect on what is happening. They evaluate its usefulness. They also attempt to arrange events to achieve their purposes. They do this both overtly and covertly. Furthermore, there is evidence that clients can creatively contribute to outcomes. In addition, clients bring together what they are learning in therapy with their everyday lives to create change.

PSYCHOTHERAPY AS A MEETING OF MINDS

On the basis of the idea of the client as an active and creative contributor, we have proposed a "meeting of minds" metamodel (Bohart & Tallman, 1999) of therapy. Psychotherapy, more so than medicine, is a meeting of two intelligences. Interventions are cocreations by the two intelligences. This model is compatible with, although somewhat different from, recent trends in the field. To quote Nissen-Lie et al. (2020), "Through the gradual shift towards a more (two-person) relational theory of psychotherapy, it is now commonly accepted to see all therapeutic interactions as interdependent, dynamic systems" (p. 1).

Our view is compatible with practice from different theoretical points of view, with some modification. The major difference is in the therapist's mindset: Is the therapist's primary focus on pathology and intervention or collaboration and dialogue? In our model, the primary focus is on collaboration and dialogue. We emphasize how a client uses an intervention more than the supposed "effects" of "applying" the intervention. For example, in one of my (ACB's) cases, the client and I were engaged in challenging dysfunctional cognitions when the client used it to branch off into a fruitful exploration of childhood experiences. The client thus creatively modified the intervention in a useful way. I went with him.

Client Contributions to the Meeting of Minds

If therapy is a meeting of minds, what does the client bring to that? First, clients can be seen as, in part, "constructing" the therapy hour through their active perceptual and search activities. A typical view of clients in psychotherapy is that their perceptions are possibly distorted (e.g., from stress, psychopathology, or transference). Therapists presumably "see" what is going on more realistically than do clients. However, research suggests that clients' perceptions are more trustworthy than once thought. Studies have repeatedly found that clients' perceptions of the relationship or alliance correlate with therapeutic outcome more highly than do therapists' or observers' perceptions, although the differences are not always statistically significant. In a recent meta-analysis, Elliott et al. (2018) found that clients' perceptions of therapist empathy correlated .27 with outcome, while observers' perceptions correlated .21, and therapists' perceptions correlated .19. Similarly, client ratings of collaboration with the therapist have a higher correlation with outcome than do therapist ratings (Orlinsky et al., 2004).

Many studies have found that clients' perceptions of what is helpful only partially overlap with the perceptions of therapists. For instance, Elliott and Shapiro (1992) and Elliott et al. (1994) found that some of the events in therapy therapists perceive as insignificant are viewed by clients as important. Levitt and Rennie (2004) studied the perspectives of therapists and clients in regard to the meaning and usefulness of what each was doing. Therapist and client perspectives only partially overlapped. They noted, "Three stories may be occurring at once: the story of the dialogue between the client and the therapist, the client's inner story, and the therapist's inner story" (p. 308). Others have found little overlap between clients and therapists regarding what was helpful (Castonguay et al., 2010; Helmeke & Sprenkle, 2000). These data suggest that clients selectively attend to and focus on aspects of the therapy environment that they see as important. What they see and how they interpret it is not necessarily what therapists think is helpful. If we assume that clients' perceptions of therapy have some veridicality in terms of what is useful, this supports the idea of their active, constructive role.

It should be noted that therapists' and clients' perceptions are not always discrepant. In fact, some recent studies have found that the degree to which therapists and clients converged in their identification of important change moments correlated with outcome (Nissen-Lie et al., 2020). In one study, clients and therapists did agree on the basic nature of the change process even if they did not identify the same change moments (Altimir et al., 2010). However, clients tended to report more successful change processes than their therapists. The authors speculated that this might be due to the fact that clients are the best informants on how the change process has operated for them.

Second, many clients bring into therapy their own ideas about what is wrong and what they need (sometimes referred to as their theories of change). In 1961, Carl Rogers (1961) wrote, "It is the client who knows what hurts, what directions to go, what problems are crucial, what experiences have been deeply buried" (p. 12). It has been suggested that therapists should be aware of and work with clients' ideas about what is wrong and their ideas about change (Duncan & Miller, 2000; Shapiro, 1986). Hamm et al. (2018) recently argued that it is important to work with clients' agendas with persons diagnosed with schizophrenia.

Before we look at the evidence, we make a conceptual clarification. Although Rogers said that it is clients who know what hurts and what directions to go in, this does not mean that they consciously know this. Not all people who come to therapy may have explicit theories of change (Knight et al., 2012), nor do they necessarily know explicitly what is wrong or what direction to go in or have explicit preferences for one form of therapy or the other. This does not mean clients have no sense of what is right for them or what would help fix what is wrong. Such knowledge may be implicit. It may take a dialogical process to discover and articulate what they implicitly know about what they need to do to change. In that sense, the process would be a coconstructive one between therapist and client (Knight et al., 2012).

Given this caveat, there is evidence that many clients enter therapy with beliefs about what they need (e.g., Philips et al., 2007). Their beliefs may influence how they interpret and use what therapists offer. Clients' motivation for the type of therapy they want can be influenced by their beliefs about the causes of their problems. Meyer and Garcia-Roberts (2007) found that clients were more motivated for interpersonal interventions when they believed their depression was caused by interpersonal issues. Similarly, clients who saw their depression as characterological wanted therapy that was personality changing. Clients who thought their problems were based on childhood issues wanted past-focused therapy, and so on. Clients did not want behavioral approaches if they thought there were more complex reasons for their depression. This was possibly because they did not believe simple behavioral interventions could fix their problems.

There is evidence that clients' views of the nature of their problems influence how therapy works. Studies have found that clients who have therapists that align with the clients' attributional theories are more satisfied with therapy and have better outcomes (Hayes & Wall, 1998; Tracey, 1988). Therapists are perceived as more credible and understanding when they align with clients' attribution of responsibility (Worthington & Atkinson, 1996).

Clients' preexisting ideas can also influence how they process therapy. Kühnlein (1999) interviewed 49 inpatients who had cognitive behavior therapy. Participants did not simply adopt what the therapist presented. Instead, they selectively focused on the parts they found helpful. They combined the helpful elements with their previously existing schemas. Mackrill (2008) found that how clients processed therapy partly depended on their preexisting beliefs about what they needed. One client believed what he needed to do was to learn to think positively. He perceived what was going on in the sessions through that lens and concluded at the end that he had learned to think positively. But helping the client to learn to think positively was not one of the therapist's goals.

However, clients sometimes do change their beliefs about the causes of their problems. Mackrill (2008) found that clients entered therapy with specific beliefs about the causes of their problems and how to solve them. Some clients stuck with their theories. Others modified their theories when confronted with a compelling alternative explanation. Valkonen et al. (2011) found that when clients' narratives about problem etiology and change did not match the therapy they were receiving, some clients stagnated, while others productively modified their narratives to fit with the therapy.

Clients' cultural backgrounds also influence how they process therapy. Their cultural backgrounds may influence their willingness to come to therapy (Bohart & Wade, 2013), as well as how they respond to what the therapist is doing. From the client's point of view, culture is one specific set of ideas that clients use in trying to solve their problems, as well as in perceiving and interpreting what therapists offer. We gave an example of that in the previous section. There is evidence that therapists who sensitively respond to clients' cultural backgrounds and who use culturally adapted interventions have more success (Soto et al., 2018).

Clients also may come in with preferences for one form of therapeutic experience or the other. A meta-analysis by Swift et al. (2018) found a positive relationship between therapists who accommodate clients' preferences and positive outcomes. This is particularly true if clients have strong preferences. One client preference of particular relevance to the idea of the client as an active self-healer is that of the degree of their therapist's directiveness. If it is true that clients are active contributors to therapy, does this mean that they should prefer therapy interactions in which they take the lead? Cooper et al. (2019) asked laypersons what kind of therapy experience they would prefer if they were clients. The majority of participants preferred to have the therapist rather than themselves direct therapy. Beutler et al. (2004) reported evidence that, on average, clients also prefer that the therapist take the lead. But there are three caveats. First, not all persons prefer that the therapist be directive. King et al. (2000) found that, for clients who wanted a choice, 60% preferred to have cognitive behavior therapy (a directive approach), while 40% chose person-centered therapy (a nondirective approach). The second caveat has to do with what Beutler and colleagues (2018) termed "client reactance." Beutler et al. found that clients with a high need for autonomy do better with client-directed treatments such as self-help than they do with more directive treatments. This is not to say that when asked, they might not say that they prefer that the therapist take the lead. But empirically, they do better in a therapy that is comparatively nondirective. The third caveat is that although the majority of clients may prefer therapists who are directive, as we shall see later, clients also want to have a say in their therapy experience. They value and treasure their agentic contributions, want therapy to be egalitarian, and like therapy to be collaborative. Therapists being controlling and paternalistic is not desirable.

The issue is not so much who directs therapy as how the therapist is directive. Therapists can be directive and still elicit and take client input seriously, be responsive and collaborative, and foster an egalitarian atmosphere (think of a good teacher, clinical or research supervisor, or a good parent). A recent study (Smoliak et al., 2021) found that therapist directiveness or, as it was called in the study, the exercise of the therapist's professional authority worked best when the therapist first elicited the client's views before implementing an intervention. Then, the intervention was implemented in a stepwise fashion that included client responsiveness and expertise.

Putting together evidence from studies of clients' perceptions of therapy, clients' theories of change, and clients' preferences, what clients bring to the meeting of minds is as follows. They are active interpreters of the therapy environment. They focus on what they need, figure out if the therapist is good for them, have preferences about what they want and need, and interpret what they are getting in terms of what they want and need. They actively seek out and focus on aspects that are important to them and assimilate what is happening to their plans, beliefs, and goals. Not all clients necessarily do all these things. Some clients, for instance, adopt the therapist's frame of reference. However, this too fits with the view of the client as an active cocontributor.

Therapy as Socially Shared Cognition and Collaboration

Moving on from the client's side, we now take a look at how therapists and clients interact. We have suggested that therapy is like the functioning of an intelligent two-person group (Bohart & Tallman, 1999)—a case of socially shared cognition (Resnick et al., 1991). An example of socially shared cognition comes from a study by Elliott (1984) of insight events in therapy. He looked at the interaction between client and therapist that led to the insight event. Elliott said,

> The complexity of these interventions, especially their interactive nature, makes it virtually impossible to fit these events into simple cause-effect explanations or easy-to-analyze "before-after" designs. In other words, the client insights that occur cannot be simply attributed to one person or the other; neither can one neatly contrast client process variables before and after the pivotal intervention. Client and therapist responses interpenetrate, forming "joint events" which are cooperatively produced. (pp. 274–275)

Similarly, Angus (1992) discussed how a rating system developed by herself and a colleague privileged therapists by labeling what they did as "interventions," while what clients said and did were labeled as "responses." Angus observed,

> It is evident that this rating system is based on the implicit assumption that the therapist's job is to provide direction and offer interventions in therapy while the client's job is to follow and respond. This assumption is challenged by the results of the qualitative study. . . . At different points in the verbal interaction, all clients and all therapists in this study were found to initiate topics, make interventions, and follow the lead of the other participant. Had the four sessions been rated on [this coding system] . . . the activity and reflexivity . . . of the clients would have been rendered invisible by the *a priori* decision to classify client statements as responses to therapists' interventions. (p. 201)

In the previously cited Bohart and Byock (2005) study in which the coauthors imagined themselves to "be" clients in three different cases of Carl Rogers, they discovered that the idea of coexperiencing, cothinking, and shared consciousness reflected their experience. To quote one of the authors in the article, "Like a good conversation, what I [Bohart] experienced was a systematic back-and-forth process where each person's responses and experiences deepened the others' and where at times it became difficult to decide just who was initiating the thinking" (p. 203).

Bohart and Byock (2005) went on to quote Clark and Brennen (1991) on human communication:

> It takes two people working together to play a duet, shake hands, play chess, waltz, teach, or make love. To succeed, the two of them have to coordinate both the content and the process of what they are doing . . . to coordinate on content [they must assume] a vast amount of shared information or common ground— that is, mutual knowledge, mutual beliefs, and mutual assumptions. And to coordinate on process, they need to update their common ground moment to moment. All collective actions are built on common ground and its accumulation. (p. 127)

We particularly like the idea of therapy as a form of "collective action" that is built on the constant and ongoing building and accumulating of "common ground." In line with this, several studies have shown that mutuality in therapy is important. Murphy and Cramer (2014) had therapists and clients rate their own experience and how they perceived the experience of the other. When therapists' and clients' ratings converged, suggesting a shared perspective, this led to a more positive outcome. This suggested that it was not merely therapist attunement to the client that mattered but mutual communicative attunement. MacFarlane and colleagues (2017) found that the creation of empathy in therapy is a mutual process between therapist and client. Finally, a meta-analysis of mutuality in therapy in relation to outcome found a moderate effect size of $d = 0.51$ (Cornelius-White et al., 2018).

The meeting of minds model views therapy fundamentally as an act of collaboration, with intervention coming from that, in contrast to the interventionist model, which sees collaboration as in service of intervention. Although many clients may want therapists to take the lead, if clients are active agents, this would imply that they would also value collaboration. We have previously pointed out (Bohart & Tallman, 1999) that what therapists often mean by collaboration is client compliance. What we mean by collaboration is something more cocreative than that. Therapists should listen to clients, respect the client's frame of reference, work to establish common ground, and coordinate what they do with clients' wisdom. Therapists should also be open to forging solutions together or to the possibility of clients creating their own solutions. A genuinely collaborative attitude invites clients' creative contributions and nurtures their agency. This does not mean every client will want a 50–50 relationship. As noted in our previous discussion of therapist directiveness, the use of professional authority (Smoliak et al., 2021) does not preclude the inclusion of client expertise and responsively listening to them. Many clients may be content to follow the therapist's lead. It means that the therapist is open to moving toward higher levels of collaboration when that is indicated.

The evidence is that collaboration and a related construct, goal consensus, are moderately positively related to outcome (effect sizes of .61 and .49, respectively; Norcross & Lambert, 2018). Other studies indicate the usefulness of collaboration. Bachelor et al. (2007) found that 26.7% of clients were active collaborators. Although they mentioned collaborating with their therapists, they emphasized their own activities in the change process. Another 36.7% were mutual collaborators. They saw what happened in therapy as a joint product of themselves and their therapists. Yet another 33.3% were classified as dependent on the therapist to provide direction, but this did not mean that they did not also see themselves as collaborating in the process.

Fitting with the idea of collaboration is research suggesting that clients want a say in decision making and value an egalitarian relationship in therapy. Noyce and Simpson (2018) found that therapists who work to reduce the power differential and establish a level of mutual respect fostered better therapeutic alliances. Katsakou and Pistrang (2018) studied therapy with clients with borderline personality disorder. They found that when participants did not feel included as equal partners—when they thought therapy was imposed on them rather than negotiated and agreed—they didn't feel motivated to make progress. When they saw the therapist as rigid or inflexible, they felt their liberty restricted. When they felt included, they felt trusted, valued, and empowered. Similarly, Sundet (2011) found that families liked having some say in what was going on.

With a focus on mutuality, dialogue, and two minds working together, therapist responsiveness becomes the single most important therapist "skill." *Effective responsiveness* (Stiles et al., 1998) consists of therapists' ability to be aware of and adjust to the evolving context. Repeatedly, studies have found that therapists who respond uniquely and sensitively to their clients are more helpful or seen as more helpful by clients. The idea of therapists applying in a blanket manner standardized protocols to clients does not fit with the emphasis on the unique therapist–client relationships that come out of these studies. Timulak and Keogh (2017) found that clients valued the willingness of the therapist to seek client perspectives, openness to hearing what clients have to say, and the ability to moderate actions. Sundet (2011) found that families valued therapists who met the families where they were at and who were flexible.

Next, we summarize the research findings we have covered so far and then move on to spell out implications for practice.

Summarizing the Research Findings

We believe the following are compatible with the available evidence:

- Clients can and often do make an active, independent contribution to outcome in therapy. They do this both by being engaged, open, and involved in the process, as well as through their own active, creative information-processing efforts.

- Clients' active ability to creatively use what they learn in therapy provides one explanation for the dodo bird verdict. It also provides one explanation for why self-help procedures often work as well or nearly as well as professionally provided therapy.

- There is evidence that client agency correlates with both outcome and facilitation of the alliance. Furthermore, clients report that their agency contributes to therapy.

- Similarly, clients value collaboration and feeling that the therapy relationship is egalitarian and that their wishes and ideas are included in therapy.

- Clients selectively focus on and emphasize parts of the therapy experience and environment as being helpful that do not always correlate with what therapists or therapists' theories select as helpful. Yet clients' perceptions predict outcome at least as well as those of professionals and typically better. This suggests that clients actively focus on parts of the therapy experience that are useful to them in their self-healing activities.

- Clients can extract and detect underlying patterns in the therapy experience that help and support their change efforts. Their interpretations of what therapists are doing and what they are getting out of therapy do not necessarily dovetail with therapists' theories.

- Clients treat therapist responses and interventions as tools they use to help them change. They interpret them and use them in ways that meet what they need. Again, this is not necessarily what the therapist intended them for. In this regard, clients creatively operate on therapists' interventions to bring out their potential for change in terms of what clients need.

- Clients actively contribute to the therapy relationship and manage to get what they need from therapy.

- Clients can creatively go beyond therapists' interventions to generate their own interventions.

- Clients actively work outside of therapy to creatively meld their learning in therapy with their everyday lives. Change does not only happen in therapy.

- Clients integrate learnings from therapy into their schemas, preexisting ideas, and goals to create outcome. What they see as change does not necessarily dovetail with what therapists think they are changing.

- Clients' theories of change, preferences, and expectations have an impact on outcome and need to be taken into account by therapists.

- Psychotherapy, therefore, can profitably be viewed as a meeting of minds or as an example of socially shared cognition, in which therapists and clients cocreate change.

IMPLICATIONS FOR PRACTICE: SUPPORTING ACTIVE SELF-HEALING THROUGH A MEETING OF MINDS

As we have said, the client as an active expert implies that therapy is a meeting of minds. In this alternative conceptualization, the therapist is not seen as simply treating or fixing the client independently, nor as the sole healer of the medical model. The therapist is not doing something to the client. Instead, in this conceptualization, the therapist is an active participant along with the client, shares ideas and perspectives, invites and contemplates ideas and experiences from clients, and responds and works with what emerges. The therapist is flexible and aims to develop a common understanding that leads to collaboration in problem solving. The therapist and client are both steering the ship. We believe the evidence suggests the following in clinical practice.

Welcome and Incorporate Client Expertise

The therapist recognizes the client's deep expertise about their beliefs, feelings, strengths, weaknesses, history, social context, preferences, and goals. The value of client expertise may seem obvious, but embracing it contributes to the overall collaborative stance toward the client. Especially important to the therapist is the client's knowledge of barriers to change and knowledge of what has helped in the past and what has not helped. This knowledge puts the client in a strong position to contribute to or craft strategies and solutions.

The Therapist Does Not Have to Be the Hero

The therapist does not have to have all the answers. The client is an active collaborator. Because of the client's deep expertise, the therapist need not feel they must identify all insights, interventions, or the solution to the client's challenges. Further, the client must contribute because they have to translate what is learned in therapy and apply it to their complex, dynamic life situation. Many adjustments may be necessary. If therapy is successful, it will be partly due to the client's ongoing creative adaptations in their life. It is the client who is the ultimate interventionist.

If the Client Is an Expert, How Does the Therapist Support the Client's Development?

The therapist is a process expert. The therapist's professional training, interpersonal skills, and techniques amplify the client's agency, which supports development. The therapist provides basic conditions that foster growth: a safe relationship and the time, space, and support to experience feelings and think through the situation. In this space, the client can put all the issues "on the table," and both participants can work on the issues together. To serve in this role, the therapist uses active listening skills—not as an intervention to remove barriers but to be supportive and begin the process of exploration and self-understanding. The effect is to create a safe workspace for review and thought. The therapist effectively extends the client's working memory and provides interventions that stimulate client thinking, exploration, and creative applications. Clients can then reflect, reevaluate life choices, revise beliefs, reimagine, craft new perspectives, and design or codesign interventions. The therapist serves both as a trusted companion and a cothinker for addressing challenges, working through different options, and deploying strengths. The client perspective incorporates some of the therapist's input, and then the client modifies it to fit their world.

Not all clients are active to the same degree. Some clients are highly agentic and active in session. Less active clients are still experts, however. Even the quietest client interprets and assimilates what they learn from the interaction with the therapist. All clients must actively develop applications to real life from what they experience in therapy (and from other elements of their lives). Some clients are happy to follow the therapist's lead but may still have to modify interventions when they return to their lives through trial and error. Life is not static; conditions change. The client adapts continually.

A Somewhat Different View of Listening and Empathy

To support the therapeutic process, listening and empathy are used to understand and build the relationship, not primarily to soften defenses or increase compliance. Without deeply understanding the client's perspective (and demonstrating that understanding with reflections and summaries), the therapist cannot be an effective collaborator. Some approaches steer therapists to focusing on interpreting and thinking about the best response or interventions to use next, based on their theories. In contrast, we believe the main moment-to-moment focus of the therapist should be on understanding the client and actively testing that understanding with reflections and summaries, then testing the new understanding again. This means the therapist may initially be off track but eventually will understand. The therapist should follow the client, not the theory. Being heard and fully understood is intrinsically healing and supports agency, development, and openness to considering new perspectives. It helps clients listen to themselves more effectively, so they can become expert observers of their own experience and be able to introduce some distance between themselves and their challenges.

Related to listening is the handling of long quiet moments in therapy. Be open to periods of silence when the client is thinking or experiencing. Often the client is "processing," making novel associations, and reexamining. This counters our usual social conditioning but can be valuable when appropriate. Interruptions break the train of thought and weaken the client's agency.

The following are two examples of the active client through the meeting of minds. First, there can be good progress in session without much therapist participation. Some clients will describe their situation and talk fluidly, presenting the challenge and attempts to change and speculate on reasons for success and failure. They may need little input from the therapist beyond some active listening responses. At some point, they realize they know a lever to pull to make an adjustment. They will express relief and thank the therapist. The therapist often feels they did not "do anything." When this happens, the therapist did do something by providing an important function: allowing the client to have a time, place, and safe relationship to explore, feel, and think. They had an opportunity to have an effective conversation with themselves and may apply that skill later when a challenge presents itself. Second, active listening reflections and summary responses can be powerful. We have had experiences in which a client describes their attitudes and behavior and responds strongly to the comments reflected back to them, saying, "When I hear you say it, I don't like what I said." Then they discuss how they wanted to modify their attitude or actions. The therapist gave no guidance but still played an essential role in challenging an attitude that didn't reflect the client's values.

Redefining Resistance as an Opportunity for Collaborative Exploration

There are clients who are not in therapy voluntarily; some of them may not be receptive to therapy. But most clients are hurting and want to improve their lives. Inevitably, clients will disagree with some interventions, interpretations, opinions, or processes. This has been interpreted as "resistance." One way the meeting of minds model differs from other approaches is the response to noncompliance or resistance. We do not view this friction as something to overcome. We believe this calls for a collaborative attitude—exploring the ideas and feelings the client is experiencing. The therapist should be open to taking a new direction. After this exploration, new perspectives are likely to unfold.

For example, hearing "yeah, but" may be frustrating for the therapist, but it is actually an opportunity. One of us was a stockbroker in a previous career. Salespersons know resistance (called objections) indicates that you lack some important data. We learned to value objections. Hearing an objection meant we missed something essential: values, ability, lack of information, resources, other players, responsibilities, fear, or something about the relationship. After further discussion, we could incorporate the newly understood element. Similarly, the therapist can explore to learn more. In therapy, the goal is not to persuade the client to the therapist's point of view but to work together to craft a common understanding, approach, or solution based on the client's history, experience, context, and preferences. The useful approach is the one that works for the client, regardless of who invented the new direction—the therapist, client, or (typically) both.

We know from change management that people are reluctant to change behavior when they don't agree on the problem and own the solution, either by creating or contributing to or agreeing with the idea. Clients may attempt to use a therapist's intervention, but if it can't be assimilated, it will not be useful. If a therapist is too attached to their own ideas about what the client needs or how to progress, therapy can be disrupted. People often resist ideas that they feel are imposed on them. Therapists can gain buy-in by exploring the viability of an intervention with the client or working with the client on their hypotheses.

Clients make lemonade out of any lemons that the therapist offers, but conflict happens. Feel free to detach from theory, specific techniques, and personal hypotheses if they get in the way of the relationship and cause conflict. Conditions for growth are present as long as there is a good relationship and the therapist is not dominating and permits clients to share in the decision-making process. Sometimes the client might simply not be ready for "interventions." They may need more time to express, understand, and explore. The therapist can then return to working in the collaborative, safe workspace before advancing to an intervention. When clients are challenging or do not seem to be progressing, search for the wisdom in client behavior. There is a rationale behind clients' strategies, beliefs, and behavior. Learning, understanding, and reflecting that rationale helps the client examine those beliefs.

Table 1.1 shows the contrast between the traditional model of therapy and the meeting of minds model, with implications for therapist actions.

TABLE 1.1. Contrasts Between Therapy Models

Component	Traditional therapy model	Therapy as a meeting of minds
Underlying framework	Like the medical model, therapist operates on client dysfunctions, using effective interventions	Therapy is a collaboration between two intelligent minds—client and therapist cothink, coexperience, and coconstruct strategies and solutions
Beliefs	Therapist interventions produce change in clients, result in symptom reduction, as long as client complies	Client is the primary source of healing
		Change is the result of creative problem solving by client, supported by therapist ideas and interventions
		Client sculpts therapist offerings to suit own life context
		Client "owns" concepts to which they contributed
Expertise	Therapist identifies the problem, what treatment is needed, and offers solutions	Client is expert on own life
		Therapist is a process expert, expert listener, and trusted companion
	Therapist is the expert healer	Client uses expertise of the therapist
Client role	Share information	Share information
	Comply with exercises and implement interventions	Collaborate with therapist in exploring experiences, thinking, feeling, constructing strategies and interventions

(continues)

TABLE 1.1. Contrasts Between Therapy Models (*Continued*)

Component	Traditional therapy model	Therapy as a meeting of minds
Therapist role	Build relationship	Support the self-healing process
	Diagnose, plan, intervene to reduce pathology and symptoms	Be a trusted companion, listening to and fully understanding client's perspective, working with the client's realities
	Choose and apply interventions	Create a safe workplace (a time and place and permission to feel, think, imagine, and solve problems)
	Overcome barriers	
		Offer education, ideas, techniques
Purpose of listening and empathy	Build relationship and soften barriers to treatment	While listening and empathy does build relationships, its main purpose is to fully understand the client's perspective and be an effective collaborator
Therapist's moment-to-moment focus	Choosing effective process, and implementing interventions	Responsively and accurately tracking the client's perceptions and perspectives
Interventions	Interventions act on client to produce change	Interventions tend to be cocreated by client and therapist
Resistance	If client does not agree or comply, therapist may perceive client is "resistant"	Conflict suggests the need to explore further—perhaps the therapist has a knowledge gap or therapist and client have conflicting goals
	Therapist needs to treat resistance	Permit and expect client to have own interpretations and codesign their own interventions

LIMITATIONS OF THE RESEARCH

Commenting on the reliability of the evidence for the conclusions cited is difficult because this is not a thorough review. We have presented only examples of the evidence, some from previous reviews and some from recent studies. Also, we have not discussed the details of how each study was conducted.

On the basis of a convergence of evidence, we have confidence in the conclusions we have drawn, particularly the overall conclusion that clients are active, creative agents. Rozin (2001) argued that in the world of science at large, conclusions are largely based on a convergence of evidence, in contrast to psychology's emphasis on experiments. Each study may be imperfect, but a convergence of evidence can lead to confidence in a conclusion. Rozin said about evolutionary theory,

> On the one hand, the theory of evolution is as basic, general, and certain as anything in the life and behavioral sciences. On the other hand, the evidence for this

theory can be described as a truly massive amount of real-world observations (and very few experiments), all of which are individually subject to other interpretations. In short, it is a very large amount of convergent evidence, each piece of which is pretty questionable. . . . It is not clear that any of the pieces of convergent evidence for the theory of evolution would have ever passed the criteria for publication in the *Journal of Personality and Social Psychology*. (p. 7)

The studies we have cited have a variety of limitations. Some are qualitative with small samples (but if you add up the samples, there is a reasonable number). Some studies are self-report (but their findings converge with non-self-report studies). Some are unpublished conference reports or dissertations (but again, their findings converge with published studies). Overall, we believe the evidence converges on the conclusion that clients are active agents in therapy who make major contributions to their recovery process. However, there are many unanswered questions. We do not know how much clients contribute and when they do so. We do not know if all clients creatively contribute. We know little about how to facilitate and work with clients' creative contributions. Further research is needed.

CONCLUSION

We conclude with a note of clarification. We have contrasted our point of view with the dominant "interventionist" model of therapy. That model privileges the therapist's efforts and interventions and minimizes, if not totally ignores, active, creative contributions of the client. This is not to say that, in practice, good therapists are not aware of clients as active, creative agents. Indeed, we believe that good therapists recognize the need to be flexible, responsive to clients, and so on. But these are talked about in terms of the pragmatics of practice. They do not make their way into theoretical models of how change occurs. In terms of theories and models of change, clients' roles are conspicuously absent. We suggest that the evidence warrants a change in this and that understanding the role of the client will enhance our ability to help our clients.

REFERENCES

Adler, J. M., Skalina, L. M., & McAdams, D. P. (2008). The narrative reconstruction of psychotherapy and psychological health. *Psychotherapy Research, 18*(6), 719–734. https://doi.org/10.1080/10503300802326020

Altimir, C., Krause, M., de la Parra, G., Dagnino, P., Tomicic, A., Valdés, N., Perez, J. C., Echávarri, O., & Vilches, O. (2010). Clients', therapists', and observers' agreement on the amount, temporal location, and content of psychotherapeutic change and its relation to outcome. *Psychotherapy Research, 20*(4), 472–487. https://doi.org/10.1080/10503301003705871

American Psychological Association. (2013). Recognition of psychotherapy effectiveness. *Journal of Psychotherapy Integration, 23*(3), 320–330. https://doi.org/10.1037/a0033179

Angus, L., & Kagan, F. (2007). Empathic relational bonds and personal agency in psychotherapy: Implications for psychotherapy supervision, practice, and research. *Psychotherapy, 44*(4), 371–377. https://doi.org/10.1037/0033-3204.44.4.371

Angus, L. E. (1992). Metaphor and the communication interaction in psychotherapy: A multimethodological approach. In S. G. Toukmanian & D. L. Rennie (Eds.), *Psychotherapy process research: Paradigmatic and narrative approaches* (pp. 187–210). SAGE.

Angus, L. E., & Kagan, F. (2013). Assessing client self-narrative change in emotion-focused therapy of depression: An intensive single case analysis. *Psychotherapy, 50*(4), 525–534. https://doi.org/10.1037/a0033358

Asay, T. P., & Lambert, M. J. (1999). The empirical case for the common factors in therapy: Quantitative findings. In M. A. Hubble, B. L. Duncan, & S. D. Miller (Eds.), *The heart and soul of change: What works in therapy* (pp. 23–55). American Psychological Association. https://doi.org/10.1037/11132-001

Bachelor, A., Laverdière, O., Gamache, D., & Bordeleau, V. (2007). Clients' collaboration in therapy: Self-perceptions and relationships with client psychological functioning, interpersonal relations, and motivation. *Psychotherapy, 44*(2), 175–192. https://doi.org/10.1037/0033-3204.44.2.175

Bekele, A., Byock, G., Mehta, S., & Bohart, A. (2004, November 4–7). Therapy from the client's perspective: A response-by-response vicarious ethnographic investigation. In A. C. Bohart & K. Clarke (Chairs), *Qualitative explorations of the context-specific nature of therapy* [Symposium]. North American Society for Psychotherapy Research Conference, Springdale, Utah, United States.

Bergin, A. E., & Garfield, S. L. (1994). Overview, trends, and future issues. In A. E. Bergin & S. L. Garfield (Ed.), *Handbook of psychotherapy and behavior change* (4th ed., pp. 821–830). Wiley.

Beutler, L. E., Edwards, C., & Someah, K. (2018). Adapting psychotherapy to patient reactance level: A meta-analytic review. *Journal of Clinical Psychology, 74*(11), 1952–1963. https://doi.org/10.1002/jclp.22682

Beutler, L. E., Malik, M., Alimohamed, S., Harwood, T. M., Talebi, H., Noble, S., & Wong, E. (2004). Therapist variables. In M. J. Lambert (Ed.), *Bergin and Garfield's handbook of psychotherapy and behavior change* (5th ed., pp. 227–306). Wiley.

Bohart, A. C. (2007). An alternative view of concrete operating procedures from the perspective of the client as active self-healer. *Journal of Psychotherapy Integration, 17*(1), 125–137. https://doi.org/10.1037/1053-0479.17.1.125

Bohart, A. C. (2015). From there and back again. *Journal of Clinical Psychology, 71*(11), 1060–1069. https://doi.org/10.1002/jclp.22216

Bohart, A. C., Bekele, A., & Byock, G. (2007, June 20–23). *How one client productively constructs a therapy interaction from within her world view: A vicarious-ethnographic examination of one client's experience* [Poster presentation]. Society for Psychotherapy Research 38th Annual Meeting, Madison, WI, United States.

Bohart, A. C., & Boyd, G. (1997, December 4–7). *Clients' construction of the therapy process: A qualitative analysis* [Poster presentation]. North American Association of the Society for Psychotherapy Research, Tucson, AZ, United States.

Bohart, A. C., & Byock, G. (2005). Experiencing Carl Rogers from the client's point of view: A vicarious ethnographic investigation. I. Extraction and perception of meaning. *The Humanistic Psychologist, 33*(3), 187–211. https://doi.org/10.1207/s15473333thp3303_2

Bohart, A. C., & Tallman, K. (1999). *How clients make therapy work: The process of active self-healing.* American Psychological Association. https://doi.org/10.1037/10323-000

Bohart, A. C., & Tallman, K. (2010). Clients as active self-healers: Implications for the person-centered approach. In M. Cooper, J. C. Watson, & D. Hölldampf (Eds.), *Person-centered and experiential therapies work* (pp. 91–131). PCCS Books.

Bohart, A. C., & Wade, A. G. (2013). The client in psychotherapy. In M. J. Lambert (Ed.), *Bergin and Garfield's handbook of psychotherapy and behavior change* (6th ed., pp. 219–257). Wiley.

Cantor, N. (2003). Constructive cognition, personal goals, and the social embedding of personality. In L. G. Aspinwall & U. M. Staudinger (Eds.), *A psychology of human strengths* (pp. 49–60). American Psychological Association. https://doi.org/10.1037/10566-004

Castonguay, L. G., Boswell, J. F., Zack, S. E., Baker, S., Boutselis, M. A., Chiswick, N. R., Damer, D. D., Hemmelstein, N. A., Jackson, J. S., Morford, M., Ragusea, S. A., Roper, J. G., Spayd, C., Weiszer, T., Borkovec, T. D., & Holtforth, M. G. (2010). Helpful and hindering events in psychotherapy: A practice research network study. *Psychotherapy, 47*(3), 327–344. https://doi.org/10.1037/a0021164

Clark, H. H., & Brennen, S. E. (1991). Grounding in communication. In L. B. Resnick, J. M. Levine, & S. D. Teasley (Eds.), *Perspectives on socially shared cognition* (pp. 127–149). American Psychological Association. https://doi.org/10.1037/10096-006

Cooper, M., Norcross, J. C., Raymond-Barker, B., & Hogan, T. P. (2019). Psychotherapy preferences of laypersons and mental health professionals: Whose therapy is it? *Psychotherapy, 56*(2), 205–216. https://doi.org/10.1037/pst0000226

Cornelius-White, J., Kanamori, Y., Murphy, D., & Tickle, E. (2018). Mutuality in psychotherapy: A meta-analysis and meta-synthesis. *Journal of Psychotherapy Integration, 28*(4), 489–504. https://doi.org/10.1037/int0000134

Cross, D. G., Sheehan, P. W., & Khan, J. A. (1980). Alternative advice and counsel in psychotherapy. *Journal of Consulting and Clinical Psychology, 48*(5), 615–625. https://doi.org/10.1037/0022-006X.48.5.615

Dreier, O. (2000). Psychotherapy in clients' trajectories across contexts. In C. Mattingly & L. Garro (Eds.), *Narrative and the cultural construction of illness and healing* (pp. 237–258). University of California Press.

Duncan, B. L., & Miller, S. D. (2000). The client's theory of change: Consulting the client in the integrative process. *Journal of Psychotherapy Integration, 10*(2), 169–187. https://link.springer.com/article/10.1023/A:1009448200244

Elliott, R. (1984). A discovery-oriented approach to significant change events in psychotherapy: Interpersonal process recall and comprehensive process analysis. In L. S. Greenberg & L. N. Rice (Eds.), *Patterns of change* (pp. 249–286). Guilford Press.

Elliott, R., Bohart, A. C., Watson, J. C., & Murphy, D. (2018). Therapist empathy and client outcome: An updated meta-analysis. *Psychotherapy, 55*(4), 399–410. https://doi.org/10.1037/pst0000175

Elliott, R., & Shapiro, D. A. (1992). Clients and therapists as analysts of significant events. In S. G. Toukmanian & D. L. Rennie (Eds.), *Psychotherapy process research: Theory-guided and phenomenological research strategies* (pp. 163–186). SAGE.

Elliott, R., Shapiro, D. A., Firth-Cozens, J., Stiles, W. B., Hardy, G. E., Llewelyn, S. P., & Margison, F. R. (1994). Comprehensive process analysis of insight events in cognitive-behavioral and psychodynamic-interpersonal psychotherapies. *Journal of Counseling Psychology, 41*(4), 449–463. https://doi.org/10.1037/0022-0167.41.4.449

Fuertes, J. N., & Williams, E. N. (2017). Client-focused psychotherapy research. *Journal of Counseling Psychology, 64*(4), 369–375. https://doi.org/10.1037/cou0000214

Garfinkel, H. (1967). *Studies in ethnomethodology*. Prentice-Hall.

Gendlin, E. T. (1980). *Focusing*. Bantam.

Gibson, J. J. (1979). *The ecological approach to visual perception*. Houghton Mifflin.

Gold, J. R. (1994). When the patient does the integrating: Lessons for theory and practice. *Journal of Psychotherapy Integration, 4*, 133–158. https://doi.org/10.1037/h0101153

Greaves, A. L. (2006). *The active client: A qualitative analysis of thirteen clients' contribution to the psychotherapeutic process* [Unpublished doctoral dissertation]. University of Southern California.

Hamm, J. A., Buck, K. D., Leonhardt, B. L., Luther, L., & Lysaker, P. H. (2018). Self-directed recovery in schizophrenia: Attending to clients' agendas in psychotherapy. *Journal of Psychotherapy Integration, 28*(2), 188–201. https://doi.org/10.1037/int0000070

Hanna, F. J., & Ritchie, M. H. (1995). Seeking the active ingredients of psychotherapeutic change: Within and outside the context of therapy. *Professional Psychology: Research and Practice, 26*(2), 176–183. https://doi.org/10.1037/0735-7028.26.2.176

Hartmann, A., Orlinsky, D., Weber, S., Sandholz, A., & Zeeck, A. (2010). Session and intersession experience related to treatment outcome in bulimia nervosa. *Psychotherapy, 47*(3), 355–370. https://doi.org/10.1037/a0021166

Hayes, J. A., & Wall, T. N. (1998). What influences clinicians' responsibility attributions? The role of problem type, theoretical orientation, and client attribution. *Journal of Social and Clinical Psychology, 17*(1), 69–74. https://doi.org/10.1521/jscp.1998.17.1.69

Helmeke, K. B., & Sprenkle, D. H. (2000). Clients' perceptions of pivotal moments in couples therapy: A qualitative study of change in therapy. *Journal of Marital and Family Therapy, 26*(4), 469–483. https://doi.org/10.1111/j.1752-0606.2000.tb00317.x

Hendricks, M. N. (2002). Focusing-oriented/experiential psychotherapy. In D. J. Cain & J. Seeman (Eds.), *Humanistic psychotherapies: Handbook of research and practice* (pp. 221–251). American Psychological Association. https://doi.org/10.1037/10439-007

Hoener, C., Stiles, W. B., Luka, B. J., & Gordon, R. A. (2012). Client experiences of agency in therapy. *Person-Centered and Experiential Psychotherapies, 11*(1), 64–82. https://doi.org/10.1080/14779757.2011.639460

Huber, J., Born, A.-K., Claaß, C., Ehrenthal, J. C., Nikendei, C., Schauenburg, H., & Dinger, U. (2019). Therapeutic agency, in-session behavior, and patient-therapist interaction. *Journal of Clinical Psychology, 75*(1), 66–78. https://doi.org/10.1002/jclp.22700

Huber, J., Nikendei, C., Ehrenthal, J. C., Schauenburg, H., Mander, J., & Dinger, U. (2019). Therapeutic Agency Inventory: Development and psychometric validation of a patient self-report. *Psychotherapy Research, 29*(7), 919–934. https://doi.org/10.1080/10503307.2018.1447707

Katsakou, C., & Pistrang, N. (2018). Clients' experiences of treatment and recovery in borderline personality disorder: A meta-synthesis of qualitative studies. *Psychotherapy Research, 28*(6), 940–957. https://doi.org/10.1080/10503307.2016.1277040

Khattra, J., Angus, L., Westra, H., Macaulay, C., Moertl, K., & Constantino, M. (2017). Client perceptions of corrective experiences in cognitive behavioral therapy and motivational interviewing for generalized anxiety disorder: An exploratory pilot study. *Journal of Psychotherapy Integration, 27*(1), 23–34. https://doi.org/10.1037/int0000053

King, M., Sibbald, B., Ward, E., Bower, P., Lloyd, M., Gabbay, M., & Byford, S. (2000). Randomised controlled trial of non-directive counselling, cognitive-behaviour therapy and usual general practitioner care in the management of depression as well as mixed anxiety and depression in primary care. *Health Technology Assessment, 4*(19), 1–83. https://doi.org/10.3310/hta4190

Knight, T. A., Richert, A. J., & Brownfield, C. R. (2012). Conceiving change: Lay accounts of the human change process. *Journal of Psychotherapy Integration, 22*(3), 229–254. https://doi.org/10.1037/a0028871

Kühnlein, I. (1999). Psychotherapy as a process of transformation: Analysis of post-therapeutic autobiographical narrations. *Psychotherapy Research, 9*, 274–288. https://doi.org/10.1093/ptr/9.3.274

Levitt, H., Butler, M., & Hill, T. (2006). What clients find helpful in psychotherapy: Developing principles for facilitating moment-to-moment change. *Journal of Counseling Psychology, 53*(3), 314–324. https://doi.org/10.1037/0022-0167.53.3.314

Levitt, H. M. (2004, November 4–7). *What client interviews reveal about psychotherapy process: Principles for the facilitation of change in psychotherapy* [Paper presentation]. North American Society for Psychotherapy Research, Springdale, UT, United States.

Levitt, H. M., & Rennie, D. L. (2004). Narrative activity: Clients' and therapists' intentions in the process of narration. In L. E. Angus & J. McLeod (Eds.), *The handbook of narrative and psychotherapy* (pp. 298–313). SAGE. https://doi.org/10.4135/9781412973496.d23

Lilliengren, P., Philips, B., Falkenström, F., Bergquist, M., Ulvenes, P., & Wampold, B. (2019). Comparing the treatment process in successful and unsuccessful cases in two forms of psychotherapy for cluster C personality disorders. *Psychotherapy, 56*(2), 285–296. https://doi.org/10.1037/pst0000217

MacFarlane, P., Anderson, T., & McClintock, A. S. (2017). Empathy from the client's perspective: A grounded theory analysis. *Psychotherapy Research, 27*(2), 227–238. https://doi.org/10.1080/10503307.2015.1090038

Mackrill, T. (2008). *The therapy journal project: A cross-contextual qualitative diary study of psychotherapy with adult children of alcoholics* [Unpublished doctoral dissertation]. Copenhagen University.

McKenna, P. A., & Todd, D. M. (1997). Longitudinal utilization of mental health services: A time line method, nine retrospective accounts, and a preliminary conceptualization. *Psychotherapy Research, 7*(4), 383–395. https://doi.org/10.1080/10503309712331332093

Meyer, B., & Garcia-Roberts, L. (2007). Congruence between reasons for depression and motivations for specific interventions. *Psychology and Psychotherapy: Theory, Research and Practice, 80*(4), 525–542. https://doi.org/10.1348/147608306X169982

Mörtl, K., & Von Wietersheim, J. (2008). Client experiences of helpful factors in a day treatment program: A qualitative approach. *Psychotherapy Research, 18*(3), 281–293. https://doi.org/10.1080/10503300701797016

Murphy, D., & Cramer, D. (2014). Mutuality of Rogers's therapeutic conditions and treatment progress in the first three psychotherapy sessions. *Psychotherapy Research, 24*(6), 651–661. https://doi.org/10.1080/10503307.2013.874051

Nissen-Lie, H. A., Solkbakken, O. A., Falkenström, F., Wampold, B. E., Holmqvist, R., Ekeblad, A., & Monsen, J. T. (2020). Does it make a difference to be more "on the same page"? Investigating the role of alliance convergence for outcomes in two different samples. *Psychotherapy Research*. Advance online publication. https://doi.org/10.1080/10503307.2020.1823030

Norcross, J. C. (2006). Integrating self-help into psychotherapy: 16 practical suggestions. *Professional Psychology, Research and Practice, 37*(6), 683–693. https://doi.org/10.1037/0735-7028.37.6.683

Norcross, J. C. (2020, April 25). *Psychotherapy relationships that work* [Presentation]. The Wright Institute, San Francisco, CA.

Norcross, J. C., & Lambert, M. J. (2011). Evidence-based therapy relationships. In J. C. Norcross (Ed.), *Psychotherapy relationships that work: Evidence-based responsiveness* (pp. 3–22). Oxford University Press. https://doi.org/10.1093/acprof:oso/9780199737208.003.0001

Norcross, J. C., & Lambert, M. J. (2018). Psychotherapy relationships that work III. *Psychotherapy, 55*(4), 303–315. https://doi.org/10.1037/pst0000193

Noyce, R., & Simpson, J. (2018). The experience of forming a therapeutic relationship from the client's perspective: A metasynthesis. *Psychotherapy Research, 28*(2), 281–296. https://doi.org/10.1080/10503307.2016.1208373

Orlinsky, D. E., Grawe, K., & Parks, B. K. (1994). Process and outcome in psychotherapy: Noch einmal. In A. E. Bergin & S. L. Garfield (Eds.), *Handbook of psychotherapy and behavior change* (4th ed., pp. 270–378). Wiley.

Orlinsky, D. E., Rønnestad, M. H., & Willutzki, U. (2004). Fifty years of psychotherapy process-outcome research: Continuity and change. In M. J. Lambert (Ed.), *Bergin and Garfield's handbook of psychotherapy and behavior change* (5th ed., pp. 307–390). Wiley.

Philips, B., Werbart, A., Wennberg, P., & Schubert, J. (2007). Young adults' ideas of cure prior to psychoanalytic psychotherapy. *Journal of Clinical Psychology, 63*(3), 213–232. https://doi.org/10.1002/jclp.20342

Prochaska, J. O., Norcross, J. C., & DiClemente, C. C. (1994). *Changing for good*. Morrow.

Ratner, H. (Director). (1986). *Three approaches to psychotherapy: III. Cognitive therapy with Aaron Beck* [Film]. Psychological and Educational Films.

Rennie, D. L. (1990). Toward a representation of the client's experience of the psychotherapy hour. In G. Lietaer, J. Rombauts, & R. Van Balen (Eds.), *Client-centered and experiential psychotherapy in the nineties* (pp. 155–172). Leuven University Press.

Rennie, D. L. (1992). Qualitative analysis of the client's experience of psychotherapy: The unfolding of reflexivity. In S. G. Toukmanian & D. L. Rennie (Eds.), *Psychotherapy process research: Paradigmatic and narrative approaches* (pp. 211–233). SAGE.

Rennie, D. L. (1994). Storytelling in psychotherapy: The client's subjective experience. *Psychotherapy: Theory, Research, & Practice, 31*(2), 234–243. https://doi.org/10.1037/h0090224

Rennie, D. L. (2000). Aspects of the client's conscious control of the psychotherapeutic process. *Journal of Psychotherapy Integration, 10*(2), 151–167. https://link.springer.com/article/10.1023/A:1009496116174

Resnick, L. B., Levine, J. M., & Teasley, S. D. (Eds.). (1991). *Perspectives on socially shared cognition*. American Psychological Association. https://doi.org/10.1037/10096-000

Richards, R. (2007). *Everyday creativity*. American Psychological Association.

Robitschek, C., Yang, A., Villalba Ii, R., & Shigemoto, Y. (2019). Personal growth initiative: A robust and malleable predictor of treatment outcome for depressed partial hospital patients. *Journal of Affective Disorders, 246*, 548–555. https://doi.org/10.1016/j.jad.2018.12.121

Rogers, C. R. (1961). *On becoming a person*. Houghton Mifflin.

Rozin, P. (2001). Social psychology and science: Some lessons from Solomon Asch. *Personality and Social Psychology Review, 5*(1), 2–14. https://doi.org/10.1207/S15327957PSPR0501_1

Selby, C. E. (2004). *Psychotherapy as creative process: A grounded theory exploration* [Unpublished doctoral dissertation]. Saybrook Graduate School.

Shapiro, J. L. (1986). The Evolution of Psychotherapy Conference: Skeptical reflections. *Family Therapy*, 209–214.

Smoliak, O., MacMartin, C., Hepburn, A., Le Couteur, A., Elliott, R., & Quinn-Nilas, C. (2021). Authority in therapeutic interaction: A conversation analytic study. *Journal of Marital and Family Therapy*. Advance online publication. https://doi.org/10.1111/jmft.12471

Soto, A., Smith, T. B., Griner, D., Domenech Rodríguez, M., & Bernal, G. (2018). Cultural adaptations and therapist multicultural competence: Two meta-analytic reviews. *Journal of Clinical Psychology, 74*(11), 1907–1923. https://doi.org/10.1002/jclp.22679

Stiles, W. B., Honos-Webb, L., & Zurko, M. (1998). Responsiveness in psychotherapy. *Clinical Psychology: Science and Practice, 5*(4), 439–458. https://doi.org/10.1111/j.1468-2850.1998.tb00166.x

Sundet, R. (2011). Collaboration: Family and therapist perspectives of helpful therapy. *Journal of Marital and Family Therapy, 37*(2), 236–249. https://doi.org/10.1111/j.1752-0606.2009.00157.x

Swift, J. K., Callahan, J. L., Cooper, M., & Parkin, S. R. (2018). The impact of accommodating client preference in psychotherapy: A meta-analysis. *Journal of Clinical Psychology, 74*(11), 1924–1937. https://doi.org/10.1002/jclp.22680

Tallman, K., Robinson, E., Kay, D., Harvey, S., & Bohart, A. (1994, August 12–16). *Experiential and non-experiential Rogerian therapy: An analogue study* [Paper presentation]. American Psychological Association Convention 102nd Annual Meeting, Los Angeles, CA, United States.

Talmon, M. (1990). *Single session therapy*. Jossey-Bass.

Timulak, L., & Elliott, R. (2003). Empowerment events in process-experiential psychotherapy of depression: An exploratory qualitative analysis. *Psychotherapy Research, 13*(4), 443–460. https://doi.org/10.1093/ptr/kpg043

Timulak, L., & Keogh, D. (2017). The client's perspective on (experiences of) psychotherapy: A practice friendly review. *Journal of Clinical Psychology, 73*(11), 1556–1567. https://doi.org/10.1002/jclp.22532

Tracey, T. J. (1988). Relationship of responsibility attribution congruence to psychotherapy outcome. *Journal of Social and Clinical Psychology, 7*(2–3), 131–146. https://doi.org/10.1521/jscp.1988.7.2-3.131

Valkonen, J., Hänninen, V., & Lindfors, O. (2011). Outcomes of psychotherapy from the perspective of the users. *Psychotherapy Research, 21*(2), 227–240. https://doi.org/10.1080/10503307.2010.548346

von der Lippe, A. L., Oddli, H. W., & Halvorsen, M. S. (2019). Therapist strategies early in therapy associated with good or poor outcomes among clients with low proactive agency. *Psychotherapy Research, 29*(3), 383–402. https://doi.org/10.1080/10503307. 2017.1373205

Wampold, B. E. (2010). The research evidence for common factors models: A historically situated perspective. In B. L. Duncan, S. D. Miller, B. E. Wampold, & M. A. Hubble (Eds.), *The heart and soul of change: Delivering what works in therapy* (2nd ed., pp. 49–81). American Psychological Association. https://doi.org/10.1037/12075-002

Wampold, B. E., & Imel, Z. E. (2015). *The great psychotherapy debate: The evidence for what makes psychotherapy work* (2nd ed.). Routledge/Taylor & Francis. https://doi.org/ 10.4324/9780203582015

Weigold, I. K., Porfeli, E. J., & Weigold, A. (2013). Examining tenets of personal growth initiative using the personal growth initiative scale-II. *Psychological Assessment, 25*(4), 1396–1403. https://doi.org/10.1037/a0034104

Worthington, R. L., & Atkinson, D. R. (1996). Effects of perceived etiology attribution similarity on client ratings of counselor credibility. *Journal of Counseling Psychology, 43*(4), 423–429. https://doi.org/10.1037/0022-0167.43.4.423

Zilbergeld, B., & Lazarus, A. A. (1987). *Mind power*. Ballantine.

2

Understanding and Enhancing Client Motivation

João Tiago Oliveira, Juan Martín Gómez-Penedo, and
Martin grosse Holtforth

Maria is a 50-year-old woman who came to psychotherapy presenting with complaints of sadness during most days and excessive worry about her health and the future, especially her daughter's future.[1] Maria has had two romantic relationships; her daughter's father abandoned them during her pregnancy. Soon after her daughter's birth, at the age of 33, she had visceral complications that recurrently resulted in episodes of acute pain that persist and present a considerable risk of intestinal perforation. Her second relationship started approximately 13 years ago; however, they broke up because "there is no more love, no more passion, not even friendship." Since graduating, she has worked at the same company, several hundred kilometers away from where her family of origin lives. Although she may experience low energy at times, she has always managed to do her work at the company's board of directors: "I think it's the only thing I do minimally well, maybe because it has to be done." She has few social relationships and said that her friends are almost always unavailable: "I look at other people's social networks and all have happy families and interesting lives." Maria says that her emotional difficulties have been going on for several years and that the previous psychotherapy she received was unsuccessful. Despite wanting to "feel happy" and "be like other people," her efforts to change are disorganized and always happening following an event causing acute suffering (e.g., hospitalization due to severe intestinal

https://doi.org/10.1037/0000303-003
The Other Side of Psychotherapy: Understanding Clients' Experiences and Contributions in Treatment, J. N. Fuertes (Editor)

[1]The identity of the client in this case example has been properly disguised to protect their confidentiality.

pain, end of a love relationship). She has repeatedly mentioned that her life will always be like this, that everything bad happens to her, and that if it weren't for her daughter, she would have given up. When the therapist asked her about her main goal for the therapeutic process, she said, "I want to stop feeling like this."

The process of change, within and beyond the therapeutic context, always involves several challenges. While there are moments when the individual clearly perceives movement toward a new reality, there are also moments when both the consequences of change and the path to achieve change are immersed in a dense fog. These climatic fluctuations may be constant, alternations may occur throughout the day, or they might happen more sporadically. Trying to help clients with problems that they failed to cope with themselves involves motivational issues at various levels and stages of therapy. In this endeavor, the therapists' principal goal is to optimally assist their clients in changing what is currently blocking them from living a satisfying life. These obstacles may be manyfold (Westermann et al., 2019) and may lie inside or outside the client. For instance, Maria's personality characteristics and learned helplessness prevent her from deviating from her problematic framework of reference (i.e., "I'm a miserable person"). In addition, the lack of social support hinders her engagement in more adaptive behaviors (e.g., going for lunch with friends). The overall goal of therapy is often to help clients regain personal control of their lives and work toward living more meaningfully. Motivational processes play an important role at various levels and stages of therapy, and motivational issues are relevant in the treatment of all patients, not only in those with obvious motivational deficits.

Clients may be more or less motivated at the start of psychotherapy, and participation may fluctuate at different stages of the psychotherapy process. This kind of motivation is what people usually associate with the term *psychotherapy motivation*. Ideally, clients are willing to work hard all through the therapeutic process and invest a lot of effort into changing their lives, behaviors, and associated experiences. In the first session, Maria was significantly distressed and was willing to do "whatever it takes to feel better." However, some patients may be "of two hearts" (i.e., ambivalent) about starting therapy. This ambivalence may be related to the difficulty of conceiving their own behaviors as part of the problem or taking the steps toward changing their behaviors or other parts of their lives in service of a more satisfying life. In Maria's case, when the therapist proposed behavioral activation interventions (e.g., engagement in adaptive activities such as going for a walk in the morning), she responded to all proposed strategies in the same way: "But I am not able to do it," "It's not worth it. I am just like that. I will never change." As shown through Maria's example, client motivation is important throughout therapy, and it is helpful for therapists to have a repertoire of skills to deal with clients whose motivation might dip.

In this chapter, we first review various motivational concepts and explain how they might become relevant in psychotherapy. Selected empirical findings on how different aspects of a client's motivation may affect the process and outcome of psychotherapy are also discussed. Finally, we address practical ways of detecting and addressing motivationally challenging situations in psychotherapy.

MOTIVATION IN PSYCHOTHERAPY: FROM BASIC TO PSYCHOTHERAPY-SPECIFIC MOTIVATIONAL CONSTRUCTS

During the last few decades, psychotherapy research has generated empirical evidence about the impact of specific factors and the nonspecific reasons underlying the healing process, as well as the possible differential efficacy across different psychotherapeutic approaches (Wampold et al., 2011). If the client contribution explains 30% of the variance in psychotherapy outcome—far from the 12% explained by therapeutic relationship, the next factor, and to which the client also contributes (Norcross & Lambert, 2011)—one could argue that the client is the key in every psychotherapeutic process. Research has shown that the client's engagement with the treatment (Constantino et al., 2010; Wampold et al., 2011) and resistance or reactance to change (Beutler et al., 2011) are crucial dimensions that influence treatment outcome. In fact, both constructs are strictly associated with the assumption that clients are active self-healing agents in therapy (Bohart, 2000). Client engagement in therapy reflects their motivation for change, readiness to change, feelings of belonging to the therapy and therapist, and the acknowledgment of the benefits of changing, as well as some objective indicators such as homework compliance (Wampold et al., 2011), all of which are closely related to treatment success in psychotherapy (Constantino et al., 2010). *Resistance to change* is defined as interpersonal tension that emerges from the dyadic interaction between client and therapist (Button et al., 2015; Miller & Rollnick, 2013), leading to poor outcomes and early dropout from therapy when it is not overcome (Beutler et al., 2011; Engle & Arkowitz, 2006). Thus, how much a client is involved in therapy or resists change is highly informed by motivational factors that can be attenuated or exacerbated throughout the therapeutic process.

Basic Motivational Constructs

Generally, people feel motivated when they pursue something positive or seek the absence of something negative. An individual may perceive the pursued positive or negative end states more or less consciously, and the more important the person deems what is at stake, the more strongly the positive or negative future states are linked to emotions (Heckhausen & Heckhausen, 2008). What is at stake may be understood as "goals" (i.e., targets of the person's striving or avoidance). In psychotherapy, clients seek help for parts of their lives that they failed to handle or cope with. The goals psychotherapy clients usually have involve learning something new to attain goals or reduce the individual sources of their suffering. For some patients, maintaining the status quo (e.g., a current relationship) may also be a goal. To better understand motivation in the psychotherapy context, it will be helpful first to introduce some basic motivational constructs: needs, motives, personal goals, and autonomous motivation.

Needs

It can be assumed that all humans have the same basic needs, and all humans must satisfy them. Apart from biological needs, such as food or sex, people also have psychological needs. There has been a long discussion in the literature about what these psychological needs are, and the lists of psychological needs tend to differ slightly among authors. For example, Deci and Ryan (1985) named relatedness, competence, and autonomy; Epstein (1998) mentioned self-enhancement, attachment, pleasure, and orientation or control; and Dweck (2017) saw acceptance, competence, and predictability as the basic human needs. Some authors assume overarching metaneeds, such as a need for meaning (Heine et al., 2006) or consistency among one's strivings (Grawe, 2004). Furthermore, theoreticians seem to agree that aversive outcomes such as diminished well-being or psychopathology might develop if the individual fails to satisfy these needs (Dweck, 2017; Grawe, 2004). Despite the considerable diversity of psychological needs, we know that they have the potential to generate goals and subsequent behaviors to achieve them. Therefore, successful psychotherapy should be associated with a client's ability to meet their psychological needs better. Maria's need for relatedness, for example, led her to remain in psychologically violent relationships. She always accepted her first husband's absence, betrayals, and verbal abuse for the sake of feeling connected. Her last relationship, which went on for several years, was characterized by a total lack of affection and care, but, according to her, "at least he was there."

In the therapy process, the therapist must be able to identify, keep in mind, and know how to manage the needs of their clients. A robust body of evidence has suggested the direct and indirect contributions of fulfilling needs to the achievement of positive outcomes (e.g., Sheldon & Filak, 2008). The results of a study with 51 clients diagnosed with major depressive disorder, who were randomly assigned to 16 weeks of cognitive behavior therapy or antidepressant medication, showed that psychological need fulfillment increased in both groups, and the increase in need fulfillment was associated with a decrease in depression severity (Quitasol et al., 2018). With a focus on daily variations of needs and well-being, Reis et al. (2000) showed that the daily variation in self-reported autonomy, competence, and relatedness predicted daily fluctuations in well-being. Other studies have suggested that there is an association between the fulfillment of psychological needs and a stronger therapeutic alliance (Keleher et al., 2019), attachment style characterized by security (La Guardia et al., 2000), self-regulation (Keleher et al., 2019), and/or self-endorsed motivation toward the end of therapy (van der Kaap-Deeder et al., 2014). With Maria, the therapist started by collaboratively identifying this need for relatedness and how that need manifested in her abusive relationships. Could it be that "being physically present" is what she considers "being there" for her? What types of behaviors did she adopt throughout her life that called into question other areas of her life (e.g., her daughter's development)?

Likewise, there was a great focus from the beginning on the construction of the therapeutic relationship with special emphasis on the bond dimension.

Personal Goals

As personal instances of what people strive for or want to avoid, personal goals are motivational constructs at a middle level of abstraction—that is, they are more concrete than needs but less concrete than (motivated) behavior (see Elliot, 2008, for a review). For example, the psychological need to strive for relatedness may be linked with a personal goal of maintaining a harmonious, loving relationship with one's partner and with the concrete behavior of inviting one's partner for a romantic dinner at a fine restaurant. The literature has suggested two kinds of motivation (and goals): approach and avoidance. In this context, *approach goals* are developed to satisfy psychological needs, whereas *avoidance goals* prevent these needs from being threatened (Grawe, 2004). In other words, they differ as a function of their valence. For example, Maria's approach goals could involve devoting efforts to forming new friendships, finding a new intimate relationship, living a more active life, or looking for a new job. However, she does not do so to avoid feeling rejected, feeling humiliated, and facing the finitude of life when some new physical symptom appears (e.g., chest pain)—her avoidance goals. grosse Holtforth and Grawe (2000) empirically identified and categorized the contents of personal goals that therapists considered to be relevant for their clients in case formulations. Personal goals are used as personal standards by the individual to compare life experiences and receive individual feedback regarding goal attainment and need satisfaction (Klinger, 1977). Taken together, all personal goals of an individual inform the future the individual strives for (Markus & Nurius, 1986), giving the person's life purpose, structure, and meaning (Klinger, 1977).

Empirical research has also shown that psychotherapy clients tend to pursue more avoidance goals than do nonclinical controls (Westermann et al., 2019) and that higher levels of avoidance goals are related to lower levels of well-being, higher severity of psychopathology, and decreased levels of goal satisfaction (e.g., grosse Holtforth & Grawe, 2000). This seems to be what happens to Maria. To avoid feeling loneliness and rejection and being unable to respond to some day-to-day challenges, such as going to the hospital in the middle of the night if she has an intestinal crisis, she has remained in abusive relationships for long periods. After the last breakup, she did not work on herself and instead avoided her problems by escaping into a new relationship. One possible explanation is that due to the elicitation of more negative cognitions and emotions, monitoring and managing the goal process is much more difficult for avoidance goals than for approach goals (Tamir & Diener, 2008). Accordingly, avoiding aversive experiences is assumed to contribute to the development and maintenance of psychological distress (grosse Holtforth, 2008). This could also partially explain why avoidant clients have more difficulty attending their initial therapy appointments (Murphy et al., 2016). Accordingly, therapists often work with their clients at establishing explicit treatment goals (Oddli et al., 2014) to promote client engagement and collaboration in treatment (Park et al., 2019).

Autonomous Motivation

Autonomous motivation, a concept of self-determination theory (e.g., Deci & Ryan, 1985, 1991), is the kind of positive motivational state psychotherapy clients ideally experience, such as having a strong interest in changing oneself, being curious about new experiences to have and new skills to learn, and feeling committed to doing whatever is necessary to accomplish one's therapy goals (Ryan et al., 2011). Stressing the autonomy aspect, Zuroff and colleagues (2007) explained *autonomous motivation* as "the extent to which patients experience participation in treatment as a freely made choice emanating from themselves" (p. 137). Therefore, autonomous motivation includes intrinsically motivated behaviors that are self-determined. However, motivation can be controlled, and this *controlled motivation* occurs when the individual's behaviors are driven by internal and/or external forces and, in this sense, although they are intentional behaviors, the client does not want to pursue them. At the extreme, *amotivation* refers to a lack of intention and motivation to change (Deci & Ryan, 1991). It is composed of unintentional and disorganized behaviors because the client is unable to regulate their actions.

Autonomous motivation has shown to be a strong predictor of outcome in different treatment approaches (Dwyer et al., 2011; Zuroff et al., 2007) and in both short- and long-term therapy. Zuroff et al. (2017) found that higher levels of therapist and client autonomous motivation and lower levels of controlled motivation predicted better outcomes. In a study of patients with depression, Taylor et al. (2020) found that lower levels of autonomous motivation for treatment along with higher levels of self-criticism were associated with higher depressive symptoms 1 year after treatment. In the same study, the effect of controlled motivation was nonsignificant. Thus, the promotion of autonomous motivation in therapy seems to be a general facilitator of good outcomes (Dwyer et al., 2011). Maria has never been intrinsically motivated, meaning her levels of autonomous motivation have always been almost absent. She recalls that the only decision she feels she wanted to make in her life was to go to university: "Although I was far from home and cried every day for being away, it was the university I wanted." Otherwise, a large part of her life felt as if she was doing things because they had to be done. The amotivational state in which she often finds herself has a bidirectional relationship with her persistent depressive disorder. Her motivation is eminently controlled, either to respond to the demands placed on her by her daughter or to escape the acute subjective suffering that she often experiences. However, given her persistent depressive disorder, she recurrently falls into an amotivational state.

Constructs Particularly Relevant for Psychotherapy

As we have discussed, even when motivation is not an explicit focus of a therapeutic process, motivational factors must always be considered by the therapist because they always influence the change processes. Not considering these factors greatly increases the likelihood of therapeutic failure (e.g., Poulin et al., 2019; Sansfaçon et al., 2020; Vitinius et al., 2018). Considering that some motivational constructs are particularly relevant for psychotherapy, in this chapter, we focus on therapy motivation, ambivalence toward change, treatment goals, and client expectations as main constructs to be considered in the therapeutic process.

Therapy Motivation

Therapy motivation is the most frequent understanding of the term *motivation* in psychotherapy. Ideally, psychotherapy clients are willing to work hard during the therapeutic process and will invest a lot in changing themselves, their behavior, and/or their lives. However, motivational issues become particularly relevant in therapy when clients seem to have an insufficient or a conflicted therapy motivation. This might be the case when patients either appear to have no motivation at all or seem to be ambivalent about psychotherapy. At worst, clients do not want to start therapy at all or terminate early, do not see themselves as having a problem, or are unwilling to invest in changing themselves. All therapists appreciate a client who is extremely motivated to change and mainly driven by autonomous motivation. These clients show higher levels of engagement in the therapeutic process, facilitating their commitment to therapeutic tasks, reducing resistance to change, and facilitating the establishment of the therapeutic relationship. Frequently, therapists hear these clients say, "I do whatever is necessary to feel good," "I really want to get better, and I believe that this is the way," or "This [the problem] has to be resolved once and for all." On the opposite side, the amotivational state is, without a doubt, what raises the most difficulties for the therapist. In these cases, the client does not recognize their problem and/or see any advantage to changing.

Typically with personality disorders and frequently in substance use disorders, clients usually come to therapy at the suggestion of their relatives, following court orders, and so forth. In these cases, the motivational process needs to be the main focus of the treatment because the probability of early dropout is extremely high. In the case of personality disorders, clients often come to therapy for reasons other than their personality characteristics (e.g., depression). When therapeutic work begins to focus on the clients' characteristics that could be changed, they often do not see the change as relevant because "the problem is other people." For example, in cases of online gambling addiction, clients often come to therapy under pressure from their partners at a time when their debts are already high. However, it is frequently the case that these clients consider themselves to be in control of the situation, and they only come to therapy to maintain their relationships.

Several empirical studies have supported the role of therapy motivation as a major predictor of therapy success (e.g., Vitinius et al., 2018). At the beginning of treatment, it is necessary to have at least minimal motivation for therapy because a lack of motivation for treatment—controlled motivation and amotivation—is linked to premature termination (Poulin et al., 2019). Recently, a meta-analytic study by Sansfaçon et al. (2020) found positive effects of pretreatment motivation on improvement in general eating disorder symptoms (weighted average of the r-index = .17, CI [.09, .24]). In addition, because the psychotherapeutic process implies a high level of client involvement in therapeutic tasks (exploration of painful events, homework completion), autonomous motivation has been consistently pointed out as the type of motivation associated with therapeutic success in different therapeutic approaches and with different psychological problems (e.g., Alfonsson et al., 2016). Along with self-determination theory, the transtheoretical model of change (TTM; Prochaska & DiClemente, 1982) is the framework usually used to conceptualize and study therapy motivation.

Departing from the assumption that clients' motivation in the different stages of the psychotherapy process may vary, TTM conceptualizes behavioral change as a process that occurs over time, throughout the progression of qualitatively different psychological stages. These psychological organizations are conceptualized in five stages of change: precontemplation, contemplation, preparation, action, and maintenance (Prochaska & Norcross, 2013; see also Chapter 3, this volume). Progression through the stages can occur linearly, but a nonlinear progression is common, and individuals often recycle through the stages or regress to earlier stages from later ones. Studies using TTM also suggest that most clients (~80%) are usually at the precontemplation or contemplation stages of change. The model has been used to predict treatment outcomes with a wide range of psychological problems, especially for problematic health-related behaviors such as alcohol abuse, smoking, or dietary behaviors (Prochaska & Velicer, 1997).

As previously discussed, when Maria is not in the amotivational state, her motivation is eminently controlled motivation, and, therefore, her behaviors tend not to be self-determined (i.e., she lacks the energy to initiate and maintain changes). According to TTM, Maria is most often in the contemplation stage, as are most of the patients who come to therapy. However, Maria remains in this state for long periods, and when she reaches the stage of action, she remains in it for a short time, resulting in oscillatory movements between changing and maintaining her current state.

Ambivalence Toward Change

Even a client who is highly motivated to change will experience moments when they have doubts about the process of change, the psychotherapeutic approach, the therapist, or the usefulness of some techniques. Accordingly, in psychotherapy, clients often express the desire for change while, at the same time, they present opposite actions that can be subtler (e.g., reduced visual contact, changing the topic) and/or more explicit opposite actions (e.g., avoiding some tasks suggested by the therapists; Hagedorn, 2011). Usually, this emerges from the client's balance between, on the one hand, the acceptance of the current condition and a desire for self-stability and, on the other hand, a desire for change (Urmanche et al., 2019). When such feelings occur simultaneously, clients experience ambivalence toward change or, in other words, they are dealing with the question "To change or not to change?" In fact, when we talk about ambivalence in psychotherapy, we are referring to a process that is expected to occur frequently in treatment, but when it is not overcome, it may turn into a potentially endless cycle between two opposed tendencies (Braga et al., 2016; Oliveira et al., 2016).

In this context, ambivalence is a client variable characterized by an intrapersonal conflict between "I want to change" versus "I don't want to change" (Button et al., 2015; Oliveira et al., 2020). Obviously, this abstraction can manifest itself in different ways—for example, "I want to feel good, but I don't want to change" or "I want to change, but I want to keep the advantages of being the same." Whatever the format, this conflict results in concurrent movements toward and away from change (Engle & Arkowitz, 2006; Oliveira et al., 2016) and produces a subjective feeling of the inability to change coupled with distress in response to being unable to achieve change (Oliveira et al., 2020). For example, in Maria's case, she arrived at psychotherapy motivated to feel better. However, to achieve the goal of "feeling better" (too ambiguous for a therapeutic process and probably more an outcome than a process), Maria had to change several behaviors associated with her depressive state. Although her suffering and the desire to feel better motivated her to seek psychological help, the change in behaviors, however simple (e.g., getting up a few minutes earlier to do stretching exercises, visiting her family more frequently), triggered an experience of ambivalence that prevented her from changing. Maria wants to stop feeling depressed, and she wants to feel better, but she feels unable to change anything in her day-to-day life, however small it may be.

Unfortunately, in contrast to the profusion of clinical and theoretical literature, ambivalence in psychotherapy is an underresearched topic. Most of the extant research has been developed considering ambivalence in the form of resistance (Engle & Arkowitz, 2006). Although these constructs are closely related (Button et al., 2015; Urmanche et al., 2019), we could benefit from differentiating between these different but related concepts and the practical approaches in dealing with them from the therapist perspective (Aviram et al., 2016). Moreover, this differentiation has the potential of boosting the research in this field. In fact, resolving ambivalence is one way of reducing resistance in therapy (Constantino et al., 2019; Westra & Norouzian, 2017), while all moments of impasse have the potential to increase resistance to others' suggestions or demands (Button et al., 2015). Whereas resistance to change is mainly contextual (i.e., it emerges from the interaction between the client and the therapist; Button et al., 2015), by definition, ambivalence is a subject's inner tension and, in that sense, much harder to identify and, consequently, to address accurately. When this intrapsychic tension of ambivalence emerges in psychotherapy, both the client and therapist can begin to feel stuck. In these moments, psychological symptoms tend to intensify (Montesano, Feixas, et al., 2017), while motivation to change (Emmons et al., 1993) and engagement with therapy tend to decrease (Feixas et al., 2014), increasing the risk of poor outcomes in therapy (Miller & Rollnick, 2002; Oliveira et al., 2021).

Given these characteristics, most studies on ambivalence have been developed using qualitative approaches (Feixas et al., 2014; Gonçalves et al., 2017; Lombardi et al., 2014). The results have suggested that ambivalence toward change (a) is present in both poor- and good-outcome cases, (b) is higher at the beginning of therapy, (c) tends to decrease in recovered cases while being consistently high in unchanged cases, and (d) is associated with clinical severity (e.g., Feixas et al., 2014; Lombardi et al., 2014; Montesano, Feixas, et al., 2017; Oliveira et al., 2021). In other words, ambivalent states are expected and even desired at the beginning of treatment (McEvoy & Nathan, 2007), but their resolution throughout therapy is crucial to achieving better outcomes (Braga et al., 2018; Oliveira et al., 2021). Moreover, evidence suggests that good-outcome cases tend to present not only more ambivalence resolution levels during treatment, but they also use qualitatively different processes to do it (Braga et al., 2016, 2018; Oliveira et al., 2016).

The TTM also considers the client's ambivalence. Although ambivalence toward change is an essential aspect of the entire process, the contemplation stage is most strongly associated with ambivalence (Engle & Arkowitz, 2006); individuals recognize the problematic nature of their behavior and have started thinking about overcoming it but have not made a commitment to change (Prochaska & Norcross, 2013). Because clients start evaluating the pros and cons of change but are still struggling with the benefits of holding on to the same old pattern, ambivalence emerges from this stage of balancing. Thus, one of the main goals with Maria focused on resolving her ambivalence between changing and facing failure and uncertainty or remaining in the same situation while maintaining the associated suffering. In the case of a client who arrives at therapy due to external pressure and does not consider that they have a problem (precontemplation stage), the initial work should focus on introducing and promoting ambivalence. That is, in a tentative and exploratory way, question whether small changes could be beneficial for the client and what treatment goals could make sense.

Treatment Goals

Treatment goals are a particular kind of personal goal in psychotherapy—that is, "intended changes in behavior and experience to be attained via psychotherapy, that patient and therapist agree upon at the beginning of treatment" (grosse Holtforth & Grawe, 2002, p. 79). They focus the client's and therapist's attention on desired outcomes of psychotherapy, guide collaborative treatment planning, provide criteria for outcome assessment during and after therapy, and thereby provide transparency and ownership to the client (Westermann et al., 2019).

Considering the difficulties often found in defining treatment goals, several authors have tried to define taxonomies that incorporate a large part of the objectives that we can identify with clients. grosse Holtforth and Grawe (2002) developed an empirically constructed list of clients' goals in psychotherapy that includes three levels of abstraction (i.e., goal types, goal categories and subcategories). Table 2.1 includes the five goal types suggested—namely, coping with specific problems and symptoms, interpersonal goals, well-being and functioning, existential issues, and personal growth, as well as residual categories. The table also includes the other two levels of abstraction (goal categories

TABLE 2.1. Clients' Goals in Psychotherapy: Goal Types, Categories, and Subcategories

Goal types	Categories and subcategories
Coping with specific problems and symptoms	**Depression** (subcategories: negative thoughts, negative moods, and loss of drive or energy)
	Suicidality (self-injurious behavior, suicidality)
	Fears or anxiety (fears or anxiety in specific situations, panic attacks and social phobic fears)
	Obsessive thoughts and compulsive behaviors (obsessions or compulsions)
	Coping with trauma (traumas)
	Substance use and addiction (somatic withdrawal, changing addictive behaviors)
	Eating behaviors (coping with problematic patterns, obesity)
	Sleep (sleep problems)
	Sexuality (sexual problems)
	Coping with somatic problems (pain, chronic illnesses, adjusting medication)
	Difficulties in specific life domains or stress (stress, housing problems, work and education, time management)
Interpersonal goals	**Current relationship** (relationship with partner, spouse, or significant other; improve sex life with partner, spouse, or significant other; expectations, feelings related to partner, spouse, or significant other)
	Parenthood (parenthood)
	Other specific relationships (other specific relationships, separating from significant others)
	Loneliness, grief (coping with loneliness, grieving loss)
	Assertiveness (assertive behaviors, cognitive and emotional readiness for assertiveness)
	Connectedness and intimacy (increase frequency and quality of interpersonal contact, permitting intimacy, prepare for new relationship)
Well-being and functioning	**Exercise, activity** (improve leisure activities, increase exercise)
	Relaxation and composure (learn to relax, increase calmness and composure)
	Well-being (mental well-being, sense of comfort with body)
Existential	**Past, present, and future** (process personal history, reflect on self and future)
	Meaning of life (spiritual, religious, or meaning issues)
Personal growth	**Attitude toward self** (improve self-confidence and self-esteem, improve self-acceptance)
	Desires and wishes (recognize desires and wishes, fulfill desires and wishes)
	Responsibility and self-control (assume responsibility or learn to make decisions, learn to delegate responsibility or decrease perfectionism)
	Emotion regulation (learn to handle emotions)
Residual categories	**No treatment goals** (no treatment goals)
	Goals that cannot be categorized (goals that cannot be categorized)

Note. From "Bern Inventory of Treatment Goals: Part 1. Development and First Application of a Taxonomy of Treatment Goal Themes," by M. grosse Holtforth and K. Grawe, 2002, *Psychotherapy Research, 12*(1), pp. 85–86 (https://doi.org/10.1080/713869618). Copyright 2002 by Taylor & Francis. Reprinted with permission.

and subcategories). For example, an interpersonal goal type includes specific goals related to intimate relationships, the current family, the family of origin, and other specific relationships. Subcategories include 52 goals that are even more specific. Examples of finer subcategories of goals related to the intimate relationship are relationships with a partner, spouse, or significant other; improving their sex life with their partner, spouse, or significant other; and change expectations and feelings related to their partner, spouse, or significant other (see grosse Holtforth & Grawe, 2002).

At first, Maria's goals mainly fell under the symptom-oriented and interpersonal and functioning categories—that is, they were centered on her depression, intimate relationships, loneliness, exercise and activity, and well-being. The collaborative work between Maria and her therapist led them to agree that one of the treatment goals should be to improve her emotional regulation skills, a personal growth type of goal. Associated subcategories for Maria could include coping with negative moods, loss of drive, separating from significant others, and loneliness, as well as improving leisure activities, increasing exercise, and learning to handle emotions.

Along with an extensive body of literature, recent meta-analytic studies have shown the importance of goal setting (Cohen's $d = .34$, CI [.28–.41]) and monitoring goal progress (Cohen's $d = .40$, CI [.32–.48]) for a wide range of behavioral outcomes (e.g., Epton et al., 2017). The positive impact on outcomes increases when the outcomes are physically recorded (Harkin et al., 2016), especially when the client and therapist agree on the goals of therapy (Tryon, 2018). In addition to the impact on outcomes, the clear and objective definition of treatment goals increases the transparency of the therapeutic process and provides the opportunity to balance power between a client and therapist (Westermann et al., 2019). An objective definition of treatment goals is also important to adjust and enhance the client expectations for the treatment.

Expectations

Client expectations are related to the individual predictions they have regarding the therapy process and/or outcome. In other words, they reflect "patient prognostic beliefs about the consequences of engaging in treatment" (Constantino et al., 2011, p. 1). Client expectations generally develop even before starting treatment. In fact, even the choice of the therapist can influence the client's expectations. For example, a client who is referred to "Psychologist X for the problem you are referring to because he is an expert in these cases and will certainly be a great help to you" is more likely to develop positive expectations regarding treatment compared with a client who searched for a reference on the internet and had limited information about the therapist. Other examples of expectations are hope for improvement of well-being, hope for improvement of relationships, fear of adverse side effects, and/or fear of being ridiculed (Schulte & Eifert, 2002). In Maria's case, although she was highly motivated, because of the high levels of psychological suffering she was experiencing, her history of previous unsuccessful psychological treatments led to low expectations that therapy could help her. At the same time, she was excited about the change in therapist: "I was with my previous therapist for 20 years, but I needed to change, and she told me this was the best option I would ever find. This change could be beneficial for me."

A recent meta-analysis integrated 81 independent samples with 12,722 patients and showed that patients' high early outcome expectations were significantly associated with greater posttreatment outcomes (weighted $r = .18$; 95% CI [.14, .22]; Constantino et al., 2018). Patients with low early treatment expectations for improvement and who perceived their therapist as higher in affiliation (warmer) had greater symptom reduction. Compared with lower levels, higher expectations for treatment outcome yielded stronger rates of symptom reduction from the beginning to the end of treatment (Constantino et al., 2007). Particularly in patients with high levels of symptom distress, positive expectations are predictive of outcome (grosse Holtforth et al., 2011).

Beyond the direct impact of expectancies on outcomes, patients with greater pretreatment expectations of improvement form better alliances with their therapist from the beginning of treatment (Connolly Gibbons et al., 2003). A recent meta-analysis led by Constantino et al. (2020) showed that stronger alliance quality mediated the relationship between greater outcome expectations and improvement (standardized difference $= -.12$, CI [$-.20$, $-.05$]). This finding is consistent with and extends previous research on treatment expectancies, the therapeutic alliance, and outcome (e.g., Johansson et al., 2011). This shows that outcome expectations are associated with a variety of individual characteristics (e.g., psychological mindedness) and in-therapy behaviors that may contribute to a patient's overall assessment of the working alliance; they are also related to whether clients portray hostility or affiliative behavior toward the therapist and treatment outcome. Ahmed et al. (2012) found that clients who went on to have low outcome expectations after resistance episodes (i.e., experiencing tension in the therapy relationship) showed reduced affiliative contact with the therapist—that is, they acted independently, stated their own ideas and beliefs, asserted beliefs that were opposite to the therapist's suggestions, and exhibited hostile behaviors. These therapist–patient dyads showed positive complementarity only about half the time. Conversely, clients who went on having high outcome expectations after resistance episodes never engaged in any form of disaffiliating behavior during the resistance episode, and the therapist–patient dyad showed positive complementarity in their interactions for the majority of the time. Low outcome expectations dyads showed substantially more evidence of relational instability and interpersonal tension over treatment.

A recent study with clients who had major depression found that having previous depressive episodes was negatively associated with initial outcome expectation, while greater well-being was positively associated with initial outcome expectation (Vîslă et al., 2018). These findings also indicate a significant linear growth in a patient's outcome expectation over therapy, although neither the early alliance nor an early change in symptoms predicted outcome expectation change (Vîslă et al., 2018). This might indicate that outcome expectation change is not a by-product of early change in alliance or symptoms.

TABLE 2.2. How Suffering, Positive, and Negative Expectations Are Experienced by Clients Who Are Highly Motivated, Ambivalent, or Amotivated

	Suffering[a]	Positive expectations	Negative expectations
Therapy motivation	Yes	Yes	No
Ambivalence	Yes	Yes	Yes
Amotivation	Maybe	No	Maybe

[a]Suffering reflects impairment, distress, hopelessness, and/or helplessness.

Interestingly, Westra et al. (2010) also found that good-outcome clients frequently reported disconfirmation of negative process expectations (e.g., surprises that therapy was collaborative), while poor-outcome clients generally failed to report such experiences. Good-outcome clients also reported disconfirmations of outcome expectations (i.e., gaining more from treatment than expected, whereas poor-outcome clients reported being disappointed).

As a summary of what has been discussed about the motivational constructs specifically relevant to psychotherapy, Table 2.2 frames therapy motivation, ambivalence, and amotivation in terms of suffering, positive expectations, and negative expectations experienced by the client undergoing treatment. Clients with high motivation for therapy have usually experienced suffering and have mostly positive expectations for the therapeutic process. Amotivated clients, however, may not be aware of their suffering or misattribute their difficulties (e.g., "The problem is not my aggressive behavior but that nobody loves me as I truly am"), which leads them not to have positive expectations for treatment but rather only negative expectations. The ambivalent client experiences suffering and has positive expectations regarding treatment; however, negative expectations are also present. It is from this balance of forces that ambivalence emerges.

Maria is often in an ambivalent state. When she tries to implement efforts that result from the suffering experienced by her current situation (avoidance goal and controlled motivation), the difficulties that she anticipates she will feel when introducing changes lead her to an impasse. As the vector toward change has less force than the vector toward maintaining the current state, the oscillatory movements characteristic of ambivalence always end in centripetal movements toward maintaining the problem. So, the remaining question is, "How do therapists deal with these issues in daily practice?"

MOTIVATIONAL INTERVENTIONS IN PSYCHOTHERAPY

Recent research suggests that when low levels of motivation or ambivalence are addressed early in therapy, clients tend to be less resistant and more engaged with treatment (Aviram et al., 2016; Constantino et al., 2019; Westra & Norouzian, 2017). Accordingly, different therapeutic modalities already include specific techniques and/or modules focused on a client's motivation in the early stages of therapy (e.g., Miller & Rose, 2015). Therapists should engage in positive behaviors (e.g., show competence, be active) and let the clients experience and use their own qualities and resources. Ryan and Deci (2000) suggested that the therapeutic relationship should focus on promoting the fundamental needs for competence, autonomy, and relatedness. In this sense, the motivational attunement approach (grosse Holtforth & Castonguay, 2005) proposes a set of strategies to focus the intervention on the patient's goals and motives. The central idea is that if therapists present motivationally attuned behaviors, the probability of fulfilling the client's approach goals regarding therapy significantly increases. Thus, a therapist's behavior should be consistent with the promotion of the essential components of the therapeutic alliance: the therapeutic bond, agreement on therapeutic tasks, and agreement on therapeutic goals (Westermann et al., 2019). For example, when the therapist suggested some behavioral activation tasks for Maria, the therapist reinforced the idea that "these tasks will finally help you feel more active and therefore enable you to help your daughter face the reality that she is starting college."

Because establishing a safe and stable therapeutic relationship between a therapist and a patient is a sine qua non condition for the development of the therapeutic process, an extremely important step in promoting client motivation and treatment success is the establishment of treatment goals. The literature suggests that therapists should seek input from patients to form and implement treatment goals and plans and regularly monitor progress with the client (Tryon, 2018). In other words, an agreement on therapy goals is considered a central ingredient of the working alliance and, consequently, of treatment success. However, in almost all therapeutic processes, clients tend to come to therapy presenting objectives that are (a) too ambitious for treatment, (b) too vague and ambiguous, and/or (c) unrealistic (e.g., "to change my partner"). Therapists should collaborate with clients to define attainable treatment goals and ways to achieve them, define more approach and intrinsic objectives instead of avoidance and extrinsic objectives, and ensure that the client is committed to the defined objectives. The objectives negotiated between the therapist and client must be physically recorded during the definition of objectives and regularly monitored for progress (Tryon, 2018).

As previously stated, Maria's goals for therapy were too vague and ambiguous (i.e., "feeling better" and "being happy"). The therapist worked collaboratively with her to define the main goals for the treatment, specific goals, and small steps to achieve them. Considering Maria's high levels of neuroticism, one of the established goals for treatment was to enhance her personal growth and, in particular, increase her emotional regulation. This clear definition allowed therapeutic tasks such as identifying thoughts, emotions, and behaviors in daily events of emotional activation to be perceived by Maria as necessary and useful for the treatment.

Both the establishment of the therapeutic relationship and the definition of goals for therapy are highly affected by the client's lack of motivation or uncertainty regarding change. But the constant motivational difficulties that the therapist and client encounter throughout the treatment are common regardless of the therapist characteristics, patient characteristics, or the treatment approach. In our day-to-day lives, we deal with the imposition of having to choose between two or more options. Sometimes the choices are less relevant (buying either Pants A or B), whereas other choices have more impact on our lives (whether to continue in an unhappy relationship). Regardless of the scenario, it is common for therapists to hear, "It seems that one part of me wants A, but there is another part that wants B." As we all know, the more balanced the weights on each side, the higher the tension of the system, the more paralyzed we feel, and the more distress is generated. In psychotherapy, regardless of the content of the problem, there are always two metapoles: "to change" or "to remain the same or keep the status quo." Therefore, the literature suggests that therapists should follow the evidence, employing research-supported treatment methods, while at the same time assessing the acceptance of the treatment by the clients, recognizing a client's resistance to change, and adapting themselves and their portfolio of techniques to the client's characteristics (Norcross & Lambert, 2011).

Bearing in mind that the variations in motivational levels are present in all processes of change, therapists must have in their repertoire strategies to deal with this effectively throughout treatment. The importance of dealing effectively with the ambivalence and lack of motivation felt by patients during the change process has been a focus of interest from different theoretical traditions (O'Hanlon & O'Hanlon, 2003). However, most of the techniques and strategies we use today to deal with motivational conflicts were developed according to the principles of the humanistic, client-centered approaches (e.g., Kelly, 1991; Perls et al., 1951). In this chapter, we only present four of them briefly: (a) two-chair work, (b) motivational interviewing, (c) the dilemma-focused intervention, and (d) the decisional cube.

Two-Chair Work

Two-chair work was initially developed in the context of humanistic psychotherapeutic interventions (Perls et al., 1951). It is one of the core techniques in emotion-focused therapy (Greenberg et al., 1993), and its use has been increasing in cognitive behavior therapy (CBT; Engle & Arkowitz, 2006). This technique allows clients to explore conflicting internal feelings about change— part of them is in favor of change, but another part is deeply hesitant about change—using two chairs to promote an in-session experiential dialogue between the selves that are in conflict, which could undermine the process of change (Greenberg & Webster, 1982). During the process, the therapist accepts the patient's perspectives and acts as a facilitator, promoting the focus on the present moment and enhancing the dialogue between the voices of each self (Greenberg et al., 1993; Greenberg & Webster, 1982). The emotional arousal during two-chair work eases the awareness of the arguments from each voice and the dialogue between them, putting the patient in a better position to resolve their ambivalence. Research has suggested that the two-chair technique not only addresses personal conflicts (Greenberg & Webster, 1982) but also works with other transdiagnostic processes (e.g., Shahar et al., 2012). For instance, Clarke and Greenberg (1986) developed a study with subjects who sought counseling to resolve conflictual decisions and were randomly allocated to two sessions of two-chair work, two sessions of CBT, or no treatment. Results suggested that the two-chair group improved more than the CBT and control groups in terms of indecisiveness. In a pilot study with seven people experiencing difficulties in making an important change in their lives, Engle and Arkowitz (2006) developed four half-hour sessions using the two-chair technique to work with the focal problem. Of the seven, just one subject presented no change at all at the end of the intervention and after a 1-year follow-up.

After identifying with Maria the presence of ambivalence toward change, the therapist invited her to think of this internal tension as two opposing voices, one in favor of change and the other against change. When she sat in the "in favor of change" chair, Maria mentioned, among other things, "I have the right to be happy at some point in my life. My daughter still needs me and that's why I have to be well for her. I want to find someone with whom I can age happily." In the chair "against change," the arguments were "But you have always been incapable; you are destined to be like that. There is no point in doing anything about your health; you cannot control anything. You can have a crisis at any time and die." With this experiential approach, the therapist hoped to promote negotiation between the two opposing voices. It was expected that this negotiation would promote the integration of the parties in conflict, thus resolving the internal tension that leaves Maria at this impasse.

Motivational Interviewing

Motivational interviewing (MI; Miller & Rollnick, 2002) is a directive and client-entered approach whose main objectives are to increase intrinsic motivation and help individuals resolve their ambivalence toward change. It is expected that when some patients realize that the focus of the change is in themselves, their agency in relation to the problem increases, and, thus, the process of change occurs naturally (Miller & Rollnick, 2013; Miller & Rose, 2015). Congruent with its humanistic roots, MI is a collaborative approach where the client is considered an expert, in contrast to the models centered on their deficits (Miller & Rollnick, 2004). The core aspect of being able to process ambivalence is to increase a client's motivation for change. In this sense, this increase can be identified by *change talk*—statements oriented to change. MI seeks to identify change talk, strengthen it, and use it to establish the subject's commitments to change. In this context, MI considers ambivalence as an expected phenomenon and suggests techniques to evoke and explore it, helping the patient resolve ambivalence in the direction of positive change (Miller & Rollnick, 2004). MI was originally developed to work with substance use disorders, and its efficacy is well established through myriad empirical studies (Steele et al., 2020), which led it to be considered an empirically supported treatment for these problems. However, its use has been increasingly extended to several other problems and diagnoses (e.g., Frost et al., 2018), both as a pretreatment component (Button et al., 2015; Lombardi et al., 2014; Westra & Norouzian, 2017) and a strategy to be used throughout the therapeutic process (Marker et al., 2020). Departing from the assumption that resistance is a possible observable manifestation of a patient's felt ambivalence, results from a clinical trial of CBT for generalized anxiety disorder showed that MI-consistent therapist behaviors were associated with lower levels of patient resistance (Aviram et al., 2016). Another study suggested that the levels of resistance in the first session of high-severity worriers were lower in the patients who received MI before the beginning of the treatment (Aviram & Westra, 2011). A recent study showed that reducing patient resistance using MI before CBT treatment promotes better long-term improvement than traditional CBT (Constantino et al., 2019).

Maria came to therapy in the contemplation stage. Her therapist asked about the importance of change and how confident she was she could make the change if she decided to do so. Using a scale from 0 to 10, she reported that the importance of changing was 8, and her confidence regarding effective change was 4. This assessment informed the therapist that the intervention should be focused mainly on her confidence in changing. At that time, one of the main focuses of suffering was associated with the love relationship that Maria considered still existed, despite the distance. Maria and her therapist started exploring the pros and cons of ending the relationship permanently. From this collaborative discussion, the arguments for ending were "My daughter will stop feeling unhappy at home because her relationship with my partner is terrible. I will be able to find someone else and have a really happy relationship." However, the arguments against were "At least there is someone, even if he is only physically present. I will probably never meet anyone again. Our relationship at the beginning was so good; I felt that we were really made for each other. I know that he is not what he has been lately." Maria began the next session by saying that she had thought more about the arguments for and against change, and more arguments had arisen in favor of changing; subsequently, she and her therapist worked on them. Next, the therapist used strategies to increase change talk, such as inviting Maria to describe how she overcame difficult situations in her life in the past and what kind of strategies she used. Progressively, the decisional balance shifted to the side of changing and, therefore, putting an end to the relationship.

Dilemma-Focused Intervention

The dilemma-focused intervention (DFI; Feixas & Compañ, 2016) was specifically developed to address the patient's implicative dilemmas drawing from the personal constructs approach (Kelly, 1991). In a nutshell, DFI aims to explore and work with the patient's personal meanings and how they can represent an inner conflict between the desire for change and the need for personal coherence (Montesano et al., 2015). The goal is to promote awareness of such personal dilemmas and help patients find a way of resolving them (Montesano, Gonçalves, et al., 2017). This approach constitutes an alternative to problem-oriented strategies and offers an identity-focused, ambivalence-sensitive intervention procedure (Feixas et al., 2018). Empirical studies have suggested that implicative dilemmas are common among different diagnoses (Montesano et al., 2015), although they may appear slightly more in depressed patients (Feixas et al., 2014). It seems that patients who resolve their inner conflicts present higher reductions of psychological distress (Paz et al., 2017). In a randomized controlled trial, 128 patients presenting with depression were allocated to a combined group CBT (eight 2-hour weekly sessions) and individual dilemma-focused therapies (eight 1-hour weekly sessions) or CBT alone (eight 2-hour group weekly sessions, plus eight 1-hour individual weekly sessions). The result showed that the groups were equivalent at the end of treatment and after a 1-year follow-up (Feixas et al., 2018).

To use this intervention, the therapist first used the repertory grid technique to study Maria's system of meanings. From this assessment, it emerged that the desired change in the "sad versus happy" construct had an unwanted implication in another construct, "cares about others versus selfishness." Thus, achieving change (becoming happy) implied an undesirable change in her self-identity (becoming selfish). In the ensuing sessions, they worked on the meanings attributed by Maria to the changes necessary to implement her goal to "be happy." The assumption that this would have a negative impact on her self-identity eventually vanished.

Decision-Cube Technique

Unlike the procedures closely linked to the robust conceptual frameworks previously presented, the decision-cube technique (DCT; Bents, 2006) is a "simple" strategy or method to be used usually at the beginning of treatment to clarify the advantages and disadvantages of changing. In this exercise, the patient is asked to think of and write down the pros and cons of changing. Although the exercise could be performed between sessions, when developed in session, the therapist should assume a neutral position and act as a facilitator. The format can have some variations (e.g., as a two-column technique or as a four-field technique), such as writing down the advantages and disadvantages of changing or staying the same. This graphic representation allows the patient to become aware of the arguments that prevent them from changing, which are potential sources of ambivalence. The characteristics of DCT make it easy to include it in different therapeutic processes and different orientations. In addition to being an exercise that can be used in MI, several components of this technique have been integrated into different manualized treatments (Barlow et al., 2004). Although not many empirical studies have analyzed the impact of its isolated use (Engle & Arkowitz, 2006), a study assessed the effectiveness of using the two-chair approach and DCT to resolve partnership ambivalence (Trachsel et al., 2010). Fifty participants were randomly allocated to one of two interventions, which were two sessions each. The results suggested an equivalent reduction of partnership ambivalence in both conditions.

The therapist presented Maria with a sheet that had a printed square divided into four equal parts. In the upper left quadrant, Maria wrote reasons in favor of changing, while in the lower left, she wrote reasons in favor of staying in the same situation. In the upper right quadrant, she put reasons against the change, and in the lower right, she put reasons for staying the same. For reasons in favor of changing, Maria wrote, "being happy, don't wake up tired, have someone to give me a hug, feeling more active and dealing with your chronic health condition." The reasons in favor of staying the same identified by Maria were "inertia, habit, difficulty in changing, and I like him at times." The motives against staying the same were "continue to suffer, my daughter will have serious consequences of the life we have lived, and I will get worse and worse." Maria identified reasons against changing as "changing all this requires a lot of effort, I will have to face the possibility of failure, I may not be able, and I will not have the strength to change." With this information, the therapist was able to deconstruct with Maria the arguments against change and those in favor of staying the same. Was what she anticipates so scary? What are the reasons that made her think that she would not be able to cope with what she anticipates? Assuming these are valid, how could she overcome these difficulties? At the same time, it presented the opportunity to think of more arguments in favor of change, expand them, and thus tip the balance toward change.

CONCLUSION AND FUTURE DIRECTIONS

In clinical practice, we repeatedly hear that "we can only help those who want to be helped." Maria arrived at psychotherapy with several motivational issues, and it was up to her therapist to respond to these difficulties. At this moment, Maria is still undergoing treatment, presenting low levels of depressive symptoms and greater well-being, but she still has a long way to go. Despite the great importance of treatment models and the mastery of their techniques in psychotherapy, the client remains the center of the therapeutic process. Thus, the study of relevant client factors and how they can be promoted remains central to increasing the effectiveness of psychological treatments. What motivational factors should the therapist be aware of? What is their impact on the psychotherapy process and outcome? How can we foster them? These were some of the questions we tried to answer in this chapter, but there is much more to explore. For example, how can we also include motivational factors in personalized treatments? At the same time, research should further investigate how these factors vary, or not, in short periods (e.g., throughout the day). What are the motivational idiosyncrasies in cases of great therapeutic success (e.g., early responders, sudden gains)? And when does the therapeutic process start to go wrong? How can we identify the associated motivational issues and act promptly? We hope the coming years will provide us with more knowledge to respond to these issues so that we can be better help clients like Maria overcome their burden.

REFERENCES

Ahmed, M., Westra, H. A., & Constantino, M. J. (2012). Early therapy interpersonal process differentiating clients high and low in outcome expectations. *Psychotherapy Research, 22*(6), 731–745. https://doi.org/10.1080/10503307.2012.724538

Alfonsson, S., Olsson, E., & Hursti, T. (2016). Motivation and treatment credibility predicts dropout, treatment adherence, and clinical outcomes in an Internet-based cognitive behavioral relaxation program: A randomized controlled trial. *Journal of Medical Internet Research, 18*(3), Article e52. https://doi.org/10.2196/jmir.5352

Aviram, A., & Westra, H. A. (2011). The impact of motivational interviewing on resistance in cognitive behavioural therapy for generalized anxiety disorder. *Psychotherapy Research, 21*(6), 698–708. https://doi.org/10.1080/10503307.2011.610832

Aviram, A., Westra, H. A., Constantino, M. J., & Antony, M. M. (2016). Responsive management of early resistance in cognitive-behavioral therapy for generalized anxiety disorder. *Journal of Consulting and Clinical Psychology, 84*(9), 783–794. https://doi.org/10.1037/ccp0000100

Barlow, D. H., Allen, L. B., & Choate, M. L. (2004). Toward a unified treatment for emotional disorders. *Behavior Therapy, 35*(2), 205–230. https://doi.org/10.1016/S0005-7894(04)80036-4

Bents, H. (2006). Entscheidungswürfel [Decision cube]. In S. Fliegel & A. Kämmerer (Eds.), *Psychotherapeutische Schätze* (Vol. 101, pp. 51–53). dgvt-Verlag.

Beutler, L. E., Harwood, T. M., Michelson, A., Song, X., & Holman, J. (2011). Resistance/reactance level. *Journal of Clinical Psychology, 67*(2), 133–142. https://doi.org/10.1002/jclp.20753

Bohart, A. C. (2000). The client is the most important common factor: Clients' self-healing capacities and psychotherapy. *Journal of Psychotherapy Integration, 10*(2), 127–149. https://link.springer.com/article/10.1023/A:1009444132104

Braga, C., Oliveira, J. T., Ribeiro, A. P., & Gonçalves, M. M. (2016). Ambivalence resolution in emotion-focused therapy: The successful case of Sarah. *Psychotherapy Research, 28*(3), 423–432. https://doi.org/10.1080/10503307.2016.1169331

Braga, C., Ribeiro, A. P., Gonçalves, M. M., Oliveira, J. T., Botelho, A., Ferreira, H., & Sousa, I. (2018). Ambivalence resolution in brief psychotherapy for depression. *Clinical Psychology & Psychotherapy, 25*(3), 369–377. https://doi.org/10.1002/cpp.2169

Button, M. L., Westra, H. A., Hara, K. M., & Aviram, A. (2015). Disentangling the impact of resistance and ambivalence on therapy outcomes in cognitive behavioural therapy for generalized anxiety disorder. *Cognitive Behaviour Therapy, 44*(1), 44–53. https://doi.org/10.1080/16506073.2014.959038

Clarke, K. M., & Greenberg, L. S. (1986). Differential effects of the Gestalt two-chair intervention and problem solving in resolving decisional conflict. *Journal of Counseling Psychology, 33*(1), 11–15. https://doi.org/10.1037/0022-0167.33.1.11

Connolly Gibbons, M. B., Crits-Christoph, P., de la Cruz, C., Barber, J. P., Siqueland, L., & Gladis, M. (2003). Pretreatment expectations, interpersonal functioning, and symptoms in the prediction of the therapeutic alliance across supportive-expressive psychotherapy and cognitive therapy. *Psychotherapy Research, 13*(1), 59–76. https://doi.org/10.1093/ptr/kpg007

Constantino, M. J., Arnkoff, D. B., Glass, C. R., Ametrano, R. M., & Smith, J. Z. (2011). Expectations. *Journal of Clinical Psychology, 67*(2), 184–192. https://doi.org/10.1002/jclp.20754

Constantino, M. J., Castonguay, L. G., Zack, S. E., & DeGeorge, J. (2010). Engagement in psychotherapy: Factors contributing to the facilitation, demise, and restoration of the therapeutic alliance. In D. Castro-Blanco & M. S. Karver (Eds.), *Elusive alliance: Treatment engagement strategies with high-risk adolescents* (pp. 21–57). American Psychological Association. https://doi.org/10.1037/12139-001

Constantino, M. J., Coyne, A. E., Goodwin, B. J., Vîslă, A., Flückiger, C., Muir, H. J., & Gaines, A. N. (2020). Indirect effect of patient outcome expectation on improvement through alliance quality: A meta-analysis. *Psychotherapy Research, 31*(6), 711–725. https://doi.org/10.1080/10503307.2020.1851058

Constantino, M. J., Manber, R., Ong, J., Kuo, T. F., Huang, J. S., & Arnow, B. A. (2007). Patient expectations and therapeutic alliance as predictors of outcome in group cognitive-behavioral therapy for insomnia. *Behavioral Sleep Medicine, 5*(3), 210–228. https://doi.org/10.1080/15402000701263932

Constantino, M. J., Vîslă, A., Coyne, A. E., & Boswell, J. F. (2018). A meta-analysis of the association between patients' early treatment outcome expectation and their posttreatment outcomes. *Psychotherapy, 55*(4), 473–485. https://doi.org/10.1037/pst0000169

Constantino, M. J., Westra, H. A., Antony, M. M., & Coyne, A. E. (2019). Specific and common processes as mediators of the long-term effects of cognitive-behavioral therapy integrated with motivational interviewing for generalized anxiety disorder. *Psychotherapy Research, 29*(2), 213–225. https://doi.org/10.1080/10503307.2017.1332794

Deci, E. L., & Ryan, R. M. (1985). The general causality orientations scale: Self-determination in personality. *Journal of Research in Personality, 19*(2), 109–134. https://doi.org/10.1016/0092-6566(85)90023-6

Deci, E. L., & Ryan, R. M. (1991). A motivational approach to self: Integration in personality. In R. A. Dienstbier (Ed.), *Nebraska Symposium on Motivation, 1990: Perspectives on motivation* (pp. 237–288). University of Nebraska Press.

Dweck, C. S. (2017). From needs to goals and representations: Foundations for a unified theory of motivation, personality, and development. *Psychological Review, 124*(6), 689–719. https://doi.org/10.1037/rev0000082

Dwyer, L. A., Hornsey, M. J., Smith, L. G. E., Oei, T. P. S., & Dingle, G. A. (2011). Participant autonomy in cognitive behavioral group therapy: An integration of self-determination and cognitive behavioral theories. *Journal of Social and Clinical Psychology, 30*(1), 24–46. https://doi.org/10.1521/jscp.2011.30.1.24

Elliot, A. J. (2008). *Handbook of approach and avoidance motivation*. Routledge. https://doi.org/10.4324/9780203888148

Emmons, R. A., King, L. A., & Sheldon, K. (1993). Goal conflict and the self-regulation of action. In D. M. Wegner & J. W. Pennebaker (Eds.), *Handbook of mental control* (pp. 528–551). Prentice-Hall.

Engle, D., & Arkowitz, H. (2006). *Ambivalence in psychotherapy: Facilitating readiness to change*. Guilford Press.

Epstein, S. (1998). Cognitive-experiential self-theory. In D. F. Barone, M. Hersen, & V. B. Van Hasselt (Eds.), *Advanced personality* (pp. 211–238). Springer. https://doi.org/10.1007/978-1-4419-8580-4_9

Epton, T., Currie, S., & Armitage, C. J. (2017). Unique effects of setting goals on behavior change: Systematic review and meta-analysis. *Journal of Consulting and Clinical Psychology, 85*(12), 1182–1198. https://doi.org/10.1037/ccp0000260

Feixas, G., & Compañ, V. (2016). Dilemma-focused intervention for unipolar depression: A treatment manual. *BMC Psychiatry, 16*(1), 235. https://doi.org/10.1186/s12888-016-0947-x

Feixas, G., Montesano, A., Compañ, V., Salla, M., Dada, G., Pucurull, O., Trujillo, A., Paz, C., Muñoz, D., Gasol, M., Saúl, L. Á., Lana, F., Bros, I., Ribeiro, E., Winter, D., Carrera-Fernández, M. J., & Guàrdia, J. (2014). Cognitive conflicts in major depression: Between desired change and personal coherence. *British Journal of Clinical Psychology, 53*(4), 369–385. https://doi.org/10.1111/bjc.12050

Feixas, G., Paz, C., García-Grau, E., Montesano, A., Medina, J. C., Bados, A., Trujillo, A., Ortíz, E., Compañ, V., Salla, M., Aguilera, M., Guasch, V., Codina, J., & Winter, D. A. (2018). One-year follow-up of a randomized trial with a dilemma-focused intervention for depression: Exploring an alternative to problem-oriented strategies. *PLOS ONE, 13*(12), Article e0208245. https://doi.org/10.1371/journal.pone.0208245

Frost, H., Campbell, P., Maxwell, M., O'Carroll, R. E., Dombrowski, S. U., Williams, B., Cheyne, H., Coles, E., & Pollock, A. (2018). Effectiveness of Motivational Interviewing on adult behaviour change in health and social care settings: A systematic review of reviews. *PLOS ONE, 13*(10), Article e0204890. https://doi.org/10.1371/journal.pone.0204890

Gonçalves, M. M., Ribeiro, A. P., Mendes, I., Alves, D., Silva, J., Rosa, C., Braga, C., Batista, J., Fernández-Navarro, P., & Oliveira, J. T. (2017). Three narrative-based coding systems: Innovative moments, ambivalence and ambivalence resolution. *Psychotherapy Research, 27*(3), 270–282. https://doi.org/10.1080/10503307.2016.1247216

Grawe, K. (2004). *Psychological therapy*. Hogrefe & Huber.

Greenberg, L. S., Rice, L. N., & Elliott, R. K. (1993). *Facilitating emotional change: The moment-by-moment process*. Guilford Press.

Greenberg, L. S., & Webster, M. C. (1982). Resolving decisional conflict by Gestalt two-chair dialogue: Relating process to outcome. *Journal of Counseling Psychology, 29*(5), 468–477. https://doi.org/10.1037/0022-0167.29.5.468

grosse Holtforth, M. (2008). Avoidance motivation in psychological problems and psychotherapy. *Psychotherapy Research, 18*(2), 147–159. https://doi.org/10.1080/10503300701765849

grosse Holtforth, M., & Castonguay, L. G. (2005). Relationship and techniques in cognitive-behavioral therapy—A motivational approach. *Psychotherapy: Theory, Research, & Practice, 42*(4), 443–455. https://doi.org/10.1037/0033-3204.42.4.443

grosse Holtforth, M., & Grawe, K. (2000). Questionnaire for the analysis of motivational schemas. *Zeitschrift Fur Klinische Psychologie-Forschung Und Praxis, 29*(3), 170–179.

grosse Holtforth, M., & Grawe, K. (2002). Bern Inventory of Treatment Goals: Part 1. Development and first application of a taxonomy of treatment goal themes. *Psychotherapy Research, 12*(1), 79–99. https://doi.org/10.1080/713869618

grosse Holtforth, M., Krieger, T., Bochsler, K., & Mauler, B. (2011). The prediction of psychotherapy success by outcome expectations in inpatient psychotherapy. *Psychotherapy and Psychosomatics, 80*(5), 321–322. https://doi.org/10.1159/000324171

Hagedorn, W. B. (2011). Using therapeutic letters to navigate resistance and ambivalence: Experiential implications for group counseling. *Journal of Addictions & Offender Counseling, 31*(2), 108–126. https://doi.org/10.1002/j.2161-1874.2011.tb00071.x

Harkin, B., Webb, T. L., Chang, B. P. I., Prestwich, A., Conner, M., Kellar, I., Benn, Y., & Sheeran, P. (2016). Does monitoring goal progress promote goal attainment? A meta-analysis of the experimental evidence. *Psychological Bulletin, 142*(2), 198–229. https://doi.org/10.1037/bul0000025

Heckhausen, J. E., & Heckhausen, H. E. (Eds.). (2008). *Motivation and action* (2nd ed.). Cambridge University Press. https://doi.org/10.1017/CBO9780511499821

Heine, S. J., Proulx, T., & Vohs, K. D. (2006). The meaning maintenance model: On the coherence of social motivations. *Personality and Social Psychology Review, 10*(2), 88–110. https://doi.org/10.1207/s15327957pspr1002_1

Johansson, P., Høglend, P., & Hersoug, A. G. (2011). Therapeutic alliance mediates the effect of patient expectancy in dynamic psychotherapy. *British Journal of Clinical Psychology, 50*(3), 283–297. https://doi.org/10.1348/014466510X517406

Keleher, B., Oakman, J. M., Capobianco, K., & Mittelstaedt, W. H. (2019). Basic psychological needs satisfaction, working alliance, and early termination in psychotherapy. *Counselling Psychology Quarterly, 32*(1), 64–80. https://doi.org/10.1080/09515070.2017.1367271

Kelly, G. (1991). *The psychology of personal constructs*. Routledge. https://doi.org/10.4324/9780203405970

Klinger, E. (1977). *Meaning and void: Inner experience and the incentives in people's lives*. University of Minnesota Press.

La Guardia, J. G., Ryan, R. M., Couchman, C. E., & Deci, E. L. (2000). Within-person variation in security of attachment: A self-determination theory perspective on attachment, need fulfillment, and well-being. *Journal of Personality and Social Psychology, 79*(3), 367–384. https://doi.org/10.1037/0022-3514.79.3.367

Lombardi, D. R., Button, M. L., & Westra, H. A. (2014). Measuring motivation: Change talk and counter-change talk in cognitive behavioral therapy for generalized anxiety. *Cognitive Behaviour Therapy, 43*(1), 12–21. https://doi.org/10.1080/16506073.2013.846400

Marker, I., Corbett, B. E., Drummond, S. P. A., & Norton, P. J. (2020). Intermittent motivational interviewing and transdiagnostic CBT for anxiety: A randomized controlled trial. *Journal of Anxiety Disorders, 75*, Article 102276. https://doi.org/10.1016/j.janxdis.2020.102276

Markus, H., & Nurius, P. (1986). Possible selves. *American Psychologist, 41*(9), 954–969. https://doi.org/10.1037/0003-066X.41.9.954

McEvoy, P. M., & Nathan, P. (2007). Perceived costs and benefits of behavioral change: Reconsidering the value of ambivalence for psychotherapy outcomes. *Journal of Clinical Psychology, 63*(12), 1217–1229. https://doi.org/10.1002/jclp.20424

Miller, W. R., & Rollnick, S. (2002). *Motivational interviewing: Preparing people for change* (2nd ed.). Guilford Press.

Miller, W. R., & Rollnick, S. (2004). Talking oneself into change: Motivational interviewing, stages of change, and therapeutic process. *Journal of Cognitive Psychotherapy, 18*(4), 299–308. https://doi.org/10.1891/jcop.18.4.299.64003

Miller, W. R., & Rollnick, S. (2013). *Motivational interviewing: Helping people change* (3rd ed.). Guilford Press.

Miller, W. R., & Rose, G. S. (2015). Motivational interviewing and decisional balance: Contrasting responses to client ambivalence. *Behavioural and Cognitive Psychotherapy, 43*(2), 129–141. https://doi.org/10.1017/S1352465813000878

Montesano, A., Feixas, G., Caspar, F., & Winter, D. (2017). Depression and identity: Are self-constructions negative or conflictual? *Frontiers in Psychology, 8*(877). https://doi.org/10.3389/fpsyg.2017.00877

Montesano, A., Gonçalves, M. M., & Feixas, G. (2017). Self-narrative reconstruction after dilemma-focused therapy for depression: A comparison of good and poor outcome cases. *Psychotherapy Research, 27*(1), 112–126. https://doi.org/10.1080/10503307.2015.1080874

Montesano, A., López-González, M. A., Saúl, L. A., & Feixas, G. (2015). A review of cognitive conflicts research: A meta-analytic study of prevalence and relation to symptoms. *Neuropsychiatric Disease and Treatment, 11*, 2997–3006. https://doi.org/10.2147/NDT.S91861

Murphy, E., Mansell, W., Craven, S., & McEvoy, P. (2016). Approach-avoidance attitudes associated with initial therapy appointment attendance: A prospective study. *Behavioural and Cognitive Psychotherapy, 44*(1), 118–122. https://doi.org/10.1017/S135246581400023X

Norcross, J. C., & Lambert, M. J. (2011). Evidence-based therapy relationships: Research conclusions and clinical practices. In J. C. Norcross (Ed.), *Psychotherapy relationships that work* (2nd ed., pp. 3–22). Oxford University Press. https://doi.org/10.1093/acprof:oso/9780199737208.003.0001

Oddli, H. W., McLeod, J., Reichelt, S., & Rønnestad, M. H. (2014). Strategies used by experienced therapists to explore client goals in early sessions of psychotherapy. *European Journal of Psychotherapy & Counselling, 16*(3), 245–266. https://doi.org/10.1080/13642537.2014.927380

O'Hanlon, W. H., & O'Hanlon, B. (2003). *A guide to inclusive therapy: 26 methods of respectful, resistance-dissolving therapy*. Norton.

Oliveira, J. T., Faustino, D., Machado, P. P. P., Ribeiro, E., Gonçalves, S., & Gonçalves, M. M. (2021). Sudden gains and ambivalence in the unified protocol for transdiagnostic treatment of emotional disorder. *International Journal of Cognitive Therapy, 14*(3), 592–611. https://doi.org/10.1007/s41811-021-00106-w

Oliveira, J. T., Gonçalves, M. M., Braga, C., & Ribeiro, A. P. (2016). How to deal with ambivalence in psychotherapy: A conceptual model for case formulation. *Revista de Psicoterapia, 27*(104), 119–137.

Oliveira, J. T., Ribeiro, A. P., & Gonçalves, M. M. (2020). Ambivalence in Psychotherapy Questionnaire: Development and validation studies. *Clinical Psychology & Psychotherapy, 27*(5), 727–735. https://doi.org/10.1002/cpp.2457

Oliveira, J. T., Sousa, I., Ribeiro, A. P., & Gonçalves, M. M. (2021). Premature termination of the unified protocol for the transdiagnostic treatment of emotional disorders: The role of ambivalence toward change. *Clinical Psychology and Psychotherapy*. Advance online publication. https://doi.org/10.1002/cpp.2694

Park, J., Swift, J. K., & Penix, E. A. (2019). The relationship between client regulatory focus and treatment use intentions, attitudes, credibility beliefs, and outcome expectations for psychotherapy. *Journal of Contemporary Psychotherapy, 49*(4), 265–272. https://doi.org/10.1007/s10879-019-09419-6

Paz, C., Montesano, A., Winter, D., & Feixas, G. (2017). Cognitive conflict resolution during psychotherapy: Its impact on depressive symptoms and psychological distress. *Psychotherapy Research, 29*(1), 45–57. https://doi.org/10.1080/10503307.2017.1405172

Perls, F., Hefferline, R. F., & Goodman, P. (1951). *Gestalt therapy*. Julian Press.

Poulin, L. E., Button, M. L., Westra, H. A., Constantino, M. J., & Antony, M. M. (2019). The predictive capacity of self-reported motivation vs. early observed motivational language in cognitive behavioural therapy for generalized anxiety disorder. *Cognitive Behaviour Therapy, 48*(5), 369–384. https://doi.org/10.1080/16506073.2018.1517390

Prochaska, J. O., & DiClemente, C. C. (1982). Transtheoretical therapy: Toward a more integrative model of change. *Psychotherapy: Theory, Research, & Practice, 19*(3), 276–288. https://doi.org/10.1037/h0088437

Prochaska, J. O., & Norcross, J. C. (2013). *Systems of psychotherapy: A transtheoretical analysis* (8th ed.). Cengage Learning.

Prochaska, J. O., & Velicer, W. F. (1997). The transtheoretical model of health behavior change. *American Journal of Health Promotion, 12*(1), 38–48. https://doi.org/10.4278/0890-1171-12.1.38

Quitasol, M. N., Fournier, M. A., Domenico, S. I. D., Bagby, R. M., & Quilty, L. C. (2018). Changes in psychological need fulfillment over the course of treatment for major depressive disorder. *Journal of Social and Clinical Psychology, 37*(5), 381–404. https://doi.org/10.1521/jscp.2018.37.5.381

Reis, H. T., Sheldon, K. M., Gable, S. L., Roscoe, J., & Ryan, R. M. (2000). Daily well-being: The role of autonomy, competence, and relatedness. *Personality and Social Psychology Bulletin, 26*(4), 419–435. https://doi.org/10.1177/0146167200266002

Ryan, R. M., & Deci, E. L. (2000). Self-determination theory and the facilitation of intrinsic motivation, social development, and well-being. *American Psychologist, 55*(1), 68–78. https://doi.org/10.1037/0003-066X.55.1.68

Ryan, R. M., Lynch, M. F., Vansteenkiste, M., & Deci, E. L. (2011). Motivation and autonomy in counseling, psychotherapy, and behavior change: A look at theory and practice. *The Counseling Psychologist, 39*(2), 193–260. https://doi.org/10.1177/0011000009359313

Sansfaçon, J., Booij, L., Gauvin, L., Fletcher, É., Islam, F., Israël, M., & Steiger, H. (2020). Pretreatment motivation and therapy outcomes in eating disorders: A systematic review and meta-analysis. *International Journal of Eating Disorders, 53*(12), 1879–1900. https://doi.org/10.1002/eat.23376

Schulte, D., & Eifert, G. H. (2002). What to do when manuals fail? The dual model of psychotherapy. *Clinical Psychology: Science and Practice, 9*(3), 312–328. https://doi.org/10.1093/clipsy.9.3.312

Shahar, B., Carlin, E. R., Engle, D. E., Hegde, J., Szepsenwol, O., & Arkowitz, H. (2012). A pilot investigation of emotion-focused two-chair dialogue intervention for self-criticism. *Clinical Psychology & Psychotherapy*, *19*(6), 496–507. https://doi.org/10.1002/cpp.762

Sheldon, K. M., & Filak, V. (2008). Manipulating autonomy, competence, and relatedness support in a game-learning context: New evidence that all three needs matter. *British Journal of Social Psychology*, *47*(2), 267–283. https://doi.org/10.1348/014466607X238797

Steele, D. W., Becker, S. J., Danko, K. J., Balk, E. M., Adam, G. P., Saldanha, I. J., & Trikalinos, T. A. (2020). Brief behavioral interventions for substance use in adolescents: A meta-analysis. *Pediatrics*, *146*(4), Article e20200351. https://doi.org/10.1542/peds.2020-0351

Tamir, M., & Diener, E. (2008). Approach-avoidance goals and well-being: One size does not fit all. In A. J. Elliot (Ed.), *Handbook of approach and avoidance motivation* (pp. 415–428). Psychology Press.

Taylor, G., Dunkley, D. M., Zuroff, D. C., Lewkowski, M., Foley, J. E., Myhr, G., & Westreich, R. (2020). Autonomous motivation moderates the relation of self-criticism to depressive symptoms over one year: A longitudinal study of cognitive-behavioral therapy patients in a naturalistic setting. *Journal of Social and Clinical Psychology*, *39*(10), 876–896. https://doi.org/10.1521/jscp.2020.39.10.876

Trachsel, M., Gurtner, A., von Känel, M. L., & grosse Holtforth, M. (2010). Keep it in or let it out? Ambivalence over the expression of emotion as a moderator of depressiveness in unemployed subjects. *Swiss Journal of Psychology/Schweizerische Zeitschrift für Psychologie/Revue Suisse de Psychologie*, *69*(3), 141–146. https://doi.org/10.1024/1421-0185/a000016

Tryon, G. S. (2018). Goals and psychotherapy research. In M. Cooper & D. Law (Eds.), *Working with goals in psychotherapy and counselling* (pp. 87–110). Oxford University Press. https://doi.org/10.1093/med-psych/9780198793687.003.0005

Urmanche, A. A., Oliveira, J. T., Gonçalves, M. M., Eubanks, C. F., & Muran, J. C. (2019). Ambivalence, resistance, and alliance ruptures in psychotherapy: It's complicated. *Psychoanalytic Psychology*, *36*(2), 139–147. https://doi.org/10.1037/pap0000237

van der Kaap-Deeder, J., Vansteenkiste, M., Soenens, B., Verstuyf, J., Boone, L., & Smets, J. (2014). Fostering self-endorsed motivation to change in patients with an eating disorder: The role of perceived autonomy support and psychological need satisfaction. *International Journal of Eating Disorders*, *47*(6), 585–600. https://doi.org/10.1002/eat.22266

Vîslă, A., Constantino, M. J., Newkirk, K., Ogrodniczuk, J. S., & Söchting, I. (2018). The relation between outcome expectation, therapeutic alliance, and outcome among depressed patients in group cognitive-behavioral therapy. *Psychotherapy Research*, *28*(3), 446–456. https://doi.org/10.1080/10503307.2016.1218089

Vitinius, F., Tieden, S., Hellmich, M., Pfaff, H., Albus, C., & Ommen, O. (2018). Perceived psychotherapist's empathy and therapy motivation as determinants of long-term therapy success—Results of a cohort study of short term psychodynamic inpatient psychotherapy. *Frontiers in Psychiatry*, *9*(660). https://doi.org/10.3389/fpsyt.2018.00660

Wampold, B. E., Hollon, S. D., & Hill, C. E. (2011). Unresolved questions and future directions in psychotherapy research. In J. C. Norcross, G. R. VandenBos, & D. K. Freedheim (Eds.), *History of psychotherapy: Continuity and change* (2nd ed., pp. 333–356). American Psychological Association. https://doi.org/10.1037/12353-011

Westermann, S., grosse Holtforth, M., & Michalak, J. (2019). Motivation in psychotherapy. In R. M. Ryan (Ed.), *The Oxford handbook of human motivation* (pp. 417–462). Oxford University Press. https://doi.org/10.1093/oxfordhb/9780190666453.013.23

Westra, H. A., Aviram, A., Barnes, M., & Angus, L. (2010). Therapy was not what I expected: A preliminary qualitative analysis of concordance between client expectations and experience of cognitive-behavioural therapy. *Psychotherapy Research*, *20*(4), 436–446. https://doi.org/10.1080/10503301003657395

Westra, H. A., & Norouzian, N. (2017). Using motivational interviewing to manage process markers of ambivalence and resistance in cognitive behavioral therapy. *Cognitive Therapy and Research*. Advance online publication. https://doi.org/10.1007/s10608-017-9857-6

Zuroff, D. C., Koestner, R., Moskowitz, D. S., McBride, C., Marshall, M., & Bagby, M. R. (2007). Autonomous motivation for therapy: A new common factor in brief treatments for depression. *Psychotherapy Research*, *17*(2), 137–147. https://doi.org/10.1080/10503300600919380

Zuroff, D. C., McBride, C., Ravitz, P., Koestner, R., Moskowitz, D. S., & Bagby, R. M. (2017). Autonomous and controlled motivation for interpersonal therapy for depression: Between-therapists and within-therapist effects. *Journal of Counseling Psychology*, *64*(5), 525–537. https://doi.org/10.1037/cou0000239

3

Patient Readiness to Change

What We Know About Their Stages and Processes of Change

John C. Norcross, Danielle M. Cook, and Jairo N. Fuertes

ental health professionals tell psychotherapy stories about their patients in one way. The patients themselves frequently tell and experience their stories quite another way.

Readiness to change or, more precisely, the stages of change, represent a compelling case in point: When asked how they changed their problems with or without psychotherapy, research participants repeatedly said that it depended on when. They employed different methods at different times, such as increasing their awareness early on in the change process and frequently reinforcing themselves, which led to the development of healthier alternatives later in the process. Patients repeatedly described the stages of change; clients experienced predictable heterogeneity in readiness to change and introduced this key notion to the mental health and addiction professions (Prochaska et al., 2020).

Forty years of research on the stages of change with dozens of behavioral disorders and life challenges have validated those client experiences (see reviews by DiClemente, 2018; Krebs et al., 2019; Prochaska & Norcross, 2018). Virtually all mental health professionals now acknowledge that a patient's readiness for change profoundly influences the process and outcome

Portions of this chapter are from *Psychotherapy Relationships That Work: Vol. 2. Evidence-Based Therapist Responsiveness* (3rd ed.), by J. C. Norcross and B. E. Wampold (Eds.), 2019, Oxford University Press (https://doi.org/10.1093/med-psych/9780190843960.001.0001). Copyright 2019 by John C. Norcross. Reprinted with permission.

https://doi.org/10.1037/0000303-004
The Other Side of Psychotherapy: Understanding Clients' Experiences and Contributions in Treatment, J. N. Fuertes (Editor)

of psychotherapy. In quant speak, readiness to change powerfully moderates the success of psychotherapy (e.g., Boswell et al., 2012; Krebs et al., 2019; Mander et al., 2014).

A favorite analogy of the process of change is a physical gym and a personal trainer. The trainer or therapist assuredly makes a profound difference in the probability of effectiveness, but it is ultimately up to the client to do the heavy lifting and the hard work in therapy (Fuertes & Williams, 2017). Clients bring motivation and personal strategies for solving problems to psychotherapy (Mackrill, 2008), as well as therapeutic ingredients, including self-knowledge and strengths that help them and their therapists achieve positive outcomes in treatment (Bohart, 2000). Decades of research convincingly demonstrated that the patient contributes the lion's share to psychotherapy success (Norcross & Lambert, 2019). Indeed, research findings have consistently revealed that client factors explain the largest portion of outcome in treatment (i.e., about 40%; Bohart & Wade, 2013; Wampold & Imel, 2015).

The transtheoretical model (TTM; Prochaska et al., 1995) explains what clients experience and work on at various points in therapy. In this model, patient change is conceptualized as a process that unfolds over time and involves progression through a series of five stages: precontemplation, contemplation, preparation, action, and maintenance. At each stage, research and practice have repeatedly confirmed that different client tasks and therapist interventions are strongly associated with treatment outcome. Adapting psychotherapy to the individual client thus requires tailoring interventions to the stage in which clients find themselves. Further, as patients progress in stages, the therapeutic relationship evolves accordingly, and the TTM prescribes different optimal relationship stances for therapists at each stage (Krebs et al., 2019).

In this chapter, we consider the voluminous research evidence and clinical experience on patient readiness to change in psychotherapy. We identify the stages of change and related readiness constructs, describe popular measures to assess them, and present two clinical vignettes.[1] We describe the processes of change—how people change—at the various stages. The following sections review the research evidence on the stages: what we know in general and what we know specifically about psychotherapy patients. The chapter concludes with training and research implications and, most important, clinical applications of the stages of change in psychotherapy. We use the terms *client* and *patient* interchangeably throughout, as well as the terms *therapy, psychotherapy,* and *treatment.*

---

[1]The identities of the individuals in this chapter's case examples have been properly disguised to protect client confidentiality.

STAGES OF CHANGE: WHEN PATIENTS CHANGE

Definitions

Readiness to change refers to the patient and their attitudes, intentions, and behaviors in therapy. Each stage reflects not only a period of time but also encompasses a set of tasks required for movement to the next stage. Although the time an individual spends in each stage varies, the tasks to be accomplished are presumed to be largely invariant.

Precontemplation is the stage at which there is no intention to change behavior in the foreseeable future. Most patients in this stage are unaware or under aware of their problems. Families, friends, neighbors, or employers, however, are often well aware that the precontemplators have problems. When pre-contemplators present for psychotherapy, they often do so because of pressure from others. Usually, they feel coerced into changing by their spouses who threaten to leave, employers who threaten to dismiss them, parents who threaten to disown them, or courts who threaten to punish them. Resistance to recognizing or modifying a problem is the hallmark of precontemplation. Individuals in this stage report being unwilling to change their behavior(s) within the next 6 months (Krebs et al., 2019).

Clients' experiences of therapy at this stage and their behavior are characterized largely by indifference or resistance to therapy, a disinterest or refusal to cooperate, avoidance, and quite possibly feeling annoyed by the clinician. Patients at this stage are likely to endorse items such as "As far as I am concerned, I don't have any problems that need changing" and/or "I guess I have faults but there's nothing that I really need to change" (Krebs et al., 2019).

In the *contemplation* stage, clients are aware that a problem exists and are seriously thinking about overcoming it, but they have not made a commitment to take action yet. People can remain stuck in the contemplation stage for long periods. Contemplators struggle with their positive evaluations of their dysfunctional behavior and the amount of effort, energy, and loss it would cost to overcome it. Serious consideration of the pros and cons of changing—ambivalence (see also Chapter 2, this volume)—is the defining feature of contemplation. Individuals in this stage report seriously considering changing their behavior(s) within the next 6 months. A readiness perspective facilitates therapists' empathy by viewing resistance (precontemplation) and ambivalence (contemplation) as natural parts of behavior change. The patient is "stuck" at a particular stage or struggling through a normal progression.

Clients' experiences of therapy at this stage and their behavior are characterized by less resistance, better reality testing, and greater consideration of the need for help. Clients begin to realize that they have a problem that needs solving, but with this realization comes trepidation about what they will have to endure, give up, or lose to overcome their problem. Clients at this stage of therapy are likely to endorse items such as "I have a problem and I really think I should work on it" and/or "I've been thinking that I might want to change something about myself" (Krebs et al., 2019).

Preparation combines intention and behavioral criteria. Individuals in this stage are intending to take action in the next month and have unsuccessfully taken action in the past year. As a group, individuals who are prepared for action report small behavioral changes, and although they reduce their problem behaviors, individuals in the preparation stage have not yet reached the criteria for effective action. They are often experiencing early stirrings or taking "baby steps." However, they intend to take action in the near future.

Clients' experiences of therapy at this stage and their behavior are characterized by increasing confidence, a greater understanding of what change entails, and a sense that change is possible. The client is likely to adopt a more collaborative stance with their therapist and typically feels like they have an ally in their clinician. While not quite ready to take action, the client is preparing and laying the groundwork for making changes in their life. A patient at this stage of change may endorse the following item: "I now realize that I can change" or "I am finally at the point where I am ready to tackle my problems."

In the *action* stage, individuals modify their behavior, experiences, and/or environment to overcome their problems. Action involves the most overt behavioral changes and requires a considerable commitment of time and energy. Behavioral changes in the action stage tend to be the most visible and externally recognized. Individuals are classified in action if they have successfully altered their dysfunctional behavior for a period spanning from 1 day to 6 months. Modification of the target behavior to an acceptable criterion and concerted overt efforts to change are the hallmarks of action (Krebs et al., 2019).

Clients' experiences of therapy at this stage are likely to include greater confidence and satisfaction with psychotherapy; beginning to feel proud of their work, even if it is unpleasant; and continuing to see their therapist as an important ally. Patients at this stage of the process are likely to endorse the following items: "I am really working hard to change" and "Anyone can talk about changing, I am actually doing something about it" (Krebs et al., 2019).

Maintenance is the stage in which people work to prevent relapse and consolidate the gains attained during the action stage. For addictive behaviors, this stage extends from 6 months to an indeterminate period past the initial action stage. For some behaviors, maintenance may last a lifetime. Remaining free of the problem and consistently engaging in a new incompatible behavior for more than 6 months are the criteria for the maintenance stage. Stabilizing behavior change and avoiding relapse are the hallmarks of maintenance (Krebs et al., 2019). The maintenance stage is also when clients learn to cope more effectively and find support outside of psychotherapy through healthier relationships. Some may continue therapy or use it as a source of support on an as-needed basis. Items endorsed by a patient at this stage would be "I may need a boost right now to help me maintain the changes I've already made" and "I'm here to prevent myself from having a relapse of my problem" (Krebs et al., 2019).

Termination of a problem occurs when a person no longer experiences any temptation to return to troubled behaviors and no longer has to make any efforts to keep from relapsing. Obviously, termination of treatment and termination of a problem are not coincidental. Psychotherapy frequently ends before serious problems terminate entirely. Consequently, for many disorders, patients will return for booster sessions, most often when they believe they may be slipping back from previous gains. Also, because treatment terminates before most problems have reached their termination, some clients tend to experience distress over the termination of therapy (Prochaska & Norcross, 2018).

Spiral or Cycle of Change

As every seasoned patient and practitioner knows, change is not a linear progression; rather, most patients move through the stages of change in a spiral pattern. People progress from contemplation to preparation to action to maintenance, but most individuals will relapse. During a relapse, individuals regress to an earlier stage. Some relapsers feel like failures—embarrassed, ashamed, and guilty. These individuals become demoralized and resist thinking about behavior change. As a result, they return to the precontemplation stage and can remain there for various periods of time. Research shows that approximately 15% of relapsers regress to the precontemplation stage. Fortunately, most— 85% or so—move back to the contemplation stage and eventually back into preparation and action (Prochaska & Norcross, 2018).

Of course, readiness to change is a behavior-specific state, not a personality trait. Clients are invariably experiencing differences in their readiness to change in the myriad difficulties they bring to treatment. A recent client, for example, presented in precontemplation for his alcohol misuse ("I don't have a problem, but my husband thinks I do"), in contemplation for his depression ("Yes, I think I should probably do something about that"), but in action for his relationship crisis and threatened divorce ("That's what I am focusing on now"). At the same time, every patient is a successful changer on some behaviors. These previous successful efforts to change and grow serve as moments to remind them of their effectiveness through the stages of change.

Clinical Vignette

Joe, 44, lived with his wife, Debbie, and two children and came to psychotherapy at his wife's urging because his drinking was causing problems at his job and interfering with his ability to be an effective spouse and parent. While resistant to admit to alcohol as being a problem, he recognized he was underperforming "a bit" at work. He was more cognizant about needing to be a better parent and spouse. He agreed that he was ready to focus on his family and wanted to show his commitment to his wife and kids. He said that if he did that, "the rest will take care of itself." The therapist suggested that Joe try to avoid people, places, and things that were closely tied to his drinking and highlighted behaviors that would be welcomed by his wife and kids.

Joe reduced drinking alcohol at home and started being more attentive and helpful to his wife and kids. He also started to put in more effort at work, but he admitted to the therapist that he was still going to his favorite bar a couple of times a week, where he would see his old friends. He said, "I don't go get drunk"; he only wanted to see his friends, with whom he felt a genuine bond. They had a great sense of humor, rooted for the same sports teams as him, and never judged him. He felt free around them. However, inevitably, Joe would end up drinking excessively.

A particularly fruitful session occurred after a night in which he arrived home visibly drunk, and his wife woke up and confronted him. She was distressed and threatened to leave him if he did not stop drinking; their kids woke up and witnessed the incident. After a couple of sessions discussing this incident and exploring his drinking, Joe mentioned to the therapist that as part of being more involved with his kids, he was transporting them twice a week to and from gymnastics classes, which were held in the same mall as his favorite bar. Each time he took his kids to gymnastics, the sight of the bar tempted him to return to his friends. Because he had promised Debbie that he would take the kids to gymnastics, he felt like he could not stop doing so. The therapist reflected how Joe was in a difficult spot, wanting to take the kids to gymnastics, wanting to see his friends and relax, and not wanting to upset Debbie, who was happy about Joe's increased attentiveness to the kids. The therapist introduced the idea of having his wife join him for a session, and Joe agreed.

The psychotherapist provided the couple with psychoeducation on alcoholism and its treatment, and as Debbie started to cry, Joe admitted for the first time that his drinking was a problem. The therapist explained to them how the mall and the bar presented Joe with overwhelming cues to drinking and the need to avoid those cues, particularly at the beginning of treatment. Debbie replied that she understood and suggested other ways that Joe could contribute to parenting their children so that he would not feel guilty for not taking them to gymnastics. Debbie also understood better that, for Joe, the bar was a social experience where he felt relaxed and connected, but it was obviously one to avoid, along with avoiding alcohol. They explored ways that Joe could see select friends at home who would be supportive of his need to avoid alcohol. They both agreed that there would never be any alcohol in the house. They also discussed planning downtime together. Joe seemed to appreciate this gesture from Debbie and cried for the first time in session while apologizing to her for his drinking.

Along with medication to curb his urges for alcohol, by avoiding the mall (and bars), and by continuing in psychotherapy to commit more to sobriety, Joe stopped drinking. Joe realized that his family meant everything to him; he continued to improve his performance at work (he was even promoted), started attending a self-help group in his community, and continued to abstain from alcohol for several months until treatment ended. He arrived at the maintenance stage on all three treatment goals (family, work, abstinence) at the end of therapy.

The case of Joe illustrates how a patient will be at multiple stages of change with respect to different problems and will likely progress through those stages over time. Joe was initially resistant to label his alcohol consumption as problematic (precontemplation), and he seemed ambivalent about his performance at work (contemplation), but he was ready to act on being a better parent and spouse (action).

The case also illustrates how stage-matching treatment helps patients more realistically evaluate their problems and circumstances, develop an abiding sense of hope about change, clarify values and beliefs, and begin to consider and plan ways of changing. The therapist helped Joe discuss conflicts, such as the desire to avoid the bar while wanting to see his friends. The therapist also helped Joe evaluate his options and make a choice and a commitment to changing. By experiencing success in one area, Joe built self-efficacy to make changes in other, more challenging areas.

The prominence of helping relationships was also evident in this case: for Joe, it was the psychotherapist; his wife, Debbie; and his self-help group. For other patients, it could be other trusted family members, a sponsor, a religious or spiritual leader, or a respected member of the community.

Finally, the case highlights the fact that Joe, as the client, did most of the work in treatment. He had to find or build the motivation and the wherewithal to trust in his therapist and himself. He benefited from having a supportive family, a good job, and access to health care, but from beginning to end, it was up to Joe whether his therapy would prove successful.

Assessment

Multiple assessment devices have been developed over the years to assess a person's stage of change or readiness to change. The measures vary in format—questionnaires, algorithms, ladders, and interviews—as well as in specificity—generic measures for multiple problems and disorder-specific measures (Krebs et al., 2019).

The most frequent measure in psychotherapy research has been the University of Rhode Island Change Assessment (URICA), more popularly known as the stages of change measure (McConnaughy et al., 1989). This 32-item questionnaire yields separate scores on four continuous scales: precontemplation, contemplation, action, and maintenance (precontemplators score high on both the contemplation and action scales). Scores for each stage range from 8 to 40, with higher scores indicating a stronger endorsement of each subscale. Psychometric evaluation of the URICA demonstrates a stable four-factor structure (Pantalon et al., 2002) and a subscale consistency (alpha's .74–.88, Petry, 2005; .88–.89, McConnaughy et al., 1983).

Other measures of change readiness include the Stages of Change and Treatment Eagerness Scales (SOCRATES), developed for measuring readiness for change with regard to problem drinking as an alternative measure to the URICA (Miller & Tonigan, 1996). This 19-item measure produces three continuous scales: Ambivalence, Recognition, and Taking Steps, which represent continuously distributed motivational processes. The SOCRATES has been found to be related to quitting attempts for smoking cessation (DiClemente et al., 1991), alcohol use (Isenhart, 1997; Zhang et al., 2004), and drug use (Henderson et al., 2004).

In clinical practice, readiness is frequently assessed using a series of questions that result in a discrete categorization for a particular problem or goal. The practitioner asks if patients seriously intend to change the problem in the near future, typically within the next 6 months. If not, they are classified as precontemplators. Clients who state that they are seriously considering changing the problem behavior in the next 6 months are classified as contemplators. Those intending to take action in the next month are in the preparation stage. Clients who state that they are currently changing their problem are in the action stage.

The stages of change are also experienced by child and adolescent clients and are assessed by simplified methods. We often describe the cycle of change to youth as a foot race: get ready (contemplation), get set (preparation), go (action), and keep running (maintenance). The practitioner sensitively inquires, for each troubling behavior, where the youth thinks they are in that race.

PROCESSES OF CHANGE: HOW PATIENTS CHANGE

The TTM features the temporal dimension of change (the stages), as well as the principal methods of change (the processes emphasized at that stage).

Each process encompasses methods traditionally associated with disparate theoretical orientations. There are literally hundreds of global theories of psychotherapy, and there are thousands of specific treatment techniques. Practitioners will rarely agree on either the superordinate theories or the moment-to-moment methods to use. By contrast, the processes of change represent a middle level of abstraction between the global theories (such as psychoanalysis, cognitive, and humanistic) and the specific techniques (such as dream analysis, progressive muscle relaxation, and family sculpting; Prochaska & Norcross, 2018). One can think of the processes as psychological experiences in recovery (or change) that are common to patients, regardless of the therapy they are receiving (Prochaska & Norcross, 2018; Wampold & Imel, 2015). It is at this intermediate level of analysis—the processes of change—that meaningful points of convergence may be found among psychotherapy systems. It is, as well, at this level that expert psychotherapists typically formulate their treatment plans—not in terms of global theories or specific techniques but as change processes for their clients (Prochaska & Norcross, 2018).

Table 3.1 summarizes seven processes of change under the stage in which they are most frequently used (DiClemente, 2018; Norcross et al., 2011). The table presents the general goal of each change process and sample therapist interventions and client tasks. The list of change processes began with an analysis of the leading systems of psychotherapy (Prochaska, 1979) and, over the years, has been verified in hundreds of studies of psychotherapy patients and self-changers (Krebs et al., 2019).

TABLE 3.1. Stages and Processes of Change

Stage and (processes)	General goal (G), sample therapist interventions (T), and sample client tasks (C)
Precontemplation (consciousness-raising)	(G) Increasing client information about self, circumstances, and problems
	(T) Open-ended questions, reflections, paraphrasing, empathy, awareness exercises, bibliotherapy
	(C) Reflection, communication, gaining awareness, concern, hope
Contemplation (self-reevaluation)	(G) Assessing how the client feels and thinks about self with respect to a problem
	(T) Value clarification, empathy, challenges, interpretations, imagery
	(C) Weighing pros and cons of change, values clarification, goal setting
(Dramatic relief or emotional arousal)	(G) Experiencing and expressing feelings about the problems and solutions
	(T) Empathy, psychodrama, cathartic work, corrective emotional experience, role-play
	(C) Working through negative affect, grieving losses, gaining awareness, experiencing greater self-efficacy
Preparation (self-liberation)	(G) Evaluating and choosing options, increased commitment, improving self-efficacy
	(T) Decision-making methods, motivational interviewing commitment-enhancing techniques, affirmations, summaries, feedback
	(C) Making a commitment to change, formulating a realistic plan, rehearsing
Action (counterconditioning)	(G) Substituting alternative or healthier behaviors for problem, better coping
	(T) Relaxation, assertion, cognitive restructuring, behavioral rehearsal and activation
	(C) Plan implementation, healthy coping, plan monitoring, resisting urges
(Stimulus control)	(G) Avoiding or controlling stimuli that elicit problem behaviors
	(T) Restructuring the client's environment, avoiding high-risk cues, fading techniques, altering relationships
	(C) Letting go of people, places, and things associated with problems, identifying new people, places, and things that promote desired behavior
(Reinforcement)	(G) Clients rewarding themselves or being rewarded by others for changing
	(T) Contingency contracts, reinforcement, self-reward
	(C) Positive reinforcement, healthy dependence, self-soothing, self-care

(continues)

TABLE 3.1. Stages and Processes of Change (*Continued*)

Stage and (processes)	General goal (G), sample therapist interventions (T), and sample client tasks (C)
(Builds on processes from previous stages)	(G) Continuation and solidification of desirable behavior(s)
	(T) Identify strategies to prevent relapse, improve and maintain self-regulation, reinforce a focus on recovery, wellness, and use of personal strengths
	(C) Sustaining new behavior and lifestyle, coping with urges, social support

Note. Data from Norcross et al. (2011) and DiClemente (2018).

The processes of consciousness raising, self-reevaluation, dramatic relief, and self-liberation evident in the earlier stages are most closely associated with insight or awareness-oriented psychotherapies, including the psychoanalytic, experiential, and cognitive traditions (Norcross et al., 2011). These psychotherapy systems focus primarily on the subjective aspects of the individual. The processes of counterconditioning, stimulus control, and reinforcement evident in action and maintenance are most closely associated with action-oriented therapies, including those in the behavioral and systemic traditions (Prochaska & Norcross, 2018).

Clients' Experiences Within Stages and Processes

Once a patient's stage of change is evident, therapists can know which processes will generally prove to be the most effective and the interventions to use to help the patient progress to the next stage of change. Rather than intervene in a haphazard or trial-and-error manner, therapists can use the knowledge of stages and processes and proceed in a more systematic and efficient style. The key is to use the right method (processes) at the right time (stages).

Here is how patients typically experience progress through the stages of change (adapted from Prochaska & Norcross, 2018).[2] During precontemplation, individuals use change processes significantly less than people do in any other stage. Precontemplators process less information about their problems, spend less time and energy reevaluating themselves, experience fewer emotional reactions to the negative aspects of their problems, are less open with significant others about their problems, and do little to shift their attention or their environment in the direction of overcoming their problems. If you do not believe you have a problem, why bother with changing it? In treatment, these patients have been historically labeled resistant, defensive, or in denial.

What do patients do and experience as they move from precontemplation to contemplation? When therapists focus on consciousness-raising methods—

---

[2]Portions of this section are from *Systems of Psychotherapy: A Transtheoretical Analysis* (9th ed.), by J. O. Prochaska and J. C. Norcross, 2018, Oxford University Press. Copyright 2018 by J. O. Prochaska and J. C. Norcross. Reprinted with permission.

such as observations, education, and interpretations—clients become more aware of the causes, consequences, and cures of their problems. In precontemplation, clients become more aware of their ineffective defenses and become more conscious of what they are defending against. The tasks for the patient at precontemplation focus mainly on increasing awareness, concern, and hope.

For the patient at contemplation, the tasks focus on weighing alternatives, options, and the pros and cons of change, building solid reasons and values to support change, and making decisions to change (DiClemente, 2018). In moving through contemplation, clients become increasingly aware of themselves and the nature of their problems and thus are freer to reevaluate themselves affectively and cognitively. The self-reevaluation process includes an assessment of which values clients will try to actualize, act on, and make real and which they will let go of. The more central problems are to clients' core values, the more their reevaluation will involve changes in their sense of self. Contemplators also use environmental reevaluation—that is, they deeply consider the effects their behaviors exert on their social environment, especially the people they care about most.

Preparation indicates a readiness to change in the near future and the incorporation of valuable lessons from past change attempts. Preparers are on the verge of taking action and need to set goals and priorities accordingly. To better prepare patients for action, progress is required in how they think and feel about their problems and how they value their destructive lifestyles. They frequently develop an action plan for how they will proceed. In addition, they will make firm commitments to follow through on the action steps. In fact, they are often already engaged in processes that would increase self-regulation and initiate behavior change.

As they prepare for the action stage, clients act from an increasing sense of self-liberation and/or willpower. Patients in preparation need to believe that they possess the autonomy and power to change their lives in key ways. Self-liberation is based in part on a sense of self-efficacy (Bandura, 1982)—the belief that one's own efforts play a critical role in succeeding in the face of difficult situations. The primary tasks for patients at the preparation stage are committing to change and creating an appropriate plan that is doable and acceptable (DiClemente, 2018).

The action stage requires a much more concerted and sustained use of behavioral and action processes—such as counterconditioning, stimulus control, and contingency management—to cope with those conditions that can coerce them into relapsing. Therapists can provide skills training, if necessary, in behavioral processes to increase the probability that clients will be successful when they do take action. In contingency management, psychotherapists serve as powerful sources of reward and help patients create their own systems of reinforcement for their desired behavior changes. Counterconditioning involves substituting healthier alternatives in conditions that normally elicit problems; for example, the client may start using relaxation to cope with anxiety or assertion to avoid problems that come with passivity. Counterconditioning entails doing the healthy opposite of the problematic behavior. Stimulus control involves managing the presence or absence of situations or cues that elicit problems, such as not driving by a favorite bar after work, as Joe did in the clinical vignette earlier. Addicted individuals, for instance, may begin to delay their use of substances each day or may control the number of situations where they rely on the addictive substances. Patients at the action stage have as primary tasks the adequate implementation of a plan or course of action, monitoring their changed behavior, continuing to engage in problem solving, healthy coping and self-regulation, and revising their plan as necessary (DiClemente, 2018).

Successful maintenance builds on each change process that has come before and encompasses a candid assessment of the conditions under which a person is likely to relapse. Clients assess their alternatives for coping with such coercive conditions without resorting to self-defeating defenses and pathological responses. Perhaps most crucial is the sense that one is becoming more of the kind of person one wants to be. Continuing to use counterconditioning, contingency management, and stimulus control is most effective when it is based on the conviction that maintaining change promotes a sense of self that is highly valued by oneself and at least one significant other. Tasks for the person at the maintenance stage include integrating new behavior into a sustainable new lifestyle, developing strategies for preventing relapse, and engaging with social support (DiClemente, 2018). When relapse occurs, the tasks for the patient include examining mistakes and problems in the change process, revising the plan, and reimplementing it.

To sum up: Effective behavior change depends on doing the right things (processes) at the right time (stages). Stage matching—aligning the change processes with the patient's stage—increases the probability of more successful and seamless psychotherapy.

Common Mismatches

We have observed two frequent mismatches in this respect. First, some clients (and clinicians) rely primarily on change processes most indicated for the contemplation stage—consciousness raising, self-reevaluation—while they are moving to the action stage. They try to modify behaviors by becoming more aware, a common criticism of classical psychoanalysis: Insight alone does not necessarily bring about behavior change. Second, other clients (and clinicians) rely primarily on change processes best suited for the action stage—contingency management, stimulus control, counterconditioning—without the requisite awareness, emotional fuel, and decision making provided in the contemplation and preparation stages. They try to modify behavior without awareness, a common criticism of radical behaviorism: Overt action without insight is likely to lead to temporary change (Prochaska et al., 1992).

Clinical Vignette

Mariela, 47, came to psychotherapy to help her cope with the sudden and unexpected loss of her 19-year-old son. She was married and had two other children: Her oldest son had recently moved out of state for graduate school, and her youngest, a daughter, was living at home and had recently begun attending a local college. At intake, she was distraught, sad, depressed, and unable to focus or to experience pleasure. She reported feeling guilty and responsible for her son's death and feeling as though she lost her sense of purpose with two of three children no longer in her care. Her husband dealt with his son's death by shutting down, a typical coping reaction for him. He seemed unable to express emotion and was not willing to grieve the loss with his wife. There had been a distance between them for some time. While a goal of therapy was not overtly discussed, the therapist noted the grief and intense negative emotions (guilt, loss, sadness) that Mariela was experiencing—and her loneliness.

The first few sessions were devoted to listening to Mariela's feelings; the psychotherapist used empathy, open-ended questions, and reflections to help her understand all that she was experiencing and provided her with support. The therapist determined early on that the work for Mariela would involve expressing and processing her grief, understanding her relationships with her remaining family members more deeply, and finding ways to help her move on. Mariela participated eagerly in the early sessions, which focused on her son, her grief, her anger, and her guilt ("I should not have let him go out that night; the weather was awful" and "Why didn't they save him? They might have tried harder if he was some rich kid"). The topic of the sessions progressed into the meaning of her loss and the context in which it occurred, including relationship problems with her husband and daughter. Mariela found that understanding her feelings and talking about her fraught relationships was much more difficult and less rewarding than the venting and expression of grief that characterized the earlier sessions. Her attendance began to dip, and she seemed less active and involved in sessions.

The therapist recognized this pattern and refocused sessions on getting Mariela to talk about what she wanted from the therapy. They discussed that, while venting felt good at the moment, it would not teach her how to cope with her family and with moving on beyond her loss. The therapist continued to be empathic but used more challenges and interpretations to focus on Mariela's difficulty with processing emotions and navigating her relationships. The therapist recognized how difficult the work was but emphasized the long-term benefits. Setting goals and planning activities allowed Mariela to get back to work, to enjoy a life she valued, and to build better relationships with her remaining family members.

After a couple of sessions discussing these options, which included goal setting, affirmation, and feedback, Mariela agreed on these general directions and tasks for treatment. Therapy progressed with a renewed energy on Mariela's part as she realized that she loved her family above all else and that her husband and kids, especially her daughter, needed her, and she needed them to get better. She also came to accept more and more that her son's death, an unimaginable loss for a parent, was an accident—a terrible accident for which she should not punish herself or others. She became more actively engaged in sessions, and her attendance improved.

After several additional sessions, Mariela shifted to action by establishing better communication with her husband and by being more attentive to and present with her kids. She allowed herself to grieve with them, and they planned time together to feel love and support. A few weeks later, she returned to work full time; she also started working out and taking better care of herself. She realized that, while she would grieve her son's death for the rest of her life, she had a renewed sense of purpose to move forward, enriched by a more tender relationship with herself and a deeper connection with her family.

The case of Mariela illustrates how, even in psychotherapy, in which a specific goal is not set at the beginning, patients will progress through the stages of change and employ the indicated processes of change. Mariela worked effectively with her grief but also gained awareness about her relationships with her family members. That awareness eventually gave way to constructive action and maintenance. In therapy, she conceived and practiced new ways of relating and coping, and she implemented a pragmatic plan to move forward.

GENERAL RESEARCH EVIDENCE ON STAGES AND PROCESSES

Decades of research have supported and shaped the core constructs of the stages and processes of change. Longitudinal studies affirm the relevance of these constructs for predicting premature termination and treatment outcome. Comparative outcome studies attest to the value of stage-matched interventions. Population-based studies highlight the need for psychosocial interventions tailored to the needs of individuals at all stages of change (see Krebs et al., 2019; Prochaska & Norcross, 2018; Prochaska et al., 1995, for reviews). We consider, first, the general research evidence on patient readiness and then summarize the research specifically on psychotherapy.

A patient's stage of change provides prescriptive as well as proscriptive information on the treatment of choice. Action-oriented therapies may prove quite effective with individuals who are in the preparation or action stage. These same programs may be ineffective or detrimental, however, with individuals in the precontemplation or contemplation stage.

For example, an intensive action- and maintenance-oriented smoking cessation program for cardiac patients was highly successful for those patients in the preparation and action stages (Ockene et al., 1992). Patients in this special-care program received personal counseling in the hospital and received monthly telephone counseling calls for 6 months following hospitalization. Of the patients who began the program in the action or preparation stage, an impressive 94% were not smoking at the 6-month follow-up. This same program failed, however, with smokers in the precontemplation and contemplation stages. For patients in these stages, less expensive and less intensive regular care did as well. Independent of the treatment received, a clear relationship emerged between the pretreatment stage and the outcome. Patients who were not smoking at 12 months included 22% of the precontemplators, 43% of the contemplators, and 76% of those in action or prepared for action at the start of the study. That is the predictable power of the stages of change. We assume all patients want therapy and are ready for action, but only some are.

As noted earlier, a consistent finding to emerge from research is that particular processes of change are more effective during particular stages of change. Forty years of research in behavior change converge in showing that different processes of change are differentially effective in certain stages of change. A meta-analysis (Rosen, 2000) of 47 cross-sectional studies examining the relationship of the stages and the processes of change showed large effect sizes (ds between 0.70 and 0.80). The studies involved smoking, substance abuse, exercise, diet, and psychotherapy. The mean effect sizes (d) were approximately .70 for variation in cognitive-affective processes by stage and .80 for variation in behavioral processes by stage, both moderate to large effects. Effect sizes for stages by processes did not vary significantly by the problem treated. Behavioral processes peaked in the action stage, while cognitive-affective processes peaked in the contemplation or preparation stages.

Stage matching—applying change processes for individuals at particular stages or readiness—has proved effective for self-changers as well as self-help programs. These tailoring efforts have primarily been population-based studies delivered via computer, mail, or phone with a focus on health behaviors. Such interventions have assessed and provided specific feedback by stage of change and other constructs, such as self-efficacy. A meta-analysis of 87 prospective, tailored interventions delivered via computer or mail across smoking cessation, physical activity, healthy diet, and mammography screening found a mean effect size (d) of .18 (95% CI = .16–.20; Krebs et al., 2010). That represents a 39% increase ($OR = 1.39$) over the nontailored intervention or minimal care conditions and indicates a small to medium-size effect for population-based interventions (Rossi, 2002). The subset of studies that intervened on smoking cessation, for instance, resulted in an absolute increase of 6% in quit rates, a rate comparable to that observed with four to eight individual in-person sessions (Fiore et al., 2008). Hence, stage matching or tailoring proved to be more effective than nontailoring for health behaviors.

SPECIFIC RESEARCH EVIDENCE ON PSYCHOTHERAPY PATIENTS

The stages of change effectively predict psychotherapy continuation and dropouts. Approximately one quarter of patients prematurely discontinue psychotherapy (Swift & Greenberg, 2012). In an early study (Brogan et al., 1999), the stages and processes of change correctly predicted 93% of premature terminators—as opposed to therapy continuers and early but appropriate terminators. The stage of change profile of the 40% who dropped out of therapy was that of precontemplators. The stage profile of the 20% who terminated quickly but appropriately was of people in the action stage. The stage profile of the therapy continuers was that of contemplators. In sum, the stage measure identifies and predicts who remains in psychotherapy (e.g., Biller et al., 2000; Derisley & Reynolds, 2000; Smith et al., 1995).

The amount of progress clients make during psychotherapy tends to be a direct function of their pretreatment stage of change. A meta-analysis of 76 studies, encompassing 21,238 psychotherapy patients, found that the stages reliably and robustly predicted outcomes in psychotherapy ($d = 0.41$; Krebs et al., 2019). The most frequent readiness measures were the URICA (46 studies) and SOCRATES (10 studies). Patients beginning in the preparation and action stages do better than those beginning in precontemplation or contemplation. To treat all psychotherapy patients as if they were in the same stage would be naive, yet that is what has been done for decades.

When therapy involves two or more clients working together, as in couple and parent–child treatment, therapy can be expected to progress most smoothly when the clients are at the same stage of change. If one member is ready for action while the other has not yet contemplated what change will mean, then treatment will be difficult at best. The therapist is then in the difficult position of being damned by one spouse for moving too slowly or resisted by the other for moving too quickly (Prochaska & Norcross, 2018).

If clients progress from one stage of change to the next during the first month of treatment, they can double their chances of taking action during the initial 6 months of treatment. Of the precontemplators who were still in precontemplation at the 1-month follow-up, only 3% took action by 6 months; of the precontemplators who had progressed to contemplation at 1 month, 7% took action by 6 months. Similarly, of the contemplators who remained in contemplation at 1 month, only 20% took action by 6 months; of the contemplators who had progressed to the preparation stage at 1 month, 41% entered the action stage by 6 months. These data demonstrate that treatments that help people progress just one stage in a month can double the chances of participants taking action on their own in the near future (Prochaska & DiClemente, 1982).

Over the past 40 years, the TTM has generated hundreds of research studies about how people change on their own and in treatment. Here we review the results of just a few of them on mental health disorders to illustrate the scope and impact of stage matching.

Several effective psychotherapies exist for depression, but there is a service gap for patients who do not receive or respond to traditional psychotherapy because of low treatment receptivity or subclinical syndromes. Three computer-assisted TTM-tailored reports and a workbook matched to the individual's stage of change addressed depression in primary care settings (Levesque et al., 2012). Primary care patients experiencing depression but not receiving treatment ($n = 481$) and primary care patients nonadherent with antidepressant medication ($n = 175$) were randomized to TTM or usual care. Patients in the TTM treatment group were more likely than the usual care group to experience a clinically significant improvement in their depression (35% vs. 25%). The odds ratio was 1.79, meaning that the patients receiving the TTM-tailored treatments were almost twice as likely to improve as the patients receiving usual care. The largest difference was found among patients suffering from major depression (22% vs. 6% improvement). Low-cost, computer-assisted, stage-matched interventions thus improved depression outcomes among primary care patients who may not be receptive to traditional treatments (Prochaska & Norcross, 2018).

In another psychotherapy study involving male perpetrators of partner violence, stage-tailored treatments were added to mandatory weekly group therapy. At the 6-month follow-up with the first 200 participants, the addition of stage matching produced a significant reduction in violence compared with weekly group counseling alone. In the stage-matched condition, only 3% of the female partners of the perpetrators had been subjected to partner violence in the past 6 months compared with 23% of the women whose partners only received group therapy (Levesque et al., 2012). In addition, about twice as many perpetrators had progressed to the action or maintenance stage during group therapy. Matching treatments to patients' stage of change has been found to decrease dropouts, improve retention, and boost outcomes in multiple disorders, including interpersonal violence. Matching treatment to stages works for a variety of problems.

As a final example, stage-matched interventions have expanded beyond individual patients to entire populations and from a single disorder to multiple domains of well-being. Adopting the World Health Organization's definition of health as more than the absence of illness, TTM studies have aimed treatments at enhancing emotional well-being, such as happiness and joy—that is, thriving rather than suffering (Prochaska et al., 2012).

One stage-tailored program reached out to nearly 4,000 people in 39 states in the United States. The adult sample averaged four chronic conditions and four risk behaviors, such as inadequate exercise, unhealthy eating, and poor stress management (Prochaska et al., 2012). They also scored well below the national averages on emotional and physical well-being, and the majority were struggling rather than thriving. The success rates for TTM-tailored telephone counseling, the TTM-tailored online program, and the control condition were, respectively, 57%, 47%, and 37% for exercise; 75%, 65%, and 53% for stress management; and 31%, 26%, and 21% for healthy eating, which was not treated. Those effectiveness patterns are clear and consistent for target behaviors.

What's more, these brief stage-matched treatments produced large impacts on overall well-being. Comparing the TTM treatments with controls showed that well-being increased about twice as much for the counselors and two thirds for the computers. Most striking was that the percentage of patients thriving almost doubled for counselors (67% vs. 34% of controls). This is an example of how psychotherapy can keep raising the bar to help more individuals feel and live better (Prochaska & Norcross, 2018).

CLINICAL APPLICATIONS

- **Assess clients' readiness to change for every goal behavior.** One cannot match what one does not know. Use the formal stage measures or informal questions to ascertain where clients "are at" for each problem or goal. In clinical practice, assessing the stage of change typically entails a straightforward question: "Would you say you are not ready to change in the next 6 months (precontemplation), thinking about changing in the next 6 months (contemplation), thinking about changing in the next month (preparation), or have you already made some progress (action)?" Stage assessment works equally well whether phrased as eliminating a disorder or reaching a goal.

- **Beware of treating all patients as though they are in action.** Professionals frequently design excellent action-oriented treatments but are then disappointed when only a small percentage of clients seek that therapy. The vast majority of patients are not in the action stage, and thus professionals offering only action-oriented programs are likely underserving or incorrectly serving the majority of their target population. The therapeutic recommendation is to move from an action paradigm to a stage paradigm.

- **Set realistic goals by moving one stage at a time.** A goal for many patients, particularly in a time-limited managed care environment, is to set realistic goals, such as helping patients progress from precontemplation to contemplation. Such progress means that patients are changing if we view change as a process that unfolds over time through a series of stages. Helping patients break out of the chronic, stuck phase of precontemplation is a therapeutic success because it almost doubles the chances that patients will take effective action in the next 6 months. If we help them progress two stages with brief therapy, we triple the chances they will take effective action.

- **Treat precontemplators gingerly.** People in precontemplation underestimate the pros of changing, overestimate the cons, feel defensive when pressured, and are not particularly conscious of their defenses (Hall & Rossi, 2008). Patients in the pre-action stages of change have lower expectations of a therapist's acceptance, genuineness, and trustworthiness (Satterfield et al., 1995). When psychotherapists pressure or try to impose action on these patients, they are likely to drive them away, consequently blaming the clients for being resistant, unmotivated, or noncompliant. Instead, match your relationships and change processes to the stage. Motivational interviewing (Miller & Rollnick, 2012) has brilliantly incorporated these lessons into its philosophical spirit and its treatment methods.

- **Tailor the processes to the stages.** The research reliably demonstrates that patients optimally progress from precontemplation and contemplation into preparation by use of consciousness raising, self-liberation, and emotional arousal. Patients progress best from preparation to action and maintenance by use of counterconditioning, stimulus control, and reinforcement management. To simplify: Use change processes traditionally associated with the insight or awareness therapies for the early stages and change processes associated with the action therapies for the later stages.

- **Avoid mismatching stages and processes.** A person's stage of change provides proscriptive as well as prescriptive information on treatments of choice. Action-oriented therapies may prove quite effective with individuals who are in the preparation or action stages. However, with individuals in precontemplation or contemplation, these same programs tend to be ineffective or detrimental.

- **Prescribe stage-matched relationships of choice.** Paralleling the notion of "treatments of choice" in terms of treatment methods, we offer "therapeutic relationships of choice" in terms of interpersonal stances (Norcross & Beutler, 1997). With patients in precontemplation, often the optimal role of the practitioner is like that of a *nurturing parent* joining with a resistant and defensive youngster who is both drawn to and repelled by the prospects of becoming more independent. With clients in contemplation, the optimal therapist stance is akin to a *Socratic teacher* who encourages clients to achieve their own insights into their condition. With clients in the preparation and action stages, the therapist's stance is more like that of an *experienced coach* who has been through many crucial matches and can provide a fine game plan or can review the participant's plan. With clients progressing into maintenance, the psychotherapist becomes more of a *consultant* who is available to provide expert advice and support when action is not progressing smoothly.

- **Practice integratively.** Psychotherapists moving with their patients through the stages of change over the course of treatment will probably employ relational stances and change processes traditionally emphasized by disparate systems of psychotherapy. That is, they will practice de facto psychotherapy integration (Norcross & Goldfried, 2019). Our research has consistently documented that psychotherapists in their consultation rooms (and self-changers in their natural environments) can be remarkably effective in synthesizing powerful change processes across the stages (Connors et al., 2013).

- **Anticipate recycling.** Most psychotherapy patients will recycle several times through the stages before achieving long-term maintenance. Accordingly, professionals and programs expecting people to progress linearly through the stages of change are likely to gather disappointing results. Be prepared to include relapse prevention in treatment, anticipate the probability of recycling patients, and minimize therapist guilt and patient shame over recycling (Prochaska et al., 2013).

- **Integrate readiness to change into treatment resources.** Readiness to change measures can be built into self-help materials, health apps, online treatments, and similar resources to enable the tailoring of interventions in ways that improve outcomes. The stages of change have been incorporated into several online assessments (e.g., ProChange, https://www.prochange.com/; InnerLife, https://www.innerlife.com/) and self-help books (*Changing to Thrive* by Prochaska & Prochaska, 2016; *Changeology* by Norcross, 2015). These resources can complement and expand psychotherapy, as well as reach underserved populations.

- **Shift to an expanded view of psychotherapy as proactive, population-based health care.** Psychotherapists need not discard effective means of assisting individuals suffering from mental disorders. Instead, they can add to these invaluable services by providing proactive recruitment and treatment of entire populations suffering from chronic biobehavioral conditions. Such an expansion could produce unprecedented impacts on the health and happiness of the populace (Prochaska et al., 2020).

RESEARCH AND TRAINING DIRECTIONS

On the basis of the research evidence and our training experience, we recommend the following training practices:

- **Train students to assess the client's stage of change.** Probably the most obvious and direct implication is to assess the stage of a client's readiness for change and tailor treatment accordingly.

- **Help students expect variability in patients' stages of change.** A useful guide is the "40–40–20 rule" in the population at large (not in action-oriented treatment programs): Approximately 40% will be in precontemplation, 40% in contemplation, and 20% in preparation or ready for action (Velicer et al., 1995).

- **Train students integratively.** Ostensibly contradictory processes become complementary when embedded in the stages of change. Specifically, change processes traditionally associated with the experiential, cognitive, and psychoanalytic persuasions prove most useful during the precontemplation and contemplation stages. Change processes traditionally associated with the existential and behavioral traditions, by contrast, are most useful during the action and maintenance stages.

- **Teach students to predicate psychotherapy more on the patient's characteristics (e.g., stage of change, culture, preferences) than on their diagnoses.** Asking the consequential questions of what the patient prefers, what matches their stage, and what the research indicates will facilitate movement toward maintenance and well-being. Remember that the largest effect sizes in psychotherapy pertain to the patient's contribution, the therapy relationship, and personalizing treatment to transdiagnostic characteristics, such as patient readiness (Norcross & Wampold, 2019).

- **Tailor supervision to the individual trainee as they simultaneously adapt psychotherapy to their clients.** As students are learning to match psychotherapy to their patient's transdiagnostic features, in a parallel process, their supervisors are tailoring supervision to multiple student characteristics (Norcross & Popple, 2017). This includes the trainee's stage of change for accepting certain feedback and learning particular skills.

- **Teach students to pursue and calculate societal impact, not only treatment efficacy.** Historically, psychotherapy outcome was evaluated by *efficacy*, the percentage of patients who were successful at posttreatment. However, treatment success is more than efficacy alone. *Impact* is defined as the participation rate times efficacy. If the best practice that produces 30% efficacy generates 5% participation, its impact is 1.5%. If an alternative practice that produces 20% efficacy generates 75% participation, its impact is 15%. The, apparently, less effective practice (in terms of efficacy) actually has 10 times as much of an impact on the population (Prochaska & Norcross, 2018).

- **Conduct client-focused research.** While a sizable amount of research on the transtheoretical model has been conducted using traditional quantitative perspectives, it would advance our understanding of change if more studies used the perspective of the patient as the primary framework of analysis. In particular, we encourage research that includes qualitative studies of the stages and processes of change as clients experience them.

Research Limitations and Future Directions

The stages of change have been found, in hundreds of studies, to apply to self-changers and psychotherapy patients of diverse ages, cultures, ethnicities, gender identities, races, religions, and sexual orientations. The meta-analyses reviewed earlier found that the stages of change evidenced similar outcome associations and predictions for patients of disparate ages, genders, and races and ethnicities. The stages are largely generalizable across cultures, disorders, and treatment settings as they represent, in our view, the underlying structure of behavior change (Prochaska et al., 1992). However, over 90% of the studies included in these meta-analyses were conducted in North America or Europe. More studies on the stages of change in psychotherapy from cultures and populations outside Western developed countries are sorely needed.

In addition, more psychotherapy studies need to directly and prospectively match and mismatch psychotherapy to the patient's stage of change. The extant research concerns the predictive utility of the stages of change in terms of outcomes and dropouts, the differential use of the processes of change at various stages of change, and the relative efficacy of assorted forms of service delivery.

Finally, in the future, proactive outreach research will markedly increase the percentage of high-risk and suffering people receiving psychosocial treatment for behavioral disorders. Because only a small minority of the population will be ready to take action, psychotherapists will increasingly design treatments for the population at every stage: the 20% or less in the preparation stage, the 40% in the contemplation stage, and the 40% in the precontemplation stage. By proactively reaching out and customizing services to readiness to change, psychotherapists can achieve a quantum increase in our ability to care for those suffering (Kazdin & Rabbitt, 2013; Prochaska et al., 2020).

CONCLUSION

The transtheoretical model highlights patient readiness or the stages of change and identifies the psychological processes that clients experience, negotiate, and resolve in modifying their behavior. Decades of research support its use as an effective guide for individual treatment, population health, and organizational change. A particular value of the model is that it privileges the inner workings of "the other side" of treatment: the client's experience and the processes by which the client and therapist collaborate to make psychotherapy successful. The model identifies the change processes and the types of interventions most likely to help the client in particular stages and outlines the tasks that clients engage in each step along the way. By attending to client heterogeneity in terms of readiness to change, the model broadens the scope of assessment and advances whole-person care beyond the client's problem or diagnosis. Matching treatment to patient readiness and other transdiagnostic characteristics demonstrably improves the efficiency and efficacy of psychological treatments (Norcross & Wampold, 2019).

REFERENCES

Bandura, A. (1982). Self-efficacy mechanism in human agency. *American Psychologist*, 37(2), 122–147. https://doi.org/10.1037/0003-066X.37.2.122

Biller, N., Arnstein, P., Caudill, M. A., Federman, C. W., & Guberman, C. (2000). Predicting completion of a cognitive-behavioral pain management program by initial measures of a chronic pain patient's readiness for change. *The Clinical Journal of Pain*, 16(4), 352–359. https://doi.org/10.1097/00002508-200012000-00013

Bohart, A. C. (2000). The client is the most important common factor: Clients' self-healing capacities and psychotherapy. *Journal of Psychotherapy Integration*, 10(2), 127–149. https://link.springer.com/article/10.1023/A:1009444132104

Bohart, A. C., & Wade, A. G. (2013). The client in psychotherapy. In M. J. Lambert (Ed.), *Bergin and Garfield's handbook of psychotherapy and behavior change* (6th ed., pp. 219–257). Wiley.

Boswell, J. F., Sauer-Zavala, S. E., Gallagher, M. W., Delgado, N. K., & Barlow, D. H. (2012). Readiness to change as a moderator of outcome in transdiagnostic treatment. *Psychotherapy Research*, 22(5), 570–578. https://doi.org/10.1080/10503307.2012.688884

Brogan, M. M., Prochaska, J. O., & Prochaska, J. M. (1999). Predicting termination and continuation status in psychotherapy using the transtheoretical model. *Psychotherapy: Theory, Research, & Practice*, 36(2), 105–113. https://doi.org/10.1037/h0087773

Connors, G. J., DiClemente, C. C., Velasquez, M. M., & Donovan, D. M. (2013). *Substance abuse treatment and the stages of change: Selecting and planning interventions* (2nd ed.). Guilford Press.

Derisley, J., & Reynolds, S. (2000). The transtheoretical stages of change as a predictor of premature termination, attendance and alliance in psychotherapy. *The British Journal of Clinical Psychology*, 39(4), 371–382. https://doi.org/10.1348/014466500163374

DiClemente, C. C. (2018). *Addiction and change: How addictions develop and addicted people recover* (2nd ed.). Guilford Press.

DiClemente, C. C., Prochaska, J. O., Fairhurst, S. K., Velicer, W. F., Velasquez, M. M., & Rossi, J. S. (1991). The process of smoking cessation: An analysis of precontemplation, contemplation, and preparation stages of change. *Journal of Consulting and Clinical Psychology*, 59(2), 295–304. https://doi.org/10.1037/0022-006X.59.2.295

Fiore, M. C., Jaén, C. R., Baker, T. B., Bailey, W. C., Benowitz, N. L., Curry, S. J., Dorfman, S. F., Froelicher, E. S., Goldstein, M. G., Healton, C. G., Nez Henderson, P., Heyman, R. B., Koh, H. K., Kottke, T. E., Lando, H. A., Mecklenburg, R. E., Mermelstein, R. J., Dolan Mullen, P., Orleans, C. T., . . . Wewers, M. E. (2008). *Treating tobacco use and dependence: 2008 update.* https://www.ncbi.nlm.nih.gov/books/NBK63952/

Fuertes, J. N., & Williams, E. N. (2017). Client-focused psychotherapy research. *Journal of Counseling Psychology, 64*(4), 369–375. https://doi.org/10.1037/cou0000214

Hall, K. L., & Rossi, J. S. (2008). Meta-analytic examination of the strong and weak principles across 48 health behaviors. *Preventive Medicine, 46*(3), 266–274. https://doi.org/10.1016/j.ypmed.2007.11.006

Henderson, M. J., Saules, K. K., & Galen, L. W. (2004). The predictive validity of the University of Rhode Island Change Assessment Questionnaire in a heroin-addicted polysubstance abuse sample. *Psychology of Addictive Behaviors, 18*(2), 106–112. https://doi.org/10.1037/0893-164X.18.2.106

Isenhart, C. E. (1997). Pretreatment readiness for change in male alcohol dependent subjects: Predictors of one-year follow-up status. *Journal of Studies on Alcohol, 58*(4), 351–357. https://doi.org/10.15288/jsa.1997.58.351

Kazdin, A. E., & Rabbitt, S. M. (2013). Novel models for delivering mental health services and reducing the burdens of mental illness. *Clinical Psychological Science, 1*(2), 170–191. https://doi.org/10.1177/2167702612463566

Krebs, P., Norcross, J. C., Nicholson, J. M., & Prochaska, J. O. (2019). Stages of change. In J. C. Norcross & B. E. Wampold (Eds.), *Psychotherapy relationships that work* (3rd ed., Vol. 2, pp. 296–328). Oxford University Press. https://doi.org/10.1093/med-psych/9780190843960.003.0010

Krebs, P., Prochaska, J. O., & Rossi, J. S. (2010). A meta-analysis of computer-tailored interventions for health behavior change. *Preventive Medicine, 51*(3–4), 214–221. https://doi.org/10.1016/j.ypmed.2010.06.004

Levesque, D. A., Ciavatta, M. M., Castle, P. H., Prochaska, J. M., & Prochaska, J. O. (2012). Evaluation of a stage-based, computer-tailored adjunct to usual care for domestic violence offenders. *Psychology of Violence, 2*(4), 368–384. https://doi.org/10.1037/a0027501

Mackrill, T. (2008). Exploring psychotherapy clients' independent strategies for change while in therapy. *British Journal of Guidance & Counselling, 36*(4), 441–453. https://doi.org/10.1080/03069880802343837

Mander, J., Wittorf, A., Klingberg, S., Teufel, M., Zipfel, S., & Sammet, I. (2014). The patient perspective on therapeutic change: The investigation of associations between stages of change and general mechanisms of change. *Journal of Psychotherapy Integration, 24*(2), 122–137. https://doi.org/10.1037/a0036976

McConnaughy, E. A., DiClemente, C. C., Prochaska, J. O., & Velicer, W. F. (1989). Stages of change in psychotherapy: A follow-up report. *Psychotherapy: Theory, Research, & Practice, 26*(4), 494–503. https://doi.org/10.1037/h0085468

McConnaughy, E. A., Prochaska, J. O., & Velicer, W. F. (1983). Stages of change in psychotherapy: Measurement and sample profiles. *Psychotherapy: Theory, Research, & Practice, 20*(3), 368–375. https://doi.org/10.1037/h0090198

Miller, W. R., & Rollnick, S. (2012). *Motivational interviewing: Helping people change.* Guilford Press.

Miller, W. R., & Tonigan, J. S. (1996). Assessing drinkers' motivation for change: The Stages of Change Readiness and Treatment Eagerness Scale (SOCRATES). *Psychology of Addictive Behaviors, 10*(2), 81–89. https://doi.org/10.1037/0893-164X.10.2.81

Norcross, J. C. (2015). *Changeology: 5 steps to realizing your goals and resolutions.* Simon & Schuster.

Norcross, J. C., & Beutler, L. E. (1997). Determining the therapeutic relationship of choice in brief therapy. In J. N. Butcher (Ed.), *Objective psychological assessment in managed health care: A practitioner's guide* (pp. 42–60). Oxford University Press.

Norcross, J. C., & Goldfried, M. R. (Eds.). (2019). *Handbook of psychotherapy integration* (3rd ed.). Oxford University Press. https://doi.org/10.1093/med-psych/9780190690465.001.0001

Norcross, J. C., Krebs, P. M., & Prochaska, J. O. (2011). Stages of change. In J. C. Norcross (Ed.), *Psychotherapy relationships that work: Evidence-based responsiveness* (2nd ed., pp. 296–328). Oxford University Press. https://doi.org/10.1093/acprof:oso/9780199737208.003.0014

Norcross, J. C., & Lambert, M. J. (Eds.). (2019). *Psychotherapy relationships that work: Volume 1. Evidence-based therapist contributions* (3rd ed.). Oxford University Press.

Norcross, J. C., & Popple, L. M. (2017). *Supervision essentials for integrative psychotherapy*. American Psychological Association. https://doi.org/10.1037/15967-000

Norcross, J. C., & Wampold, B. E. (Eds.). (2019). *Psychotherapy relationships that work: Vol. 2. Evidence-based responsiveness* (3rd ed.). Oxford University Press.

Ockene, J., Kristeller, J. L., Goldberg, R., Ockene, I., Merriam, P., Barrett, S., Pekow, P., Hosmer, D., & Gianelly, R. (1992). Smoking cessation and severity of disease: The Coronary Artery Smoking Intervention Study. *Health Psychology, 11*(2), 119–126. https://doi.org/10.1037/0278-6133.11.2.119

Pantalon, M. V., Nich, C., Frankforter, T., Carroll, K. M., & the University of Rhode Island Change Assessment. (2002). The URICA as a measure of motivation to change among treatment-seeking individuals with concurrent alcohol and cocaine problems. *Psychology of Addictive Behaviors, 16*(4), 299–307. https://doi.org/10.1037/0893-164X.16.4.299

Petry, N. M. (2005). Stages of change in treatment-seeking pathological gamblers. *Journal of Consulting and Clinical Psychology, 73*(2), 312–322. https://doi.org/10.1037/0022-006X.73.2.312

Prochaska, J. O. (1979). *Systems of psychotherapy: A transtheoretical analysis*. Dorsey.

Prochaska, J. O., & DiClemente, C. C. (1982). Transtheoretical therapy: Toward a more integrative model of change. *Psychotherapy: Theory, Research, & Practice, 19*(3), 276–288. https://doi.org/10.1037/h0088437

Prochaska, J. O., DiClemente, C. C., & Norcross, J. C. (1992). In search of how people change. Applications to addictive behaviors. *American Psychologist, 47*(9), 1102–1114. https://doi.org/10.1037/0003-066X.47.9.1102

Prochaska, J. O., Evers, K. E., Castle, P. H., Johnson, J. L., Prochaska, J. M., Rula, E. Y., Coberley, C., & Pope, J. E. (2012). Enhancing multiple domains of well-being by decreasing multiple health risk behaviors: A randomized clinical trial. *Population Health Management, 15*(5), 276–286. https://doi.org/10.1089/pop.2011.0060

Prochaska, J. O., & Norcross, J. (2018). *Systems of psychotherapy: A transtheoretical analysis* (9th ed.). Oxford University Press.

Prochaska, J. O., Norcross, J. C., & DiClemente, C. C. (1995). *Changing for good*. HarperCollins.

Prochaska, J. O., Norcross, J. C., & DiClemente, C. C. (2013). Applying the stages of change. In G. P. Koocher, J. C. Norcross, & B. A. Greene (Eds.), *Psychologists' desk reference* (3rd ed., pp. 176–181). Oxford University Press. https://doi.org/10.1093/med:psych/9780199845491.003.0034

Prochaska, J. O., Norcross, J. C., & Saul, S. F. (2020). Generating psychotherapy breakthroughs: Transtheoretical strategies from population health psychology. *American Psychologist, 75*(7), 996–1010. https://doi.org/10.1037/amp0000568

Prochaska, J. O., & Prochaska, J. M. (2016). *Changing to thrive*. Hazelden.

Rosen, C. S. (2000). Is the sequencing of change processes by stage consistent across health problems? A meta-analysis. *Health Psychology, 19*(6), 593–604. https://doi.org/10.1037/0278-6133.19.6.593

Rossi, J. S. (2002). *Comparison of the use of significance testing and effect sizes in theory-based health promotion research* [Paper presentation]. Society for Multivariate Experimental Psychology 43rd Annual Meeting, Charlottesville, VA, United States.

Satterfield, W. A., Buelow, S. A., Lyddon, W. J., & Johnson, J. T. (1995). Client stages of change and expectations about counselling. *Journal of Counseling Psychology, 42*(4), 476–478. https://doi.org/10.1037/0022-0167.42.4.476

Smith, K. J., Subich, L. M., & Kalodner, C. (1995). The Transtheoretical Model's stages and processes of change and their relation to premature termination. *Journal of Counseling Psychology, 42*(1), 34–39. https://doi.org/10.1037/0022-0167.42.1.34

Swift, J. K., & Greenberg, R. P. (2012). Premature discontinuation in adult psychotherapy: A meta-analysis. *Journal of Consulting and Clinical Psychology, 80*(4), 547–559. https://doi.org/10.1037/a0028226

Velicer, W. F., Hughes, S. L., Fava, J. L., Prochaska, J. O., & DiClemente, C. C. (1995). An empirical typology of subjects within stage of change. *Addictive Behaviors, 20*(3), 299–320. https://doi.org/10.1016/0306-4603(94)00069-B

Wampold, B. E., & Imel, Z. E. (2015). *The great psychotherapy debate: The evidence for what makes psychotherapy work* (2nd ed.). Routledge. https://doi.org/10.4324/9780203582015

Zhang, A. Y., Harmon, J. A., Werkner, J., & McCormick, R. A. (2004). Impacts of motivation for change on the severity of alcohol use by patients with severe and persistent mental illness. *Journal of Studies on Alcohol, 65*(3), 392–397. https://doi.org/10.15288/jsa.2004.65.392

4

Therapist and Client Facilitative Interpersonal Skills in Psychotherapy

Timothy Anderson and Matthew R. Perlman

Both therapist and client interpersonal skills play important roles in psychotherapy. Therapist skills have been widely studied and recognized as core competencies for therapists (e.g., Castonguay & Hill, 2017); however, clients also bring individual relational skills into therapy that play significant roles in the course and outcome of treatment. For example, a client who is verbal, psychologically minded, and insightful may have a head start in treatment because those interpersonal skills aid many tasks in psychotherapy. The client's preexisting set of interpersonal skills and traits can even influence the therapist's expression of interpersonal skills and aid in unlocking effective therapist skills. By understanding and utilizing the client's interpersonal talents, the therapist can synergistically enhance their interpersonal skills and these interactive processes can yield benefits throughout treatment.

We begin this chapter by describing aspects of a traditional approach to studying interpersonal dynamics in therapy, focusing on therapist input (i.e., interpersonal skills) and client output (i.e., reactions). Understanding the client's skill development thus involves an appreciation for how therapist interpersonal skills are implicated in the client's improvement in interpersonal skills. Although we begin with a focus on the unique role of therapists' skills, we also continually ask, "How is the client contributing?" We build on this question by highlighting unique, client-directed interpersonal skills that are strengths, and we showcase individual differences in how clients respond to different therapists' interpersonal skills and therapeutic situations. Client interpersonal skills might

https://doi.org/10.1037/0000303-005
The Other Side of Psychotherapy: Understanding Clients' Experiences and Contributions in Treatment, J. N. Fuertes (Editor)

even aid therapists in overcoming treatment obstacles and thus are a possible catalyst to the effectiveness of therapist interpersonal skills. This chapter concludes by considering interpersonal skills bidirectionally, accounting for the input and interplay of both therapist and client interpersonal skills, each having important independent influences that add to more than the sum of their parts.

THERAPIST FACILITATIVE INTERPERSONAL SKILLS AND CLIENT REACTIONS

Clients are acutely aware of the interpersonal attributes that therapists bring into the room, such as warmth, hopefulness, and a general ability to be involved with the client. These characteristics have long been recognized in practice settings and have also been a focus of research on therapist effects (Castonguay & Hill, 2017). *Therapist effects* refers to findings that individual psychotherapists differ from each other in client outcomes, prompting a search to identify the therapist characteristics that account for these outcomes (Baldwin & Imel, 2013; Wampold & Imel, 2015). Researchers have identified interpersonal skills and characteristics of therapists that are independent from their interactions with clients; regardless of therapists' skills, the interactive processes are also shaped by clients' contributions. Even so, therapists' interpersonal skills and characteristics have proven to be important factors in treatment (Anderson et al., 2009). Heinonen et al. (2014) found that self-reported therapist basic interpersonal relational styles, particularly engaged relational styles, were predictive of client-rated alliances. Heinonen et al. used ratings on a measure of therapist skill that were collected before treatment, and they assessed skill independence from any effects of client interactions during therapy. Schöttke et al. (2017) measured therapists' interpersonal characteristics through a group format as well as with expert interviews. They found that group ratings of positive therapist interpersonal dispositions were predictive of client outcomes, above and beyond techniques used, over the 5-year period after the therapist assessments.

The influence of therapists' interpersonal characteristics on clients has been studied with research methods designed to isolate the therapist's performance from interactions with a client. The Facilitative Interpersonal Skills (FIS) task (Anderson et al., 2009) is performance based and rates therapists' responses to brief, challenging client situations (see Table 4.1). The FIS approach comprises a collection of therapist skills, including common facilitative conditions first recognized by Rogers (1957), such as warmth, acceptance, understanding, and empathy. The FIS also includes the therapist's individual skill-based contributions to the therapeutic alliance and being responsive to clients' interpersonal problems. Facilitative interpersonal skills include persuasiveness and hopefulness, which are common across most treatment approaches and also indicate therapists' vocal expressiveness. These particular characteristics of therapist facilitative interpersonal skills are central to our approach, and we consider them in depth next and later in relation to client skills and characteristics.

TABLE 4.1. Therapist Facilitative Interpersonal Skills and Associated Client Skills

Skill set	Therapist facilitative interpersonal skills	Client skills activated and/or developed in therapy
Voice skills	*Verbal fluency*: vocal cadence and good tonality that engages the listener. Vocal expression that "approaches" the listener with a coherent interpersonal message that is responsive to the situation and may result in calming and reassuring the listener.	Develops from the therapist a model and practice of verbal communication skills
		Discovers identity, speaking in their own "voice"
		Gains an internalized therapist voice (or other important person)
	Emotional expression: vocal energy of the therapist's speaking voice that can be heard in the pace, frequency, and amplitude of verbal expression. Emotional expression is sometimes described as animated, especially for emphasizing emotional experiences. In contrast, speech that is flat and monotone is often lacking emotional expression. The therapist includes language that accesses emotion, feelings, and the emotional effect of topics on the client.	Gains increased emotional awareness and expression
		Learns to verbalize emotional expression with more depth and range
		Synchronizes vocal expressions to match emotional vocabulary and intensity
		Discerns emotive expressions with specific emotions (guilt vs. anger)
		Develops tolerance and trust in expressing emotions
		Learns to separate emotion from cognition
		Learns to express positive emotions (e.g., care, love)
Encouragement skills	*Hope and positive expectations*: the ability to facilitate client beliefs of hopefulness is core to client engagement. The interpersonal skills needed for hope involve (a) encouraging personal agency within the client and (b) helping to build the pathways for reaching goals. Hope focuses on building client agency for actions that will facilitate meeting the client's goals (and less on building a plausible explanation).	Increases hope and optimism in the future
		Participates in therapeutic work (and alliance)
		Sparks and enhances client resilience and hardiness
		Offers new (corrective) experience and insight into understanding problem
		Gains assertiveness to contribute their own insights to the therapist's contributions
		Builds confidence in expressing wishes and desires

(continues)

TABLE 4.1. Therapist Facilitative Interpersonal Skills and Associated Client Skills (*Continued*)

Skill set	Therapist facilitative interpersonal skills	Client skills activated and/or developed in therapy
	Persuasiveness: a core common characteristic of most psychotherapeutic work, persuasion involves the ability to provide a clear, organized understanding about the meaning of a client's distress. This skill involves an ability to conceptualize an understanding that might include a rationale and explanation for the problem. Effective persuasion can be subtle too, but it has to be plausible to the client. Persuasion is based on providing a plausible explanation (and not necessarily positive expectations, which is hope).	Develops agency and self-advocacy skills Learns to work with people in a more planful and strategic manner; can think in terms of immediate, short-term, and longer term goals
Emotion skills	*Warmth, acceptance, and understanding*: the therapist's ability to care for and appreciate the other and their situation without blame. Openness, high regard for, and noncritical awareness of the client are involved. Indications of weaker skill include a judgmental attitude, condescension, rudeness, disapproval, guilt induction, exasperation, or annoyance. The nonspecific expressions are mostly independent from what the therapist is doing (e.g., giving advice) but more about how the therapist is appreciating the client. *Empathy*: an awareness and expression of the subjective experiences of the client (i.e., thoughts and emotions). Included is some ability to accurately identify these experiences.	Expands experiential awareness Increases interest in experiences of self and others Gains greater self-acceptance, and acceptance of others Decreases self-criticism and increases self-forgiveness Increases internal awareness (see emotional expression) Expands mindfulness capacity and habits Expands capacity for empathy for self and others Increases compassion for self and other

TABLE 4.1. Therapist Facilitative Interpersonal Skills and Associated Client Skills (Continued)

Skill set	Therapist facilitative interpersonal skills	Client skills activated and/or developed in therapy
Alliance skills	*Alliance bond capacity*: the therapist's skill or capacity to engage in a collaborative environment. The therapist may invite the client to work jointly on problems. This may come in the form of direct and overt requests for shared effort with the client or may be apparent through subtler gestures for mutual work with the client. *Alliance rupture repair and responsiveness*: the therapist's ability to be responsive to the unique interpersonal issues, unique expressions, and changing context of the client. Sometimes the client makes direct requests, or there is clear tension in the relationship, implying a more obvious focus for responsiveness. At other times there are subtler but more meaningful shifts in the therapy context, or clients may be less engaged, which also implies a different responsiveness.	Experiences direct support in relationship with therapist Activates or develops more secure attachments Develops capacity for cooperation and collaboration as an interpersonal ability Gains in disposition to trust others Learns self-assessment, self-monitoring Expands interpersonal problem-solving ability Initiates or expands relationship-seeking and building outside of therapy Develops a capacity to deal with conflict and tension in a more direct and healthy manner Uses less withdrawal and less provocative confrontation to address needs, issues, and conflicts with self, therapist, and others Learns to move past differences, forgive, and understand without necessarily accepting Learns and develops the value and ability to compromise Learns to set and maintain boundaries in a flexible and adaptive manner

The FIS approach is used, in part, to isolate the independent contributions of therapists' skills from their clients and the therapy setting. The reason for separating therapist facilitative interpersonal skills is to better understand what the therapist uniquely contributes to their client's outcome. Studies have shown that the FIS task significantly predicts therapist effects. For example, in a sample of 25 therapists and 1,141 clients, the FIS predicted the extent to which the individual therapists were contributing to their clients' outcomes (Anderson et al., 2009). In a prospective design, higher FIS ratings of therapists on the performance task were associated with predicted decreases in client symptoms across sessions (Anderson, McClintock, et al., 2016). A third outcome study (Anderson, Crowley, et al., 2016) used a randomized controlled trial design in which therapists were selected and assigned to roughly equal-sized independent groups based on interpersonal skill (weak vs. strong) and training status (trained vs. untrained). Therapists with strong interpersonal skills had better alliances and client outcomes compared with therapists with weaker interpersonal skills. Furthermore, the effect of therapists' interpersonal skill occurred regardless of their training status. In fact, some therapists who did not have formal training but had strong interpersonal skills even displayed equal levels of good experiential and narrative processes (Anderson et al., 2021). Clients did not seem to be aware of, or clinically respond to, therapist training status, although it is likely that trained doctoral clinicians were utilizing evidence-based psychotherapeutic interventions and research-supported language to describe psychopathology and the clinical process. Clients typically do not have the same training or educational background as their therapists; however, they do have a similar understanding of the importance of a personal connection. Clinicians who can tap into this shared, human experience of interpersonal relating seem more likely to find pathways that ultimately lead to client improvement or healing. In summary, evidence from several different laboratories and from investigators using a variety of methods implicates therapist interpersonal skills, above and beyond technique, as an active agent in client change over the course of therapy. Therapist interpersonal skills are vital in effective therapy in that clients notice and respond positively to therapists' skills.

We now describe how specific therapist interpersonal skills are used to influence the client. Clients may react to each of these skills in different ways, and it is helpful to understand these differential reactions. Although a discussion of separate therapist skills is conceptually useful, we recognize that there are other conceptual schemes and theories for organizing and understanding therapeutic interpersonal skills. However, the FIS construct has been well researched and empirically supported by research studies from different investigators who examined conceptually similar therapist characteristics, such as facilitative interpersonal skills (e.g., empathy, warmth, management of criticism, cooperation), using different methods but finding similar results on therapist effectiveness (e.g., Schöttke et al., 2017). Thus, we use the therapist FIS framework here but recognize the important contributions of other researchers, not to mention the myriad findings on similar therapeutic processes that consistently have been shown to predict therapy outcomes (Norcross & Lambert, 2019).

We begin with a description of how each therapist's facilitative interpersonal skills are expressed, the purported effects on clients, and the synergetic influence of activating significant relational processes. Table 4.1 provides a summary of how therapist interpersonal skills correspond to client interpersonal skills. To make more broad-based statements about relationships between therapist skills and client reactions, we have organized the eight therapist facilitative interpersonal skills into four interrelated skill clusters: (a) *voice skills* comprise verbal fluency and emotional expression, (b) *convincing skills* comprise hope and persuasion, (c) *emotion skills* comprise warmth (encompassing warmth, acceptance, and understanding) and empathy, and (d) *alliance skills* comprise alliance bond capacity (ABC) and alliance rupture repair and responsiveness. Furthermore, grouping the skills into clusters provides a translatable way to link FIS concepts to the extant literature and to identify empirical trends in how client interpersonal skills and characteristics are implicated.

Voice Skills: Verbal Fluency and Emotional Expression

A therapist's voice may aesthetically resonate with the client, and the tones of their voice can even be compared to the singing of a therapeutic "song." The therapist's FIS approach to voice focuses on the skills of verbal fluency and emotional expression, which we generically group together as "voice skills." Voice skills are based on the foundational work of Rice and Kerr's (1986) model of therapeutic voice. Rice and Kerr identified four therapist vocal patterns that provided insight into aspects of the therapy process and interaction: focused, externalizing, emotional, and limited. An optimal voice in therapy conveys *focus*, which conveys that a speaker is attentive to internal affective experience. Poor vocal engagement (e.g., limited speech, timidity) may indicate that the speaker has difficulty accessing their inner experience through *limited* or constricted vocal expressions and withdrawn vocal energy. However, more emotional expression is not necessarily better, because an *overly emotional voice* results when emotional overflow disrupts or distorts attempts to access experiences. Finally, a voice that is *external* has an outward attention and may involve a rehearsed, disingenuous, or premonitored quality. As Rice and Kerr described, patterns of a therapist's vocal quality can skillfully match specific therapeutic tasks and goals, which might include a *softened voice* to create intimacy and focused client exploration, whereas a *definitive voice* may aid in expressing some specific interventions, tasks, and persuasiveness (although this approach has a risk of the client potentially experiencing it as overbearing). Findings from Tomicic et al. (2015) were consistent with this form of the therapeutic use of voice as an *affirmative* voice that may express committed speech and confidence as well as the use of full pauses that may serve to punctuate meanings and direct the rhythm of conversation.

Voice ratings within facilitative interpersonal skills focus on particularly challenging moments that spotlight the *interpersonal problems* conveyed within a voice. Clients expressing distressing emotions with an interpersonal target have unique uses of voice. In challenging client moments used in FIS stimulus videos (Anderson et al., 2020), clients conveyed various vocal disruptions that included extreme inhibition (e.g., Bethany, a client who was stuck and had problems talking), situation inhibition (e.g., Sean, a client who was not able to find a job), and emotional overflow (e.g., Suzie, an exasperated client who loudly proclaimed that nothing was working in therapy).[1] In each FIS situation, the interpersonal use of voice is highlighted because each situation involves a client vocally expressing and targeting the therapist with their interpersonal request.

---

[1]The identities of the individuals in this chapter's case examples have been properly disguised to protect client confidentiality.

Thus, a client who is angry at a therapist conveys a unique interpersonal vocal expression because that message is interpersonal and targets the other person in the room.

The therapist's skillful use of voice is essential in (a) demonstrating to the client that they have an adequate and appropriate understanding of the client's internal world and (b) enhancing the use of other vital skills in resolving the client's concern. In the earlier example, a therapist with strong facilitative interpersonal skills would be wise to not overwhelm Bethany with an overly emotional voice or dominate the interpersonal space with an overbearing response. By providing a calm and reassuring vocal tone, however, the therapist can vocally express an interest in helping overcome the barriers that prevented Bethany from being able to talk in the session. Through the appropriate expression of their voice, therapists convey beyond words ways that help clients identify and modify their own disruptions in experiential awareness and expressiveness, thus enhancing future communication. The therapist's ameliorative voice plays an essential role in the opening phases of therapy in which many levels of therapist exploratory skills are needed to help clients unlock thoughts and feelings that may be difficult for them to access or express clearly (Hill, 2019). Furthermore, in all examples from the FIS task, the client voice conveys an *interpersonal disruption* because it communicates information and meanings that are directed to the therapist and includes attitudes about the therapeutic relationship. When therapists coordinate their use of voice to match subtle client verbal experiences, clients are provided the maximum opportunity for expressing their experiences through their own voice.

The benefits of a therapist's voice in promoting client participation and expression are realized when the client's vocal skills are enhanced too, ideally leading to the harmonizing and cocreative cadences of client and therapist voices. As described by Tomicic et al. (2015), the productive expression of therapist and client voices is obvious to the listener and is "perceived as capable of transmitting its potential for innovation and transformation due to its aural quality" (p. 11). This vocal transformation is more likely to occur and have a lasting impact on the client when the therapist's voice is emotionally expressive. Kim et al. (2019) exposed participants to brief 1-minute sounds of voices with varying levels of emotional expressiveness and found that voices that were emotionally expressive were more likely to be remembered 1 week later. Thus, even a brief 1-minute exposure to novel voices can result in long-term memory and acquired familiarization when the new voice is emotionally expressive. Knox et al. (1999) found that clients acquire memories for their therapist's voice and increasingly rely on this as part of an internal representation for their therapist (including visual and felt sense memories). Such internal representations of the therapist were used by clients to create a sense of comfort outside of sessions and increased through therapy.

As the therapist's voice is increasingly remembered and relied on for comfort (Knox et al., 1999), clients can gain access to similar aspects of their psychological selves in which many client problematic experiences reside (e.g., cognitive beliefs, maladaptive emotion schemes). Mosher and Stiles (2009) described the process of therapeutic change as including the entry of the therapist's "voice" into conversation with the client's preexisting collection of multiple other voices and signs that sustain their problematic experiences. Clients can change when the new representation of voices, including the therapist's, facilitates the assimilation of problematic experiences.

Convincing Skills: Hope and Persuasion

Psychotherapy has been conceptualized as a process of interpersonal persuasion (Beutler, 1979), so the therapist's skill in convincing clients to strive for change may be central to treatment success. Therapists' interpersonal skills in building hope are linked to the client's parallel experiences of feeling hopeful and trait hopefulness. In fact, Fuertes and Williams (2017) indicated that client hope was one of the major client characteristics most promising for future research, so it is especially important to consider the link between the therapist's skills and client hope. Clients who feel hopeful and engaged in therapeutic work seem more likely to gain outlook as an interpersonal skill when repeatedly encouraged by a therapist with the facilitative interpersonal skills of hope and persuasion.

There are considerable obstacles in defining hope. Hope sometimes seems like other abstract concepts, like courage, truth, or faith, and thus is difficult to define or think about as a skill. Yet the fact that therapists are so highly engaged in building and maintaining client hope suggests that hope is a skill that can be learned and practiced. Snyder (2002) identified hope as including two components: (a) a feeling of positivity and optimism in the future as well as (b) identified pathways by which optimism can be achieved—a course of action that can be taken in order to achieve one's desired goals. Therapists who can effectively express these two components of hope with clients are modeling and facilitating clients in acquiring these skills and inviting collaborative discussions about creating the pathways, which is itself definitional to hope.

Research findings on therapist effects lend support to hope being a core feature of effective therapists. Therapists who have demonstrated more improved outcomes (i.e., relative to other therapists) tend to exhibit more personal resilience compared with therapists who are less effective (Pereira et al., 2017). Client interactions with therapists who are likely to be resilient and effective in conveying hope are likely corrective experiences themselves and antidotes to hopelessness. We return to considering the unique aspects of client hope and resilience in the next section.

Part of therapists' skill of hope is linked to their persuasive abilities to enhance client expectations and to spark hope within clients. This therapist skill often involves multiple facilitative interpersonal skills, including skillful listening, understanding, and empathizing with clients. A therapist's ability to talk with clients about hopelessness, ironically, can be an encouraging sign. Building hope is integrated within most forms of treatments too, and this is also why the therapist skill of persuasion is essential for building hope. For example, in emotion-focused therapy (Greenberg, 2017), hopelessness and sickness are one fundamental pole of therapeutic work; this pole is necessary because it also defines the opposite pole, which often involves hope, growth, and health. For the treatment to be successful, therapists must persuasively engage the client in the search for the other pole of the treatment dialectic, which often involves the discovery of experiencer-voiced hopefulness.

Case Example of Therapist Facilitative Interpersonal Skills and Client Reactions

Nancy, a 63-year-old retired clerk, is an example of a client experiencing therapist vocal expression, hope, and persuasion and responding in kind. At the beginning of therapy, Nancy demonstrated little emotional expression and mostly a sense of despair and hopelessness. She was aware that her restricted, anxious sense of her experience was partly the result of having experienced militaristic and hostile parenting during childhood, which had left an ominous mark even though Nancy had little contact with her family since breaking off relations after she completed high school. Although Nancy initially spoke with little emotion, she appeared insightful about her lifelong resentment, and she was certain that this chapter in her life was resolved. The therapist facilitated Nancy in identifying her emotions by commenting on nuanced behaviors and other subtle indicators, but the therapist's search for this missing emotional expression became a guessing game. The therapist frequently guessed that the client "must have" felt angry and frustrated, and yet the client seemed confused, reacting as one might when attempting to discern the intent of a speaker of a foreign language. For example, the therapist had noticed that Nancy had been twitching her leg while talking about her father. In contrast with the client, the therapist became highly energized with emotional expression at this moment and shared her own fantasy that her leg movements reminded her of wanting to angrily kick the person she was speaking about. Later in the session, the client cognitively tried to identify with the therapist's construction by adding, "I never put that together. High price to pay for getting to kick him. But I guess I had to find a way to kick him somehow or other." This simple facilitative interpersonal skill of persuasion with exaggerated emotional expression seemed a bit forced and artificial, but Nancy independently returned to the moment in several future sessions. The success of this moment apparently was not an accurate empathy of emotion, since the client continued to insist that she was not expressing anger. Still, the therapist's vocal expressions, emotional involvement, and attempts at persuasion mattered more. The client referred to the kicking metaphor during a later session:

> You had mentioned that I was kicking. . . . You could have let it go by, but you pointed it out to me. You could have known it as a therapist yourself, but you told it to me, and I was able to try it on for myself.

For Nancy, the expression and involvement mattered much more than the accuracy of her therapist's persuasive interpretations.

Emotion Skills: Warmth and Empathy

Both therapist empathy and warmth have been emphasized from the beginning of psychotherapy practice and training and are recognized as core competencies in therapist training. While the central role of therapist warmth and empathy are recognized as independent skills, it is the client experience of warmth and empathy that ultimately matters. For example, client ratings of empathy are more relevant to whether the client improves during therapy than to the therapist's perceptions of empathy (Elliott et al., 2019). Traditional models of empathy (e.g., Barrett-Lennard, 1981) locate the beginning of the empathic skill as residing within the therapist. However, clients also exhibit skills in warmth and empathy that provide an independent contribution to therapy processes and outcomes. Warmth and empathy are highly interactive variables in practice; thus, separating therapist and client skills is particularly challenging. As Elliott et al. (2019) noted, part of the interpersonal expression of empathy is beyond the skillful expression to a specific client response—but at a metarelational level, the therapist must recognize the client's needs for manifest reflections of their experience from the therapist. As described by Orlinsky et al. (2004), empathy extends beyond the mere expression of therapist and client individual skills and involves a mutual communicative attunement within the relationship.

Recognizing these differences in client needs for warmth and empathy involves other interpersonal skills, particularly in the therapist's ability to be responsive (Stiles et al., 1998) and to be sensitive to and accommodate the client's defensiveness or rupture in response to expressions of empathy and warmth. Thus, interpersonally skilled therapists respond by fitting their empathic expression to the client's unique interpersonal skills and characteristics. Interpersonally skilled therapists understand their client's needs in order to modulate the amount and quality of empathy needed to maximize the therapeutic impact. For example, although all clients may require some level of therapist empathy, clients who are prone to externalize, to be distrustful, or to be highly reactant are less likely to benefit from high levels of therapist empathic expression, regardless of how skillful the expression is (Beutler & Consoli, 1993). There are other interpersonal differences among clients in how therapist empathy is received. Some clients may experience empathy as it has been traditionally described in more emotional terms, whereas other clients may resonate with more cognitive and problem-solving communications from their therapists (MacFarlane et al., 2017).

It may not be surprising that therapists are more capable of being warm with clients who are perceived by others as more likable. As Farber et al. (2019) noted, clients who are themselves "warm, empathic, and disclosing, are more easily liked and likely elicit more affirmation than others" (p. 311), whereas clients who express negative and disaffiliative characteristics present a more difficult challenge for therapists. Because it is generally more difficult to remain warm with interpersonally cold and hostile clients, a high number of these interpersonally thorny situations within client situation videos are used to measure facilitative interpersonal skills (Anderson et al., 2020). It is difficult for therapists to summon skillful expressions of warmth, acceptance, and understanding when clients are detached or not very friendly. Not surprisingly, clients who express a desire to be valued and prized by their therapist are more likely to draw out their therapists' skillful expressions of positive regard toward them (Farber et al., 2019). Similarly, clients who are more disclosive and open about their experiences make it easier for therapists to express the skills of empathic expression (Elliott et al., 2019).

In terms of practice, the previous case of Nancy also illustrated the facilitative interpersonal skills of warmth, acceptance, and understanding. As Nancy continued in therapy, she gained confidence in expressing how much she felt valued by the therapist and how important it was for her to feel valued for her emotional struggle. At one point, Nancy became tearful in response to hearing the therapist express how much she valued her. Nancy, filled with tears, opened up to express how meaningful the therapist's acceptance had been:

> To hear you say that I've done magnificently. You see, you're a very important person in my life. . . . But to hear a person, to hear you, say that I've done magnificently. . . . That sounded fantastic. . . . My God, I didn't know anyone would think that about me. It's almost more acceptance than I can stand.

Alliance Skills: ABC and Alliance Rupture Repair and Responsiveness

The working alliance is a dyadic process variable, including the unique synergy of reactions that takes place when two or more people interact. The nature of that reaction depends on each person in the relationship. Therapists who have a capacity to form cooperative bonds with others will bring that property into their therapeutic alliances too. Therapists who skillfully express ABC can encourage clients to reciprocate in trustful, cooperative therapeutic work. Therapists' ABC and their warmth, acceptance, and understanding are similar skills, which likely form a common factor that also includes therapist expressions of openness and experiential awareness (Kolden, 1996). However, clients also bring their own alliance skills into therapy. Clients bring a capacity to bond with their therapists, to make up with them when ruptures occur, and to be responsive to them. ABC may itself be one aspect of a strong therapeutic attachment relationship in which a client's attachment system is activated to seek proximity and safety within a functioning therapeutic relationship. The skillful use of ABC was described by Mallinckrodt (2010), who suggested a model for how therapists might somewhat strategically regulate the bond by activating client attachments or deactivating them through therapeutic distance (see Chapter 5, this volume).

However, a therapist's skills in ABC are some of the most relationally interactive of all therapist facilitative interpersonal skills, which implies that the client's response is particularly important. Regardless of how strong a therapist's ABC skills might be, it is impossible to engage in a collaborative relationship with a client who is not collaborative and relationally capable (Fuertes & Williams, 2017). Client capacities, then, are important to understand in order to maximize the effectiveness of the therapist's ABC skills. The client's interpersonal skill, which is often apparent through preexisting attachment styles, is an especially important aspect of how therapists regulate ABC and warmth. Considering the client's interpersonal characteristics is thus a necessary component of therapists' ABC because some clients may have, at least initially, aversive reactions to friendly and affiliative offers of support (e.g., Benjamin, 2018; Horowitz, 2004). In other words, a skillful therapist is *responsive* to the client's attachment style and also to the full context of the treatment, other client characteristics, and the unique aspects of the situation. The ability to modulate ABC, as well as most any other therapeutic skill, is worth noting as a separate skill, referred to as *therapist responsiveness* (Stiles et al., 1998). Therapist ABC is not "one size fits all." Clearly, the ability to address stress points, resistances, and repair ruptures is itself a skill (Muran & Eubanks, 2020), requiring therapist responsiveness to identify and address the natural consequences of fluctuations in collaborative therapeutic work.

Client interpersonal characteristics play a significant role in a client's ability to form a working alliance with their therapist and, by implication, this likely suggests some responsiveness (or lack thereof) to therapists' expression of ABC and warmth. Clients who have a pretherapy history of support from others, such as through parental care, are more likely to form positive working alliances with therapists (e.g., Hersoug et al., 2009). Client interpersonal characteristics also can make it more challenging to form an alliance, especially with clients who are socially avoidant, cold, or detached (Hersoug et al., 2009). Meta-analytic evidence implicates client attachment style in outcomes more generally (Levy et al., 2018) and that clients with an insecure attachment style, more specifically, are less successful in forming therapeutic alliances (Bernecker et al., 2014). One possibility is that clients with insecure attachments are less interpersonally capable of making use of therapists' ABC skills.

General conclusions about the role of client skills in response to therapist-offered skills are not possible at this point because of the lack of controlled studies. However, available evidence on these variables seems to suggest that clients who have fewer social supports, disaffiliative interpersonal characteristics, and insecure attachment styles will have challenges in receiving their therapists' offering of warmth and ABC. It also seems likely that the role of client skills in working with therapist ABC may be complicated by context and the interaction of these variables. For example, Coyne et al. (2018) found that clients with avoidant attachments do not benefit from having relatively higher levels of social support and satisfactory relationships, at least in terms of the development of the therapeutic alliance. Interestingly, high levels of social support, which would normally facilitate the alliance and therapeutic engagement, tend to negatively influence the alliance for these avoidant clients (Coyne et al., 2018). Thus, therapists may expect a positive alliance based on the client's satisfactory external relationships, and therapists may struggle with their own reactions when they unexpectedly find themselves struggling to form an alliance with a client who has satisfactory attachments but avoids new relationships (including with the therapist). Therapists with weaker alliance and responsiveness skills may be more easily enticed into blaming the client or fixating on their social avoidance instead of becoming attuned to interpersonal opportunities to solve the dilemma. Therapist responsiveness to these complications of context is also implicated in a study by Errázuriz and Zilcha-Mano (2018), who found that the nature of feedback tended to exacerbate increased symptomatic change (i.e., high symptom feedback made things worse in the future). Overall, therapists who provide generic warmth and ABC may be helpful, but they may have significant limitations too, mostly because these therapists' unwavering positivity may not be skillfully responsive to some clients' unique interpersonal styles and needs (especially clients who might be negatively reactive to strong displays of warmth).

The complexity of maintaining an alliance bond involves a separate but related skill of remaining responsive to shifts in interpersonal tensions and being skillful in repairing alliance ruptures. Client and therapist skills both likely play a central role in the process of resolving alliance ruptures (known as rupture repair). While significant research shows that repairing alliance ruptures results in enhanced therapeutic outcomes (Eubanks et al., 2018), the impact of therapist responsiveness and rupture-repair skills on clients is mostly unclear at this time. Recent studies show that in-session processes, especially changes in the working alliance and implementation of common factor techniques (e.g., appropriate responsiveness to general attachment patterns), predict the successful resolution of ruptures (Ben David-Sela et al., 2021). One possibility is that therapist rupture-repair skills affect multiple relational client characteristics and may also depend on external supports, client interpersonal styles, and the cultural context in which therapy takes place. More research is needed in this important area.

Case Example of Empathy and Alliance Interpersonal Skills

The role of empathy and alliance interpersonal skills is present throughout the case of Janice. Janice presented to therapy after experiencing repeated interpersonal frustration in her marriage to a more reserved, less emotionally attuned partner. The voice skills mentioned earlier were already especially strong and powerful. As a professor of humanities, Janice was amazingly verbally expressive; as a near-constant performer in the lecture hall, she could overwhelm her therapist with dramatic and enticingly interesting narratives from her personal life. Janice was also quite persuasive, so she was open to appeals to persuasive logic from her therapist. However, what was painfully missing was emotional connection and trust that others could meet her strong needs for attachment. Janice had seemed to place nearly insatiable demands for emotional fealty on her partner, but she was not very prepared to maintain a secure and emotional presence. It was also relevant that Janice had a childhood history of emotional deprivation and trauma from caregivers, which she was intellectually aware of as influencing her marriage. The need for alliance as well as warmth, acceptance, and understanding always seemed to be part of the therapeutic interpersonal relationship. While she was able to provide generally adequate empathy and warmth, Janice would often respond with a mountain of facts and information, even in response to basic emotional reflections. Janice, while appreciative of receiving compassion and concern from her therapist, often felt like she had to lead in-depth, emotionally focused conversations in session. This played into a major enactment in Janice's life in which she, despite her exceptional insight and ability to articulate, found herself yet again unable to connect with a close other (her therapist) on the level she craved. Janice's interpersonal issues seemed influenced by her prior experiences (many of them traumatic) in which she needed to use a keen intellect and strong communication skills to receive attention from suboptimal caregivers. This pattern, which in many ways was adaptive in early life, was heavily reinforced and only became maladaptive in Janice's marriage to a partner who became quickly overwhelmed by her interpersonal approach. The pattern continued in the therapeutic relationship when the client's difficulties in extending and deepening skills in warmth and empathy appeared limited by logical explanations for how others fell short of her trust.

Integrating Therapist and Client Interpersonal Skills

Therapists vary in their interpersonal skill sets. Much like their clients, therapists possess unique combinations of different skills. Although individual therapists have relative strengths and weaknesses in their skills, the overall correlation of these skills is high; therefore, it is more helpful to think of how combinations of these therapist skills work together. In fact, the ability to synchronize sets of skills may itself involve interpersonal skills in self-awareness, metacognition, and responsiveness (Stiles & Horvath, 2017).

To illustrate the importance of integrating the variety of therapist interpersonal skills, a simple case of unresolved trauma is used with different hypothetical options in order to show how multiple facilitative interpersonal skills are separate but often integrated. The client experienced long-standing posttraumatic stress disorder and presented to therapy with an emotive but ironically disengaged interpersonal style. The client focused on external events and storytelling with self-negating attributions. A therapist who is effective with cognitive behavior therapy might be successful in beginning to identify some of this client's negative self-attributions, enhanced by the facilitative interpersonal skill of persuasion. As therapy progressed, the therapist detected that the pattern of stories had an external, detached quality. While the cognitive insights were productive, the therapist recognized some experiential limitations. Therapists with highly developed facilitative interpersonal skills, particularly warmth, acceptance, and understanding, are better able to identify these interoceptive forms of client expressions of experience. The ability to absorb and tolerate these states when client anxiety and stress are activated in momentary reactions allows these therapists to access a larger stage at which other interpersonal skills may unfold. Even so, evocative exposure work often stalls if clients become discouraged and do not engage in in-between session exposures as homework, which requires a therapist's use of hope and positive expectations.

Therapists with empathy are equipped to influence the client's emotional avoidance. Therapists who employ a narrative or experiential approach to trauma might draw on the facilitative interpersonal skills of empathy, emotional expression, and warmth, acceptance, and understanding as ways to engage with the client's more volatile and problematic interoceptively experienced emotional states from the trauma. For example, being aware of subtle, trauma-activated stress reactions in clients allows therapists with strong facilitative interpersonal skills to express more broad-based responsiveness (Stiles & Horvath, 2017) and maintain emotional attunement with the client for longer periods of time. Maintaining presence is useful in accessing and repairing the client's attachment system and can be observed in terms of the therapist's high levels of ABC.

In summary, a confluence of therapist interpersonal skills is usually involved in effective treatment, and the mix and emphases of different therapist facilitative interpersonal skills may depend on the treatment, the client's interpersonal availability, and the collaborative aims (ABC). Therapists who can draw on strong facilitative interpersonal skills and integrate them responsively are more likely to assist clients in uncovering and deepening their expression or at least to move more quickly to the more salient aspects of the client's story, whereas therapists with weaker interpersonal skills are more likely to practice less effectively with externally surfaced material.

THE UNIQUE ROLE OF CLIENT INTERPERSONAL SKILLS

Although it is clear that clients play a major role in psychotherapy (Bohart & Wade, 2013), relatively little attention has been given to the diffuse effects that they exert on the process and outcome of therapy. The source of change has frequently been linked to client ratings of outcome and process measures. Even so, the client frequently has been characterized as a more passive recipient of the therapist's interventions, rather than a contributor. To the extent that clients are described more actively, their agency is regularly depicted not as skillful coactors but as compliant to a treatment enacted by their therapist; deficiencies are replaced with new skills, enhanced patterns of thinking and behavior, and a more genuine sense of personal agency.

Because of the traditional focus on the role of therapist skill (both technical and relational) and its effect on client change, some members of the psychotherapy community have lost sight of the role that clients actively play in generating these effects. This therapist-centric view is obvious in the medical model of psychotherapy as applications of specific treatments and techniques. Mostly, psychotherapy has been conceived to comprise therapist actors and clients as recipients of those actions. Although there is plenty of psychotherapy theory aimed toward the client (for an example, see Rogers & Wood,

1974), it is disproportionally thin and underresearched compared with the therapist literature.

Although most of the client interpersonal skills discussed in this chapter have been either parallel forms of therapist facilitative interpersonal skills or described in response to therapist skills, there are several skills clients bring to therapy that are mostly unique to them. Client skills can even play a strong, independent role in shaping the effectiveness of the core therapist facilitative interpersonal skills discussed earlier. Here, we consider a model for how the client is the driving force in how skills are expressed. Clients express many similar interpersonal skills that influence how therapists respond. Table 4.2 provides a model of client skills and corresponding therapist reactions that we have formulated for this chapter. This table is based on our research on therapist facilitative interpersonal skills, our reading of the current literature on clients' influence on therapists, and our clinical experience. The model is presented here for future empirical attention.

Novel laboratory research by Moors and Zech (2017) points toward the unique contributions of clients and therapists in enhancing treatment satisfaction. These researchers examined two major facets of interpersonal behaviors: warmth and agency. Participants imagined themselves in the role of a therapy patient and watched videos of several different therapists who varied on interpersonal traits of warmth and agency. The results showed that clients universally responded more positively to warm therapist behaviors, but their responses to agentic presentations varied based on the clients' own interpersonal profiles. Highly agentic (dominant) clients reported greater satisfaction to the dominant and warm therapist video, whereas less agentic (more submissive) clients responded more positively to the warm, nondominant video. These findings suggest that there are more than simply pretreatment attributes at work. Beyond the specific workings of clients and the specific workings of therapists lies something greater: their interaction.

Clients can also take a leading role in shaping the use of interpersonal skills in subtle but powerful ways. For example, recent research has shown that even nonverbal social mimicry (i.e., a client or therapist's unconscious physical imitation of the other) can have measurable, interactive qualities in client–therapist dyads, and client contributions to these behaviors have unique, predictive effects on the development of the working alliance (Salazar Kämpf et al., 2021). We believe that clients' interpersonal skills impact treatment in conjunction with therapists' interpersonal skills. Clients demonstrate underappreciated interpersonal abilities in disclosing interpersonal messages, which often requires considerable fortitude and courage for them to disclose these aspects of themselves. Clients express themselves using many forms of interpersonal messaging; in order to be responsive, therapists often discover that their clients have interpersonal abilities that are discovered through their therapy. In some cases, these interpersonal skills can be abilities that are underused strengths. Surprisingly, it is sometimes the clients who must compensate for their therapist's limitations (albeit even minor) in understanding client interpersonal messages.

TABLE 4.2. Proposed Model of Client Interpersonal Skills and Therapist Reactions

Skill set	Client facilitative interpersonal skills	Therapist skills activated and/or developed in therapy
Voice skills	The client speaks in an engaging, approachable matter. Their tone, cadence, and other vocal qualities match the content of their speech. Client presents an appropriate, digestible amount of information with each communication.	Is easier to attend to and attune to client communications Requires less cognitive energy to identify and decipher potential content-affect splits Is better able to respond to core client issues without becoming bogged down or distracted by less pertinent detail Reduces the chance to miss important communications due to misinterpretations
Encouragement skills	Despite obstacles, setbacks, or challenges, the client is open to the possibility of (some level of) recovery, change, or improvement. Experiences agency and control in aspects of everyday life. Believes themselves to be worthy of treatment and improvement. Feels guided by larger meaning or values. Can access and communicate some parts of these beliefs to others. The client is able to effectively self-advocate and navigate systems that are challenging or can provoke frustration.	Is better able to provide targeted, persuasive messages of hope and improvement Feels more likely to go above and beyond to help the client (both in session and in meeting other basic needs, when appropriate) Promotes more regular, genuine communications of support, motivation, and belief in the client's ability to achieve goals Reduces the likelihood of feeling unfairly blamed for setbacks or barriers to goal attainment
Emotion skills	The client has strong access to internal states and is able to communicate at least the essential components of these states. At very high levels, client also shows warmth, openness, and consideration for their therapist both in response to (a) potentially difficult disclosures and (b) the therapist as a person. The client is able to provide feedback on or correct inaccurate or incomplete therapist statements about the client's emotional states.	Contributes to more accurate reflections, empathy, and summary statements Enhances conceptualization and helps to be better able to provide impactful, appropriate interventions Has an easier time accessing, experiencing, and expressing warmth, acceptance, and understanding Is more likely to engage in emotionally focused content in sessions

TABLE 4.2. Proposed Model of Client Interpersonal Skills and Therapist Reactions (*Continued*)

Skill set	Client facilitative interpersonal skills	Therapist skills activated and/or developed in therapy
Alliance skills	The client possesses abilities to form a collaborative relationship with the therapist. If the therapist ruptures the alliance or causes some form of process disruption, the client is able to recognize and communicate about it in such a way that does not trigger excessive therapist defensiveness. When presenting challenges or changes to the relational configuration, the client does so in a respectful, reasonable, and interpersonally considerate way.	Enhances ability to form, maintain, and repair alliance with client Increases comfort with, and higher frequency of, discussions of the status of the therapeutic relationship Reduces defensiveness and, relatedly, increases focus on client and unfolding process in the session Imparts greater awareness of ruptures and "mistakes"; also offers a chance for meaningful interpersonal improvement (both with this client and others)

Client Interpersonal Skills of Convincing: Hope and Resilience

As discussed by Fuertes and Williams (2017), an example of a client skill is the ability to remain hopeful. Although we discussed hope earlier as a core interpersonal skill of therapists that catalyzes change, a large portion of hope is also an independent client interpersonal skill. Without some measure of client hope, the work of therapy cannot be done. Some flicker of hope must be present for a client to hire a therapist and attend the first session.

Success in building client hope has a few prerequisites, especially when a client presents with minimal hopefulness. For example, Padesky and Mooney (2012) stated that clients must have some capacity for trust in others and the ability to form an attachment in order to develop resilience. We are reminded of numerous suicidal clients who can find no reason to live except for their attachment to a pet—any route to activating attachment systems can be a lifeline. In addition, Padesky and Mooney described client-defining prerequisites for hope as including basic good health, cognitive competency to engage in planning, emotional competency to identify and express feelings, emotion regulation, and a belief or "faith" that life has meaning.

In one study, clients who expressed greater hope were found to make symptomatic improvements, but they did so in later sessions, after signs of hope first appeared (Abel et al., 2016). A paradox of the client's interpersonal skill of hope is that building hope is often the first task of therapy, and yet the requirements of hope involve several other client interpersonal skills. For example, building basic attachments and trust often requires sustained therapeutic work. When clients present with little hope, therapists can feel lost without "a foothold in hope" until other client interpersonal skills emerge or can be learned. Clients without cognitive competency and emotion regulation skills often struggle to build hopefulness too, because cognitive planning is needed to identify pathways for meeting goals and any experiences of optimism are fleeting and impermanent. Therefore, hope is an advanced client interpersonal skill and is built through the development of other client interpersonal skills.

A somewhat separate aspect of the client's interpersonal skill of hope is the ability to direct hope into meaning making and action. Imagining pathways for improving one's problem does not imply that the route imagined is meaningful to the client or that any substantive movement toward it will be made. Setting the experience and optimism of hope into action relates to additional client skills. First, hope can only be effective and mature when it is meaningfully integrated within the client's personal construct system and sense of self. *Meaningful hope* is achieved through assistance from a therapist who is both persuasive and empathic. Clients may express this skill through using metaphors and developing reflexive, meaningful narratives about themselves.

A client's ability to self-advocate is a learnable skill, which allows clients to influence the process and speed at which they receive adequate care and attention for their concerns. Self-advocacy has been noted as an important aspect of care for a host of physical and behavioral health concerns across diverse populations (e.g., Cuenca-Carlino & Mustian, 2013; Hagan et al., 2017). Increasingly, self-advocacy has been identified as a critical client skill in transforming hope into achieving therapeutic goals. The importance of self-advocacy as a client skill has been long recognized when working with clients with disabilities (e.g., Gerber et al., 1996). For example, Kimball et al. (2016) recognized that self-advocacy skills among clients with disabilities are associated with skills of relational attachment skills, partly acquired through parents, but actualized through storytelling and collaborative activism with peers. The same need for self-advocacy and perseverance is an important client skill for psychological and emotional problems as well. Thus, client skills in self-advocacy not only require hope, but they are also frequently combined with other client skills such as the therapeutic bond and meaningful autobiographical narratives.

INTERPLAY BETWEEN CLIENT AND THERAPIST SKILLS

Clients' interpersonal expressions and responses have a profound impact on important therapeutic processes. The therapeutic construct of empathy provides a perfect example. As originally conceptualized by Barrett-Lennard (1981), empathy represents a multistage cycle that involves critical contributions from both the client and therapist. First, a client must share a feeling, then a therapist must perceive and attempt a responsive understanding. Finally, the client can elect to receive and acknowledge this communication. Further elaboration by MacFarlane et al. (2015) confirmed the multidimensional, interactive nature of empathy. Collaboratively formed processes, such as the expression and reception of empathy, represent the heart of clinical intervention, and they ultimately rely on client input as much as on therapist input to be successful.

More extensive examples can be found in the alliance rupture-repair literature, in which detecting, unpacking, and negotiating client contributions to the therapeutic process is deemed central to change. Indeed, entire theories of psychotherapy, such as control mastery theory (CMT; Weiss, 1993; Weiss et al., 1986), are built around these client-focused premises. CMT holds that clients enter the relational space with particular "pathogenic beliefs" about themselves and the world around them (Weiss et al., 1986). In CMT-based interventions, clients are understood to be offering "tests" of their beliefs about the therapist, and clients understand the therapist's response accordingly. Having high regard for how clients are active interpersonal agents who are making sense of the others, including the therapist, is one step toward appreciating clients as bringing valuable interpersonal skills into the treatment. Making use of clients' interpersonal strengths in this way allows for a more complete appreciation for the client and for their capacity to exercise interpersonal strengths toward the therapeutic goal in a truly collaborative engagement with their therapist. Even when the source of symptomatic distress seems to be from blind spots in other domains, clients often have learned to compensate through interpersonal strengths in other areas. Thus, even when clients are in a severely damaged state, the ability to form productive therapeutic work can develop within and around the zone of these client capacities. In these interactions, which might appear as markers in rupture-repair work (Eubanks et al., 2018), clients are the gatekeepers by which "tests" are introduced into the relationship.

Case Example of Client Interpersonal Skills

Some clients present with such high intra- and interpersonal skills that they could effectively work with any clinician and achieve progress. This situation is not too far from the idea of "bowling with bumpers," whereby almost any (therapist) action ends up achieving a positive result, regardless of delivery or technical ability. Of course, there are also situations in which clients may present with such significant skills that they may "overwhelm" unprepared or inexperienced therapists.

One such example is Darryl, a Black, heterosexual male college student who presented to therapy with depression. Darryl began therapy shortly after transferring colleges. He experienced a significant rupture in his primary peer group, which led him to have a drug overdose, take medical leave, and, ultimately, withdraw from his first university. Darryl wanted to prevent this from happening again at his new school. Darryl routinely reported severe depressive symptoms on standard outcome measures (e.g., the Beck Depression Inventory–II or Outcome Questionnaire–45) but masked these symptoms with humor in session. Darryl's therapist, a White, male postdoctoral clinician, found these high symptom scores concerning, but his concern was routinely assuaged by Darryl's easygoing charm in the therapy room. Darryl easily conveyed interpersonal warmth, which often initiated and "unlocked" the therapist's strong facilitative interpersonal skills such as warmth, acceptance, and understanding as well as emotional expression and ABC. Believing their strong rapport to be indicative of a good process, Darryl's clinician continued to approach the case from the same straightforward cognitive approach for months.

As Darryl's clinician continued to monitor his outcomes, he noticed that Darryl was not reporting any progress. Over the course of many sessions, Darryl and his clinician "pulled back the veneer" of Darryl's distress, moving beyond their initial shared high interpersonal skills of verbal and emotional bonding—mostly through a shared sense of humor. Partly, this revelation to Darryl's distress occurred through a therapist-led skill (alliance rupture-repair responsiveness), in which the therapist persuasively invited further consideration of how their shared humor might serve to mask those hidden self-devaluations and negative feelings. Indeed, behind the laughter, deep-seated but hidden experiences of guilt and pain were slowly revealed. Darryl had grown up in a privileged, upper-class community. He was acutely aware of the suffering of other people of color and felt constant guilt over his self-perceived lack of achievement. This self-perception led to a kind of paralysis that prevented him from changing his circumstances (and reinforced the negative, self-critical beliefs). The one interpersonal skill that seemed lacking was hope; Darryl seemed to rely on his therapist for more influence of the facilitative interpersonal skills of hope and positive expectations. Yet Darryl displayed an inner resilience and determination that kept him engaged through a strong ABC. Darryl and his clinician were able to harness Darryl's strong grasp of language and communication through metaphors (and shared verbal fluency with his therapist), which he deftly used to describe his experiences with depression. Phrases like "sitting in the pigsty" of depression became markers for a conversation about important topics in session. Given Darryl's early discomfort with direct self-disclosure, using extensive metaphors provided a vehicle for "safe" but genuine self-exploration. In this case, Darryl was able to better understand and improve his self-perceptions, which opened up the therapist's use of persuasion and also aided in building hope and positive expectations.

By the end of treatment, Darryl had a new, supportive group of friends, started his first-ever long-term romantic relationship, and was on track to graduate with honors and pursue graduate training in a helping field (to fulfill his dream of giving back to underserved and culturally marginalized communities). This process was gradual and took well over 2 years to reach. In this case, because the clinician was unaware of how Darryl was using communication to effectively mask deeper concerns, therapy was stagnant for an excessive period and could have easily resulted in premature termination.

CONCLUSION AND FUTURE DIRECTIONS

Therapist interpersonal skills clearly influence clients to experience less distress, and there is plenty of research that implicates the role of client's interpersonal skills in these changes. Clients are affected by a wide swath of their therapists' interpersonal imprints, including voice, warmth, bonding, and hopefulness. These qualities have common associations with each other, and yet by definition, they are expressed by each therapist in highly unique and personalized ways. The client's perspective and experience of the unique impact of their therapist's skills is suggested by the research findings. The extent of the clients' interpersonal skill as a unique factor in treatment, even as an initiative influence for "unlocking" therapists' facilitative interpersonal skills, is an underappreciated and potent force in treatment. While we believe that implications from the mostly correlational findings and clinical observations are compelling, future research is sorely needed on how therapist interpersonal skills interact with client interpersonal skills and capacities.

For example, matching client–therapist research strategies (and related actor–partner interdependence modeling analyses) would greatly expand our understanding of clients and therapists as interdependent dyads. Even less empirical research has been conducted on the role that clients play in activating their therapists' skills. There is evidence that supports the role of therapist interpersonal skills as influencing the client, likely by facilitating client development of interpersonal skills. Clearly, therapist effectiveness, expressed through therapist interpersonal skills, appears to interface with client characteristics and skills in several ways. Furthermore, the literature reviewed here suggests that clients also bring extraordinary, even gifted, interpersonal skills to bear in therapeutic work in ways that can positively impact their therapeutic experiences, sometimes even helping therapists to unlock their own influential interpersonal skills.

REFERENCES

Abel, A., Hayes, A. M., Henley, W., & Kuyken, W. (2016). Sudden gains in cognitive-behavior therapy for treatment-resistant depression: Processes of change. *Journal of Consulting and Clinical Psychology, 84*(8), 726–737. https://doi.org/10.1037/ccp0000101

Anderson, T., Crowley, M. E., Himawan, L., Holmberg, J. K., & Uhlin, B. D. (2016). Therapist facilitative interpersonal skills and training status: A randomized clinical trial on alliance and outcome. *Psychotherapy Research, 26*(5), 511–529. https://doi.org/10.1080/10503307.2015.1049671

Anderson, T., Finkelstein, J., & Horvath, S. (2020). Facilitating therapist facilitative interpersonal skills through responsiveness. *Counselling & Psychotherapy Research, 20*(3), 463–469. https://doi.org/10.1002/capr.12302

Anderson, T., McClintock, A. S., Himawan, L., Song, X., & Patterson, C. L. (2016). A prospective study of therapist facilitative interpersonal skills as a predictor of treatment outcome. *Journal of Consulting and Clinical Psychology, 84*(1), 57–66. https://doi.org/10.1037/ccp0000060

Anderson, T., Ogles, B. M., Patterson, C. L., Lambert, M. J., & Vermeersch, D. A. (2009). Therapist effects: Facilitative interpersonal skills as a predictor of therapist success. *Journal of Clinical Psychology, 65*(7), 755–768. https://doi.org/10.1002/jclp.20583

Anderson, T., Stone, S. J., Angus, L., & Weibel, D. T. (2021). Double trouble: Therapists with low facilitative interpersonal skills and without training have low in-session experiential processes. *Psychotherapy Research.* Advance online publication. https://doi.org/10.1080/10503307.2021.1913293

Baldwin, S. A., & Imel, Z. E. (2013). Therapist effects: Findings and methods. In M. J. Lambert (Ed.), *Bergin and Garfield's handbook of psychotherapy and behavior change* (6th ed., pp. 258–297). John Wiley and Sons.

Barrett-Lennard, G. T. (1981). The empathy cycle: Refinement of a nuclear concept. *Journal of Counseling Psychology, 28*(2), 91–100. https://doi.org/10.1037/0022-0167.28.2.91

Ben David-Sela, T., Dolev-Amit, T., Eubanks, C. F., & Zilcha-Mano, S. (2021). Achieving successful resolution of alliance ruptures: For whom and when? *Psychotherapy Research, 31*(7), 870–881. https://doi.org/10.1080/10503307.2020.1862432

Benjamin, L. S. (2018). *Interpersonal reconstructive therapy for anger, anxiety, and depression: It's about broken hearts, not broken brains.* American Psychological Association. https://doi.org/10.1037/0000090-000

Bernecker, S. L., Levy, K. N., & Ellison, W. D. (2014). A meta-analysis of the relation between patient adult attachment style and the working alliance. *Psychotherapy Research, 24*(1), 12–24. https://doi.org/10.1080/10503307.2013.809561

Beutler, L. E. (1979). Values, beliefs, religion and the persuasive influence of psychotherapy. *Psychotherapy: Theory, Research, & Practice, 16*(4), 432–440. https://doi.org/10.1037/h0088370

Beutler, L. E., & Consoli, A. J. (1993). Matching the therapist's interpersonal stance to clients' characteristics: Contributions from systematic eclectic psychotherapy. *Psychotherapy: Theory, Research, & Practice, 30*(3), 417–422. https://doi.org/10.1037/0033-3204.30.3.417

Bohart, A. C., & Wade, A. G. (2013). The client in psychotherapy. In M. J. Lambert (Ed.), *Bergin and Garfield's handbook of psychotherapy and behavior change* (6th ed., pp. 219–257). John Wiley and Sons.

Castonguay, L. G., & Hill, C. E. (Eds.). (2017). *How and why are some therapists better than others? Understanding therapist effects.* American Psychological Association. https://doi.org/10.1037/0000034-000

Coyne, A. E., Constantino, M. J., Ravitz, P., & McBride, C. (2018). The interactive effect of patient attachment and social support on early alliance quality in interpersonal psychotherapy. *Journal of Psychotherapy Integration, 28*(1), 46–59. https://doi.org/10.1037/int0000074

Cuenca-Carlino, Y., & Mustian, A. L. (2013). Self-regulated strategy development: Connecting persuasive writing to self-advocacy for students with emotional and behavioral disorders. *Behavioral Disorders, 39*(1), 3–15. https://doi.org/10.1177/019874291303900102

Elliott, R. E., Bohart, A. C., Watson, J. C., & Murphy, D. (2019). Empathy. In J. C. Norcross & M. J. Lambert (Eds.), *Psychotherapy relationships that work* (3rd ed., pp. 245–287). Oxford University Press. https://doi.org/10.1093/med-psych/9780190843953.003.0007

Errázuriz, P., & Zilcha-Mano, S. (2018). In psychotherapy with severe patients discouraging news may be worse than no news: The impact of providing feedback to therapists on psychotherapy outcome, session attendance, and the alliance. *Journal of Consulting and Clinical Psychology, 86*(2), 125–139. https://doi.org/10.1037/ccp0000277

Eubanks, C. F., Muran, J. C., & Safran, J. D. (2018). Alliance rupture repair: A meta-analysis. *Psychotherapy: Theory, Research, & Practice, 55*(4), 508–519. https://doi.org/10.1037/pst0000185

Farber, B. A., Suzuki, J. Y., & Lynch, D. A. (2019). Positive regard and affirmation. In J. C. Norcross & M. J. Lambert (Eds.), *Psychotherapy relationships that work* (3rd ed., pp. 288–322). Oxford University Press. https://doi.org/10.1093/med-psych/9780190843953.003.0008

Fuertes, J. N., & Williams, E. N. (2017). Client-focused psychotherapy research. *Journal of Counseling Psychology, 64*(4), 369–375. https://doi.org/10.1037/cou0000214

Gerber, P. J., Reiff, H. B., & Ginsberg, R. (1996). Reframing the learning disabilities experience. *Journal of Learning Disabilities, 29*(1), 98–101, 97. https://doi.org/10.1177/002221949602900112

Greenberg, L. S. (2017). Emotion-focused therapy of depression. *Person-Centered and Experiential Psychotherapies, 16*(2), 106–117. https://doi.org/10.1080/14779757.2017.1330702

Hagan, T. H., Rosenzweig, M., Zorn, K., van Londen, J., & Donovan, H. (2017). Perspectives on self-advocacy: Comparing perceived uses, benefits, and drawbacks among survivors and providers. *Oncology Nursing Forum, 44*(1), 52–59. https://doi.org/10.1188/17.ONF.52-59

Heinonen, E., Lindfors, O., Härkänen, T., Virtala, E., Jääskeläinen, T., & Knekt, P. (2014). Therapists' professional and personal characteristics as predictors of working alliance in short-term and long-term psychotherapies. *Clinical Psychology & Psychotherapy, 21*(6), 475–494. https://doi.org/10.1002/cpp.1852

Hersoug, A. G., Høglend, P., Havik, O. E., von der Lippe, A., & Monsen, J. T. (2009). Pretreatment patient characteristics related to the level and development of working alliance in long-term psychotherapy. *Psychotherapy Research, 19*(2), 172–180. https://doi.org/10.1080/10503300802657374

Hill, C. E. (2019). *Helping skills: Facilitating exploration, insight, and action* (5th ed.). American Psychological Association.

Horowitz, L. M. (2004). *Interpersonal foundations of psychopathology.* American Psychological Association. https://doi.org/10.1037/10727-000

Kim, Y., Sidtis, J. J., & Van Lancker Sidtis, D. (2019). Emotionally expressed voices are retained in memory following a single exposure. *PLOS ONE, 14*(10), e0223948. https://doi.org/10.1371/journal.pone.0223948

Kimball, E. W., Moore, A., Vaccaro, A., Troiano, P. F., & Newman, B. M. (2016). College students with disabilities redefine activism: Self-advocacy, storytelling, and collective action. *Journal of Diversity in Higher Education, 9*(3), 245–260. https://doi.org/10.1037/dhe0000031

Knox, S., Goldberg, J. L., Woodhouse, S. S., & Hill, C. E. (1999). Clients' internal representations of their therapists. *Journal of Counseling Psychology, 46*(2), 244–256. https://doi.org/10.1037/0022-0167.46.2.244

Kolden, G. G. (1996). Change in early sessions of dynamic therapy: Universal processes and the generic model of psychotherapy. *Journal of Consulting and Clinical Psychology, 64*(3), 489–496. https://doi.org/10.1037/0022-006X.64.3.489

Levy, K. N., Kivity, Y., Johnson, B. N., & Gooch, C. V. (2018). Adult attachment as a predictor and moderator of psychotherapy outcome: A meta-analysis. *Journal of Clinical Psychology, 74*(11), 1996–2013. https://doi.org/10.1002/jclp.22685

MacFarlane, P., Anderson, T., & McClintock, A. S. (2015). The early formation of the working alliance from the client's perspective: A qualitative study. *Psychotherapy: Theory, Research, & Practice, 52*(3), 363–372. https://doi.org/10.1037/a0038733

MacFarlane, P., Anderson, T., & McClintock, A. S. (2017). Empathy from the client's perspective: A grounded theory analysis. *Psychotherapy Research, 27*(2), 227–238. https://doi.org/10.1080/10503307.2015.1090038

Mallinckrodt, B. (2010). The psychotherapy relationship as attachment: Evidence and implications. *Journal of Social and Personal Relationships, 27*(2), 262–270. https://doi.org/10.1177/0265407509360905

Moors, F., & Zech, E. (2017). The effects of psychotherapists' and clients' interpersonal behaviors during a first simulated session: A lab study investigating client satisfaction. *Frontiers in Psychology, 8*, 1868. https://doi.org/10.3389/fpsyg.2017.01868

Mosher, J. K., & Stiles, W. B. (2009). Clients' assimilation of experiences of their therapists. *Psychotherapy: Theory, Research, & Practice, 46*(4), 432–447. https://doi.org/10.1037/a0017955

Muran, J. C., & Eubanks, C. F. (2020). *Therapeutic performance under pressure: Negotiating emotion, difference, and rupture.* American Psychological Association. https://doi.org/10.1037/0000182-000

Norcross, J. C., & Lambert, M. J. (Eds.). (2019). *Psychotherapy relationships that work* (3rd ed.). Oxford University Press.

Orlinsky, D. E., Rønnestad, M., & Willutzki, U. (2004). Process and outcome in psychotherapy. In M. J. Lambert (Ed.), *Bergin and Garfield's handbook of psychotherapy and behavior change* (5th ed., pp. 307–389). Wiley.

Padesky, C. A., & Mooney, K. A. (2012). Strengths-based cognitive-behavioural therapy: A four-step model to build resilience. *Clinical Psychology & Psychotherapy*, *19*(4), 283–290. https://doi.org/10.1002/cpp.1795

Pereira, J. A., Barkham, M., Kellett, S., & Saxon, D. (2017). The role of practitioner resilience and mindfulness in effective practice: A practice-based feasibility study. *Administration and Policy in Mental Health*, *44*(5), 691–704. https://doi.org/10.1007/s10488-016-0747-0

Rice, L. N., & Kerr, G. P. (1986). Measures of client and therapist vocal quality. In L. S. Greenberg & W. M. Pinsof (Eds.), *The psychotherapeutic process: A research handbook* (pp. 73–105). Guilford Press.

Rogers, C. R. (1957). The necessary and sufficient conditions of therapeutic personality change. *Journal of Consulting and Clinical Psychology*, *21*(2), 95–103. https://doi.org/10.1037/h0045357

Rogers, C. R., & Wood, J. K. (1974). Client-centered theory: Carl R. Rogers. In A. Burton (Ed.), *Operational theories of personality* (pp. 211–258). Brunner/Mazel.

Salazar Kämpf, M., Nestler, S., Hansmeier, J., Glombiewski, J., & Exner, C. (2021). Mimicry in psychotherapy—An actor partner model of therapists' and patients' non-verbal behavior and its effects on the working alliance. *Psychotherapy Research*, *31*(6), 752–764. https://doi.org/10.1080/10503307.2020.1849849

Schöttke, H., Flückiger, C., Goldberg, S. B., Eversmann, J., & Lange, J. (2017). Predicting psychotherapy outcome based on therapist interpersonal skills: A five-year longitudinal study of a therapist assessment protocol. *Psychotherapy Research*, *27*(6), 642–652. https://doi.org/10.1080/10503307.2015.1125546

Snyder, C. R. (2002). Hope theory: Rainbows in the mind. *Psychological Inquiry*, *13*(4), 249–275. https://doi.org/10.1207/S15327965PLI1304_01

Stiles, W. B., Honos-Webb, L., & Surko, M. (1998). Responsiveness in psychotherapy. *Clinical Psychology: Science and Practice*, *5*(4), 439–458. https://doi.org/10.1111/j.1468-2850.1998.tb00166.x

Stiles, W. B., & Horvath, A. O. (2017). Appropriate responsiveness as a contribution to therapist effects. In L. G. Castonguay & C. E. Hill (Eds.), *How and why are some therapists better than others? Understanding therapist effects* (pp. 71–84). American Psychological Association. https://doi.org/10.1037/0000034-005

Tomicic, A., Martinez, C., & Krause, M. (2015). The sound of change: A study of the psychotherapeutic process embodied in vocal expression. Laura Rice's ideas revisited. *Psychotherapy Research*, *25*(2), 263–276. https://doi.org/10.1080/10503307.2014.892647

Wampold, B. E., & Imel, Z. E. (2015). *The great psychotherapy debate: The evidence for what makes psychotherapy work.* Routledge. https://doi.org/10.4324/9780203582015

Weiss, J. (1993). *How psychotherapy works: Process and technique.* Guilford Press.

Weiss, J., Sampson, H., & the Mount Zion Psychotherapy Research Group. (1986). *The psychoanalytic process: Theory, clinical observations, and empirical research.* Guilford Press.

5

Clients' Experiences of Attachment in the Psychotherapy Relationship

Brent Mallinckrodt

John Bowlby (1988), in one of his last scholarly writings, asserted that the adult client–therapist relationship could be understood as a form of attachment. In the decades following his seminal work, a large body of research has accumulated to support this position (for reviews, see Levy et al., 2019; Mikulincer & Shaver, 2016). It is perhaps understandable that much of this attention has focused on the therapist's role in facilitating client change through providing and regulating a secure therapeutic attachment (e.g., Teyber & Teyber, 2017). However, the goal of this chapter is to reexamine this literature from the client's perspective of experiencing attachment in the psychotherapy relationship. We begin this exploration from outside the therapeutic setting by considering the elements of all healthy child–caregiver attachments.

HEALTHY CHILD–CAREGIVER ATTACHMENTS

Summarizing a large body of theory and research, Mikulincer and Shaver (2016, pp. 15–16) identified five key functions that secure attachment to caregivers serve for a developing child. Attachment figures provide (a) a target for *proximity seeking*, (b) a *safe haven* when children feel threatened, and (c) a *secure base* that permits children to explore the environment and develop growing mastery. Together, these first three elements promote a sense of "felt security."

I thank Merry Capozzolo, Patrick Grzanka, Cheri Marmarosh, Joe Miles, and Meifen Wei for their comments on previous drafts of this chapter.

https://doi.org/10.1037/0000303-006
The Other Side of Psychotherapy: Understanding Clients' Experiences and Contributions in Treatment, J. N. Fuertes (Editor)

As a capacity for appraisal becomes more developed, children regard attachment figures as (d) *stronger and wiser*. If comfortable proximity cannot be maintained, children experience (e) *separation anxiety* until a sense of connection is reestablished. These five elements are considered essential features of child–caregiver attachment. For infants, physical proximity is paramount, but as children are able to internalize mental representations of an attachment figure, a sense of emotional connection can be maintained through internal representation, even in the caregiver's physical absence.

Researchers who apply adult attachment theory to understand psychotherapy processes argue that each of these five essential elements has a close corollary in many therapeutic relationships (Daniel, 2006; Mallinckrodt, 2010; Obegi & Berant, 2009). For example, clients who experience their therapist as a safe haven are able to process past traumatic experiences more effectively (Kinsler et al., 2009). Research suggests that clients' secure base of attachment to their therapist is associated with greater client depth of in-session exploration in the middle phase of time-limited counseling (Mallinckrodt et al., 2005; Romano et al., 2008). The client's process of reaching out for help, then self-disclosing in counseling is a form of proximity seeking. Studies of help-seeking preferences suggest clients approach therapists because the latter are regarded stronger and wiser (Vogel & Wei, 2005). Finally, of course, many clients experience separation anxiety as termination nears (Joyce et al., 2007; see also Chapter 12, this volume).

Although it is clear that each of the five essential features of child–caregiver attachment can reemerge as a recognizable aspect of many adult client–therapist relationships, not all therapy relationships manifest each of these features. Among those that do, the particular character of attachment varies greatly. The reemergence in psychotherapy of these five essential features of early attachment is perhaps best understood through the lens of Mikulincer and Shaver's (2016, pp. 27–41) model of adult attachment system activation and functioning. This model begins with the premise that the set goal of attachment behavior for both children and adults is the perception of *felt security*. When a threat is perceived, if an attachment figure (i.e., caregiver in childhood or relationship partner in adulthood) is believed to be available and responsive in times of need, and the individual's proximity-seeking attempts are rewarded, then one perceives the world as generally safe and attachment figures as generally likely to be helpful if summoned. The resulting sense of felt security promotes positive working models of self and others and a "secure base script" (Mikulincer & Shaver, 2016, p. 19) that features a series of if–then propositions similar to these:

> If I encounter a threat or experience distress, then I can approach one of my attachment figures to seek help, and they are likely to be sensitive and to respond in ways that serve to resolve the problem. As a result, I will experience relief and comfort because I drew close to this person and sought help.

Thus, according to Mikulincer and Shaver's model, if a significant threat is perceived, an individual's attachment behavioral system is activated and proximity-seeking to an attachment figure is the preferred "security-based" primary strategy.

However, according to Mikulincer and Shaver's (2016) model, if an individual has learned through repeated experience that attachment figures are not likely to be sensitive or responsive when first approached, this person will activate one or both of two possible *secondary strategies*. If experience suggests that attachment figures are sometimes responsive, but not reliably so, the distressed individual might engage in the secondary strategy of attachment *hyperactivation*. In this strategy, individuals intensify proximity-seeking efforts and magnify their communication of distress. Hyperactivation strategies involve hypervigilance for perceived threats and signs of abandonment, appraisal of objectively modest threats as catastrophic, and rumination about past experiences of threat. Individuals who hyperactivate their attachment behavioral repertoire may plead for assistance, be unable to engage in autonomous efforts to self-soothe or problem solve, and redouble bids to solicit supportive responses from attachment figures. Because this strategy is occasionally rewarded with some relief from distress, the intensity and persistence of these behaviors despite frequent disappointments can be understood as the powerful byproduct of intermittent reinforcement. Alternatively, if repeated experience has shown that efforts to obtain comfort and support from an attachment figure are almost never successful, such an individual might engage in a secondary strategy of attachment *deactivation*. In this strategy, proximity-seeking efforts are abandoned. Individuals engage in what Bowlby (1969/1982) termed "compulsive self-reliance." They eschew soliciting support and try to avoid becoming dependent on others. These individuals fear intimacy and deny needs for emotional connection. They expend great effort to suppress threat-related cognition, thoughts of tenderness, or other mental representations that, in others, evoke the primary secure attachment system. The deactivating strategy can be understood as the result of primary attachment behaviors that have been extinguished through consistent lack of reinforcement from caregivers.

Tendencies toward hyperactivation or deactivation are maintained in adulthood due to the enduring nature of working models. *Working models* are cognitive–affective structures that develop through repeated childhood experiences of caregivers responding (or failing to respond) to a child's attempt to solicit comfort. Bowlby (1973) described working models of others as involving judgments about whether attachment figures are generally likely to respond consistently and positively to bids for comfort and protection, whereas the model of self involves beliefs about whether one is "the sort of person towards whom anyone, and the attachment figure in particular, is likely to respond in a helpful way" (p. 204). Initially, writers followed Bartholomew and Horowitz (1991) in describing adult attachment prototypes in terms of positive/negative dichotomies for models of self and others, yielding four attachment styles: Secure, Preoccupied, Dismissing, and Fearful (see Figure 5.1). However, subsequent research suggests the data do not support sharp qualitative distinctions (Fraley & Waller, 1998). Thus, it is useful to think of the

FIGURE 5.1. Attachment Style, Dimensions of Adult Attachment, and Working Models

	Low ECR Anxiety (positive model of self)	High ECR Anxiety (negative model of self)
Low ECR Avoidance (positive model of others)	**Secure**	**Preoccupied** *hyperactivating*
High ECR Avoidance (negative model of others)	**Dismissing** *deactivating*	**Fearful** *alternating hyperactivating and deactivating*

Note. ECR = Experiences in Close Relationship scale dimensions; *Italics* = secondary attachment strategies.

working model of others as a continuum anchored at the positive pole by beliefs that attachment figures are generally trustworthy, dependable, and likely to respond positively if solicited for support; in contrast, the negative pole is anchored by beliefs that attachment figures are unreliable, self-interested, often malevolent, and not likely to be helpful if approached. A positive working model of self is distinguished by self-affirming beliefs that one is lovable and deserving of care from attachment figures, whereas the negative pole is characterized by low self-worth and a sense of oneself as being deeply flawed. Thus, a client with a positive model of others might believe that counselors (as attachment figures) are benevolent and likely to be helpful in general to other clients. However, if this client has a negative working model of self, they may believe they are a deeply flawed individual uniquely underserving of help. Therefore, they must go to extraordinary lengths to gain and maintain their counselor's support. The concept of unconditional positive regard may be quite alien to clients with a negative working model of self.

Although the term "working" suggests a provisional nature, in practice, working models are resistant to change because the cognitive–affective structures involve expectations about self and others that tend to be self-confirming (Bartholomew & Horowitz, 1991; Mikulincer & Shaver, 2016). For example, those with a negative model of self are hypervigilant for signs of impending abandonment. Their need for frequent reassurance may become wearisome to friends and lovers, who then, in exasperation, actually terminate the relationship. Persons with a negative model of others scan the social landscape for signs of less than total dependability in friends. These individuals tend to find the very disappointments they are looking for even in the most loyal relationships.

A study of undergraduates early in their first-ever college experience conceptualized the college transition as an adult version of Ainsworth's Strange Situation (Jeong et al., 2021). Both anxiety and avoidance were positively correlated with defects in affect regulation, but the patterns differed. Attachment anxiety, but not avoidance, was negatively correlated with a dimension of emotional intelligence based on capacity for self-soothing ("repair" of negative emotions).

Avoidance, but not anxiety, was negatively correlated with recognizing the value of paying attention to feelings. Thus, hyperactivation and deactivation may be associated in the general population with unique affect regulation deficits (Mikulincer & Shaver, 2019), and these deficits have important implications for clients' experiences in therapy.

HYPERACTIVATION AND DEACTIVATION OF ATTACHMENT IN THE THERAPY RELATIONSHIP

Because secondary attachment strategies are deeply ingrained in clients' fundamental help-seeking strategies, they are likely to emerge in a developing therapeutic relationship, especially if clients perceive a significant threat, and they fear the therapist or other attachment figures will not be available or responsive. Secondary strategies are derived from working models and are a combination of unconscious automatic reactions and conscious strategies (Mikulincer & Shaver, 2016). Thus, hyperactivation and deactivation may be viewed as forms of psychotherapy transference to the extent they involve reactions to a therapist based on a client's previous attachment relationships and to the extent they have not been "earned" by the therapist's actual behavior (Woodhouse et al., 2003).

But, specifically, how do clients manifest hyperactivation or deactivation with their therapist? Mallinckrodt (2010) observed that clients who hyperactivate their attachment system often magnify the intensity of all five fundamental elements of secure attachment in the therapeutic relationship. For example, clients with hyperactivating tendencies may (a) seek especially close emotional proximity by accelerating the depth of their self-disclosure in early sessions and press for significant therapist personal self-disclosures; (b) seek safe havens through magnified expressions of distress and intensified pleas for the therapist's help or direct advice, although any sense of comfort derived from a positive therapist response is only fleeting; (c) desperately desire a secure base in the psychotherapy relationship but experience pervasive anxiety that prevents deep exploration in sessions, combined with a markedly limited sense of personal agency for achieving change outside of therapy; (d) regard their therapist as far stronger and wiser, especially in contrast to their own sense of powerlessness; and (e) experience panic when the therapist seems unavailable, coupled with dread in anticipation of termination. The negative working model of self and positive working model of others that characterize adults with hyperactivating tendencies may prompt clients to idealize their therapist (at least initially), fear abandonment, and sometimes experience jealousy toward the therapist's other clients.

In contrast, clients with deactivating attachment tendencies tend to downregulate these five critical elements and resist their emergence in the psychotherapy relationship—just as they resist these aspects of attachment in any close relationship. In therapy, these clients may (a) resist emotional proximity by missing sessions or arriving late and by keeping conversations superficial in sessions; (b) refuse to allow the relationship to become a safe haven by avoiding self-disclosures that might expose vulnerability or weakness; (c) reject the relationship as a secure base for exploration as part of a general unwillingness to introspect; (d) refuse to acknowledge the therapist as stronger and wiser, or as having anything much of value to contribute, while questioning (more than a typical client) the therapist's experience and training; and (e) refuse to allow the therapeutic relationship to become significant enough to prompt any grief or anxiety at the prospect of its end. The combination of a positive working model of self and negative model of others held by many clients with deactivating strategies prompts them to feel resentful or humiliated at the need to seek help. They invest considerable effort in warding off attachment-related feelings and cognitions (Mikulincer & Shaver, 2016). In therapy, they may experience a strong need to appear as though all is well and—to the extent there is a problem at all—that the fault lies entirely with others instead of acknowledging any personal responsibility.

The Client Attachment to Therapist Scale (CATS; Mallinckrodt et al., 1995) captures each of these five essential features of attachment relationships, although it was not specifically designed for this purpose. The initial CATS item pool was generated by a panel of nine experienced therapists. They were asked to consider descriptions of the three infant attachment types (secure, avoidant, and ambivalent) identified by Ainsworth et al. (1978) in the Strange Situation laboratory protocol. The panel was then told,

> Research suggests these patterns may be relatively enduring and may determine, for example, adult patterns of attachment in romantic relationships. We hope to pilot test a measure which would be able to detect patterns of secure, ambivalent, and avoidant attachment of clients to their counselors. (Mallinckrodt et al., 1995, p. 308)

Panelists were asked to generate Likert-type items to tap clients' experiences of these attachment dynamics. The initial CATS item pool contained 100 relatively nonredundant items, which were completed by a pool of 138 clients solicited from a hospital-based outpatient clinic, a university counseling center, and a university in-house graduate student training clinic. As Mallinckrodt (2010) observed, the final 36 client self-report items selected for the CATS—although not intentionally designed to do so—tapped each of the five essential features of attachment identified later by Mikulincer and Shaver (2016). Here are some examples:

- *Proximity seeking*: "I wish there were a way I could spend more time with my counselor."
- *Safe haven*: "My counselor is a comforting presence when I am upset."
- *Secure base*: "My counselor helps me to look closely at the frightening or troubling things that have happened to me."
- *Stronger and wiser*: "I feel that somehow things will work out OK for me when I am with my counselor."
- *Separation anxiety*: "I think about calling my counselor at home."

Although the CATS was not developed specifically to assess hyperactivation and deactivation of the five essential attachment ingredients, its 36 items provide a valuable window into clients' experience of relating to their therapist in these ways. Exploratory analyses identified three CATS factors that, for convenience, I will refer to as Secure, Avoidant, and Preoccupied. Recall that secondary strategies are only activated if the primary secure strategy is perceived to not be viable because attachment figures are unavailable or not responsive (Mikulincer & Shaver, 2016). Perhaps many items of the Secure CATS subscale, together with reverse-keyed items from the Avoidant subscale, reflect clients' subjective experience of comfortable attachment to their therapist through successful activation of the primary secure strategy. In contrast, items identified by the original factor analysis (Mallinckrodt et al., 1995) as belonging to the Preoccupied and Avoidant subscales capture clients experience of hyperactivation and deactivation, respectively. Appendix 5.1 presents a reconfiguration of the CATS items according to this new conceptualization. Note that many CATS items in the Secure Base domain tap perceptions of therapist responsiveness, dependability, and unconditional acceptance, together with perceptions of safety and perceived comfort in sessions. As noted previously, themes of secure base and safe haven are also evident in this cluster of items.

Regarding secondary strategies, the second domain of CATS items, shown in Appendix 5.1, spotlights how clients might experience hyperactivation in their therapy relationship, including an intense yearning for closeness, complaints and resentment about a lack of therapist responsiveness, jealousy directed toward other clients, and a willingness to cross professional boundaries. The final domain of CATS items, arranged in Appendix 5.1, highlights how client attachment deactivation might manifest in the therapy relationship, with themes of reluctance to self-disclose, feelings of humiliation and shame to be in therapy, and a perception of the therapist as deceitful and condescending.

Hyperactivation and deactivation are not mutually exclusive strategies. The Experiences in Close Relationship scale (ECR; Brennan et al., 1988) is a widely used self-report measure of adult attachment. Its two relatively orthogonal factors, Anxiety and Avoidance, can be arrayed to form a two-dimensional cartesian space. ECR dimensions are associated with combinations of positive and negative working models of self and others, as shown in Figure 5.1. The four attachment styles of Secure, Preoccupied, Dismissing, and Fearful are regarded by most contemporary researchers mainly as useful labels for regions defined by two continuous dimensions of anxiety and avoidance and not as four qualitatively different forms of attachment. The region labeled Fearful denotes high scores on both Anxiety and Avoidance ECR subscales, implying negative working models of both self and others. Mikulincer and Shaver (2016) described these individuals as intensely insecure and unable to decide whether proximity seeking is a viable option. This intense adult ambivalence about attachment resembles the "disorganized" infant attachment classification observed in children from abusive or highly dysfunctional families (Main & Hesse, 1990), with its characteristic alternating displays of approach and avoidance behavior toward attachment figures. Adults with a Fearful attachment style are unable to achieve any of the goals of the three other attachment strategies, namely, "[a] safety and security following proximity seeking (the primary, secure strategy), [b] defensive deactivation of the attachment system (the avoidant strategy), or [c] intense and chronic activation of the attachment system until security-enhancing proximity is attained (the anxious strategy)" (Mikulincer & Shaver, 2016, p. 41). In psychotherapy, clients with a Fearful attachment style may manifest their ambivalence toward the therapist by rapidly alternating—possibly in the same session—between withdrawal and denial of a need for support characteristic of the dismissing style and a craving for connection, proximity, and support characteristic of the preoccupied style.

Specific configurations of working models of self and of others may be associated with differing willingness of an individual to seek counseling. If so, then clients might represent a different mix of adult attachment styles than found in the general adult population. Analyses were conducted specifically for this chapter using archival data to explore this question. Study 1 from Wei et al. (2021) provided a normative sample of 459 college students drawn from education and psychology courses at a large public university in the Midwest who completed the ECR. Two samples with a combined total of 94 clients were drawn from Mallinckrodt et al. (2005) and Mallinckrodt et al. (2015). These clients were seen at two university counseling centers. The 2005 sample of clients ($n = 38$) was drawn from the same university as the Wei et al. normative sample, whereas the 2015 sample of clients ($n = 56$) was drawn from a large public university in the southeast. To calculate gender-specific norms, only students or clients who reported either a male or female gender identity were included in the current analyses. Table 5.1 shows that female clients reported significantly more Anxiety and Avoidance than females in the normative sample and that male clients reported significantly more Anxiety, but not Avoidance, than males in the normative sample.

Because comparisons of central tendency can obscure patterns of data distribution, a scatter plot was constructed to supplement Table 5.1. In Figure 5.2, z-scores were calculated based on separate norms for men and women and plotted for both the normative sample and client sample. The scatterplot x-axis depicts Anxiety. The y-axis depicts Avoidance with scores inverted (i.e., scores

TABLE 5.1. Adult Attachment Anxiety and Avoidance Differences Between Clients and Undergraduate Norms

	Normative sample		Clients		Cohen's	
	M	*SD*	*M*	*SD*	*t*	*D*
Women						
N	278		64			
Avoidance	2.84	1.20	3.35	1.53	2.54*	0.41
Anxiety	3.68	1.20	4.20	1.29	2.98*	0.43
Men						
N	181		30			
Avoidance	3.04	1.11	3.11	1.21	0.26	0.05
Anxiety	3.79	1.05	4.54	0.95	3.96**	0.73

Note. Equal variances are not assumed for *t*-test comparisons.
*$p < .05$, **$p < .01$

FIGURE 5.2. Scatterplot Distribution of Client and Undergraduate Normative Samples on Adult Attachment Style, Anxiety, and Avoidance

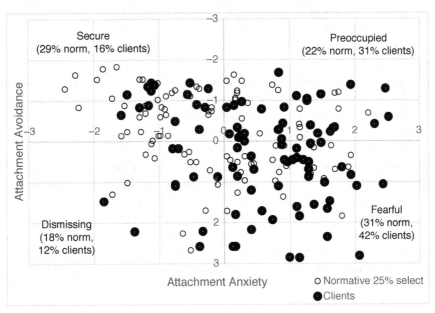

increasing from top to bottom) to match Bartholomew and Horowitz's (1991) configuration of four adult attachment styles (see Figure 5.1). Only 25% of the normative data points are shown, selected at random, to roughly equalize the number of points in both groups and make the graph in Figure 5.2 more readable. Axes intersect at the z-score 0–0 point for the normative sample and create four regions corresponding to adult attachment styles. Note that clients were relatively overrepresented in the Preoccupied and Fearful regions and relatively underrepresented in the Secure and Dismissing regions. These differences were significant, χ^2 (3, $N = 553$) = 11.78, $p = .008$. The most extreme outlier data points in the Preoccupied, Fearful, and Dismissing regions (but not Secure) in nearly all cases were clients. The findings shown in Figure 5.2 and Table 5.1 suggest that, for college students, both male and female clients tend to have higher attachment anxiety, more negative working models of self, and greater tendencies toward hyperactivation than their nonclient counterparts. Female clients, but not male clients, also appear to have significantly higher attachment Avoidance, corresponding to more negative models of others and perhaps a great tendency toward deactivation than their female student peers.

RESEARCH INSIGHTS INTO CLIENT EXPERIENCES OF ATTACHMENT IN THERAPY

A growing body of research has linked clients' adult attachment security to development of an effective working alliance (for reviews, see Bernecker et al., 2014; Diener & Monroe, 2011). A more recent meta-analysis of 36 studies and over 3,000 clients reported that clients with secure pretherapy adult attachment generally achieve better psychotherapy outcomes then those with insecure attachment. Findings also suggest that improvement in attachment security over the course of therapy parallel better treatment outcomes (Levy et al., 2018). In a study of university training clinic clients that tracked symptom levels with a brief report after each session for up to 12 sessions, Sauer et al. (2010) found that clients' attachment anxiety at intake predicted improvement during treatment, but attachment avoidance at intake did not. The specific trajectory of change for clients was related to their initial level of attachment anxiety. Not surprisingly, clients with higher anxiety exhibited a much higher level of distress at intake than those with low anxiety. The regression line for symptom change showed a steady and significant decline across sessions for clients 1 *SD* below the mean in attachment anxiety, whereas for those 1 *SD* above the mean, symptoms exhibited a sharp decline in the first three to four sessions, followed by a period of relatively little change through the middle sessions and, finally, a renewed trend toward improvement in the final sessions. Perhaps clients with high levels of anxiety experience some prompt relief from high levels of distress in the first few sessions—which Sauer et al. termed a "honeymoon" phase—but then plateau for the next five to six sessions with little self-reported improvement. The resumption of improvement in the last three sessions is puzzling because considerable termination anxiety might be expected. Perhaps this finding is partially an artifact of client attrition and missing data. Only 50% of the clients completed five or more session ratings, and only 11% completed all 12 ratings.

Other research has linked client avoidant attachment to therapists with difficulties developing a productive real relationship with the therapist, defined as "the personal relationship existing between two or more people as reflected in the degree to which each is genuine with the other and perceives the other in ways that befit the other" (Gelso, 2004, p. 6). Fuertes et al. (2007) reported that secure attachment to therapist was positively associated with client ratings of real relationship quality. In another study, client self-reported real relationship quality was also negatively related to general client attachment avoidance (assessed with the ECR) but not anxiety (Marmarosh et al., 2009).

Adult Attachment Styles and Client Interpersonal Problems

Not long after Bowlby's (1988) influential writing about attachment and psychotherapy, researchers began to investigate how adult attachment factors might influence client presenting problems. Circumplex models of personality had previously been applied to develop the 64-item client self-report, the Inventory of Interpersonal Problems (IIP; Horowitz et al., 1988). This instrument conceptualizes client perceptions of interpersonal problems in a circumplex structure formed by orthogonal dimensions of affiliation–hostility (depicted on the x-axis) and dominance–submission (depicted on the y-axis). Four regions of the circumplex are defined by the poles of these two dimensions, in clockwise order from 12 o'clock, dominance, affiliation, submission, and hostility.

The IIP instrument yields eight more fine-grained octant dimensions of interpersonal problems defined in this two-dimensional circumplex space. By convention, two-letter codes are used to label the eight octant positions of the IIP as follows, beginning at the 12 o'clock position of the circumplex and moving counterclockwise: Domineering (PA), Vindictive (BC), Cold (DE), Socially Avoidant (FG), Nonassertive (HI), Exploitable (JK), Overly Nurturant (LM), and Intrusive (NO; see Figure 5.3).

In a highly influential study (cited over 250 times in the American Psychological Association PsycInfo database), Horowitz et al. (1993) used trained interviewers to assign one of four adult attachment styles to 77 college students. Subjects then completed the IIP. Results suggested that the interpersonal problems of those classified with a Preoccupied style were centered in the Affiliative–Dominant region, centered on the NO octant of the circumplex. Those classified by interviewers with a Dismissing style reported problems in the hostile half of the circumplex centered on the Cold (DE) octant and including the Vindictive (BC) and Socially Avoidant (FG) octants. Participants classified

FIGURE 5.3. Interpersonal Problems Profiles in Circumplex Space

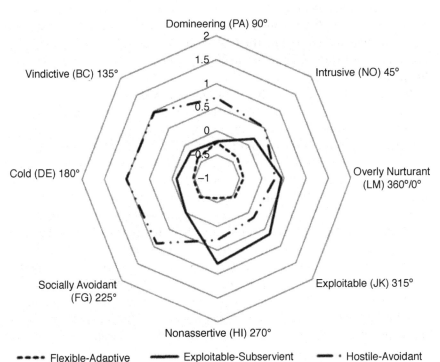

Note. Based on factor scores with a mean = 0 and *SD* = 1. From "Latent Profile Analysis of Interpersonal Problems: Attachment, Basic Psychological Need Frustration, and Psychological Outcomes," by M. Wei, B. Mallinckrodt, B. J. Arterberry, S. Liu, and K. T. Wang, 2021, *Journal of Counseling Psychology*, *68*(4), p. 474 (https://doi.org/10.1037/cou0000551). Copyright 2021 by the American Psychological Association.

as Fearful reported interpersonal problems in three octants centered on the Submissive domain: Socially Avoidant (FG), Nonassertive (HI), and Exploitable (JK). Persons classified as Secure had no extreme octant elevations but tended to have somewhat higher scores on the affiliative half of the circumplex. Note that the sample size for some attachment styles in this study was quite small (Preoccupied, $n = 11$; Dismissing, $n = 14$; Fearful, $n = 16$; Secure, $n = 36$). A recent study (Wei et al., 2021) attempted to build upon this foundation by collecting data from two independent samples of more than 400 undergraduates each. A 32-item version of the IIP was used (Soldz et al., 1995). Latent profile analysis identified three distinct patterns of self-reported interpersonal problems in Study 1 and replicated these profiles in Study 2. Figure 5.3 shows the interpersonal problem patterns in the circumplex factor space found in Study 1 for the three profile groups that Wei et al. (2021) labeled: (a) Flexible-Adaptive, (b) Exploitable-Subservient, and (c) Hostile-Avoidant.

Although Figure 5.3 presents results only for Study 1 ($N = 469$), the pattern was closely replicated in Study 2 ($N = 423$). In both samples, persons with a Flexible–Adaptive profile reported fewer interpersonal problems in every octant; those classified as Exploitable–Subservient reported problems with elevations on the Exploitable and Nonassertive octants, and those classified as Hostile–Avoidant report elevations on the Vindictive, Cold, and Socially Avoidant octants. Although only IIP octant scores were used to classify students into profile groups, correlate variables of the Study 1 students included adult attachment dimensions assessed by the ECR. Using means from the sample data, the attachment configuration of each interpersonal problem profile is plotted in Figure 5.4.

It is reasonable to assume that clients present with the same three profiles of interpersonal problems that Wei et al. (2021) identified, although probably not in the same proportions as in their sample. Taken together, these findings provide some new insights about the interpersonal problems that may be presented by clients with different attachment configurations. Interpersonal theorists (e.g., Kiesler, 1983; Tracey, 1993) emphasize that healthy, adaptive functioning requires flexibility and the capacity to function at times in any sector of the circumplex as circumstances require. (Even hostile responses are necessary for self-protection in some contexts.) Interpersonal problems stem from a rigid inflexibility and limited range of interpersonal responses (Horowitz et al., 1997; Tracey, 2005; Tracey & Rohlfing, 2010). Accordingly, items of the IIP-32 (Soldz et al., 1995) are presented in terms of behaviors clients find too hard to perform and behaviors they perceive engaging in too much. College students with an Exploitable–Subservient profile combine a negative working model of self with a model of others near the border of negative and positive. The distinctive characteristics of this profile identified by Wei et al. include the belief one is too easily persuaded by others, too often taken advantage of by others, and tries too hard to please others. The student also finds it too difficult to express anger, tell others to stop bothering them, be assertive with others, or attend to their own welfare when others are needy. In contrast, students with the Hostile–Avoidant profile of interpersonal problems combine a strongly

FIGURE 5.4. Attachment Configuration of Students With Three Distinct Interpersonal Problems Profiles

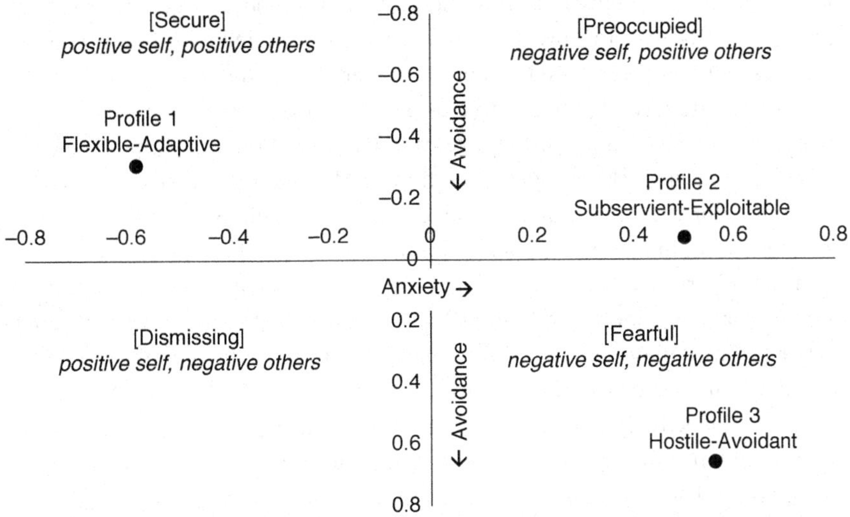

[Secure]
positive self, positive others

[Preoccupied]
negative self, positive others

← Avoidance

Profile 1
Flexible-Adaptive

Profile 2
Subservient-Exploitable

Anxiety →

[Dismissing]
positive self, negative others

[Fearful]
negative self, negative others

← Avoidance

Profile 3
Hostile-Avoidant

Note. From "Latent Profile Analysis of Interpersonal Problems: Attachment, Basic Psychological Need Frustration, and Psychological Outcomes," by M. Wei, B. Mallinckrodt, B. J. Arterberry, S. Liu, and K. T. Wang, 2021, *Journal of Counseling Psychology, 68*(4), p. 476 (https://doi.org/10.1037/cou0000551). Copyright 2021 by the American Psychological Association.

negative working model of self and negative model of others. The distinctive characteristics of this profile, according to Wei et al. are nearly polar opposite on the circumplex from the Exploitable–Subservient profile. Students with a Hostile–Avoidant profile reported that they find it difficult to show affection, experience feelings of love, join groups, introduce themselves to others, be supportive of others, or feel good about another's happiness; and they too often keep others at a distance, seek revenge, and are suspicious of others. Note that the IIP is a self-report instrument. Therefore, clients with high intake scores on subscales such as Cold or Vindictive begin treatment with the realization that they have problems in these areas. Those who are largely oblivious to their interpersonal problems will not exhibit elevated IIP scores.

The recognition that interpersonal perceptions of some individuals, even graduate students in a counseling training program, may differ from the perceptions of peers about the same target person, was the basis for a study (Mallinckrodt & Chen, 2004) that collected "round-robin" data and applied Kenny's (2019) actor–partner social relations model. Although these 76 students were not clients, they were participants in 12 bona fide Yalom-style groups intended to promote interpersonal growth. Participants completed confidentially coded pre-group instruments to assess attachment (ECR) and parental bonds. The Impact Message Inventory-Octant Form (Kiesler & Schmidt, 1991) was used by each group participant to evaluate every other participant in their group at termination (10–12 sessions) with regard to general interpersonal communication style on the circumplex. Variability in perceptions was partitioned into target and perceiver variance and then correlated with self-reports of attachment. According to Kenny's social relations model, target variance is an index of consistency in how a person is perceived by fellow group members. Mallinckrodt and Chen (2004) reported that graduate students who rated their attachment anxiety higher, relative to other graduate trainees in the sample, were perceived as significantly more friendly–dominant and significantly less hostile in their impact messages. (The Impact Message Inventory uses the label "Friendly" for the same quadrant space labeled "Affiliative" by the IIP.) Perceiver variance in Kenny's model is an index of how an individual's perception of target others systematically differs from the group consensus perception of the same targets. Mallinckrodt and Chen suggested that in growth groups, perceiver variance may indicate a kind of transference in which a group member systematically perceives others as, for example, more hostile than other group members collectively perceive the same target. In their study, higher attachment avoidance in a group member, relative to other graduate trainees, was associated with a tendency of that member to perceive all other members as less friendly–submissive, less friendly–dominant, and less dominant than fellow group members viewed the same target members. In practical terms, this suggests that to the extent actual group clients' behavior parallels the graduate students in this study, clients with attachment avoidance may systemically fail to perceive friendly overtures made by fellow members.

Adult Attachment and Client Attachment to Therapist

A meta-analysis of 16 studies published after development of the CATS in 1995 through 2015 reported that the three CATS subscales were significantly associated in expected directions with their general adult attachment dimension counterparts. Specifically, CATS Secure was negatively associated with pretherapy attachment Anxiety and Avoidance, CATS Preoccupied–Anxious was positively associated with pretherapy Anxiety, and CATS Fearful–Avoidant was positively associated with adult attachment Avoidance—but unexpectedly also with adult attachment Anxiety (Mallinckrodt & Jeong, 2015). Thus, there is strong evidence to conclude that clients' pretherapy general orientation toward adult attachment forms a template for their initial attachment to their therapist, as interpersonal approaches to therapy predict (e.g., Teyber & Teyber, 2017). In research linking CATS dimensions with psychotherapy outcome, Sauer et al. (2010) found that CATS Secure scores (but not the other two CATS subscales) were significantly but moderately associated with client symptom improvement at two university training clinics. Wiseman and Tishby (2014) reported that, for clients at a university counseling center in Israel, CATS Preoccupied and Avoidant scores were positively associated with client distress at the 15th week of therapy. Over the first 32 sessions of therapy in this study, CATS Avoidant scores were negatively associated with client improvement. CATS Secure and Preoccupied subscales were unrelated to improvement. Petrowski et al. (2013) gathered CATS and outcome data from over 400 inpatients treated at a university hospital in Germany. At the end of treatment that lasted an average of 62.5 days, CATS Secure scores were positively associated with improvement, whereas both Avoidant and Preoccupied scores were negatively associated with improvement. Differences in the findings of these three studies may have been due to the settings, clinical population, training level of therapists, or the measures of outcome used. The Outcome Questionnaire (Lambert et al., 1996) was used by Sauer et al. (2010) and by Wiseman and Tishby (2014), whereas Petrowski et al. used the German version of the Symptom Check List 90-R (SCL 90-R; Franke, 1995).

Pseudosecure Versus Individuated–Secure Attachment to Therapist

To provide a further explanation for different patterns of CATS subscale correlations with client improvement, Mallinckrodt et al. (2017) distinguished *pseudosecure* from *individuated–secure* attachment to the therapist, the latter of which refers to a genuinely secure attachment. Levy et al. (2006) discussed pseudosecurity in patients who generated seemingly secure attachment narratives that were emotionally contained and coherent, with clear supporting examples when assessed with the Adult Attachment Interview (Main et al., 1985); however, these narratives also manifested multiple less integrated mental models of attachment figures, particularly a lack of forgiveness and deep valuing of the relationship that is characteristic of truly secure adult attachment. Levy et al. (2010) noted the difficulty in distinguishing idealization of the therapist from genuinely positive working alliances in clients with borderline personality features.

Mallinckrodt et al. (2017) speculated that many clients with hyperactivating attachment tendencies also engage in pseudosecure idealization of their therapist, perhaps especially in the early sessions. Pseudosecure clients could be distinguished from other clients though examination of the Preoccupied CATS subscale score in combination with the Secure subscale. Mallinckrodt et al. also indicated that individuated–secure clients cannot be distinguished from pseudosecure clients by the CATS Secure subscale alone because both types of clients report high CATS Secure scores. However, pseudosecure clients also report high Preoccupied CATS subscale scores, whereas individuated–secure clients do not. Perhaps a failure to distinguish these two types of clients explains the low correlations sometimes found between the CATS Secure subscale and measures of client improvement. Items of the CATS Preoccupied scale may capture some of clients' insecure idealization of their therapist. If so, examination of CATS Preoccupied scores as a regression suppressor variable would help disentangle the two types of clients—at least statistically. Specifically, relative to the simple bivariate correlation, the correlations between CATS Secure and client improvement should be significantly higher if the variance due to CATS Preoccupied is removed. In other words, by controlling for CATS Preoccupied scores, "noise" variance due to pseudosecure idealization of the therapist is removed from Secure scores. Mallinckrodt et al.

reanalyzed data from the four available studies of client outcome and CATS subscale scores (Mallinckrodt et al., 2015; Petrowski et al., 2013; Sauer et al., 2010; Wiseman & Tishby, 2014) to investigate these regression suppressor effects. Because the CATS was assessed at multiple time points, there were a total of seven correlations with client improvement reported in these four studies. In six of these seven, significant regression suppressor effects were observed for CATS Preoccupied, lending strong support for distinguishing pseudosecure from individuated–secure client experience of attachment to therapist.

In practical terms, these findings suggest that it is important to distinguish between two types of clients who self-report a highly secure attachment to their therapist. Clients with pseudosecure tendencies idolize their therapist, whereas individuated–secure clients have a more realistically balanced perception. The types can be differentiated by the higher scores pseudosecure clients report on the CATS Preoccupied subscale, relative to individuated–secure clients. The distinction may be important because Mallinckrodt et al.'s (2017) findings suggest that individuated–secure clients may achieve better treatment outcomes. These findings also suggest a further reason for therapists to be alert to signs they are being idealized (at least for the present) by a client. Familiarity with items of the CATS Preoccupied scale may help distinguish between genuine client appreciation and unproductive idealization.

CLIENT CHANGE AND ATTACHMENT-RELATED CORRECTIVE EMOTIONAL EXPERIENCES

This section begins by examining how some experienced therapists respond to clients who hyperactivate or deactivate attachment in the psychotherapy relationship. Next, this section turns to a consideration of how clients might respond to these therapist strategies and perhaps gain a corrective emotional experience.

Therapist Responses to Client Hyperactivation and Deactivation

Daly and Mallinckrodt (2009) interviewed 12 experienced therapists from three widely separated communities who were nominated by their peers as especially effective in working with adult interpersonal relationship concerns. The therapists were presented with two brief case vignettes constructed by converting self-report items of the ECR Anxiety and Avoidance subscales into two sets of client descriptive statements. Thus, the vignettes presented the quintessential features of clients with hyperactivating and deactivating attachment tendencies. To remain gender neutral, the vignettes did not use personal pronouns. In this qualitative study, therapists were asked to report how they would conceptualize each client's presenting issues, engage the client in therapy, manage the therapeutic relationship, and approach working with the client. They were also asked to indicate any specific techniques that might be especially helpful with each client.

Therapeutic Distance

A key feature in the approach described by the experienced therapists in this study was strategic regulation of what Daly and Mallinckrodt (2009) termed *therapeutic distance*, defined as "the level of transparency and disclosure in the psychotherapy relationship from both client and therapist, together with the immediacy, intimacy, and emotional intensity of a session" (p. 559). Therapists acknowledged that in the initial sessions, in order to engage clients and prevent premature termination, they often indulge clients' preferred level of therapeutic distance—very close for attachment hyperactivating clients, quite distant for attachment deactivating clients—although the therapists understood that, ultimately, their stance must change if clients are to benefit from therapy. The therapists interviewed by Daly and Mallinckrodt described gently insisting on less therapeutic distance as markers of progress gradually emerge for clients with deactivating tendencies. For example, therapists pushed for more client self-disclosure and direct focus on presenting problems, invited clients to consider their own role in contributing to these painful patterns, and began to supportively confront clients who only superficially engaged in the sessions. For clients with hyperactivating tendencies, after markers of progress begin to emerge, these therapists described insisting on more therapeutic distance, for example, by gently refusing requests for direct advice and empowering clients to act with more personal agency. This description of therapist strategies is intentionally brief, to maintain a focus on client experience in this chapter. (Note that 10 of the 12 therapists generously allowed the full transcript of their interview to be published as an online supplement to Daly and Mallinckrodt's, 2009, article.)

To understand how clients might experience a therapist who regulates therapeutic distance as described by Daly and Mallinckrodt (2009), I developed a model of the moment-to-moment process in these therapy sessions. The therapeutic gratification, relief, anxiety, and frustration (T-GRAF) model is necessarily reductionistic, but it provides a useful heuristic to understand how clients with hyperactivating and deactivating attachment tendencies might subjectively experience change in therapy (Mallinckrodt, 2010). The model divides client in-session experience into two broad categories involving (a) a desire that the therapist will provide something in the next moments or (b) a fear that the therapist will initiate something in the next moments. Assuming that the therapist is aware of these client hopes and fears, the model allows for two broad categories of therapist responses to these client states: (a) decisions to initiate an in-session activity and (b) decisions to refrain from initiating a possible activity. The 2 × 2 combination of client and therapist categories yields the T-GRAF model, shown in Figure 5.5.

The cells of (A) Gratification and (B) Relief represent in-session moments of low tension because the therapists' decisions are congruent with the clients' wishes. These cells correspond to the initial *engagement* phase of therapy identified by Daly and Mallinckrodt (2009), in which therapists choose to accede to many clients' wishes in the early sessions—close proximity for hyperactivating clients, relative distance for deactivating clients—in order to maintain

FIGURE 5.5. Therapeutic Gratification, Relief, Anxiety, and Frustration Model (T-GRAF)

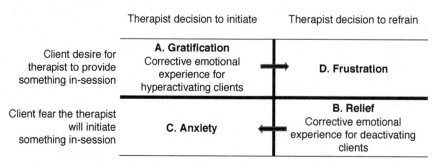

Note. From "The Psychotherapy Relationship as Attachment: Evidence and Implications," by B. Mallinckrodt, 2010, *Journal of Social and Personal Relationships, 27*(2), p. 268 (https://doi.org/10.1177/0265407509360905). Copyright 2010 by SAGE. Reprinted with permission.

enough comfort to prevent premature termination. However, very little change may be possible if clients are never able to move outside these initial, relatively safe positions.

For clients with hyperactivating tendencies, the direction of change involves a shift from Cell A to Cell D in the T-GRAF model—that is, from Gratification (of desires for dependency) toward Frustration—as therapists increasingly refrain from providing direct advice and gradually promote (and insist) on more client autonomy. Interestingly, some of the experienced therapists interviewed by Daly and Mallinckrodt (2009) identified growing client tolerance for frustration as one of the emerging markers signaling that a transition from the engagement phase to the working phase of therapy was now possible. The shift from Cell A to D—that is, from Gratification to Frustration—promotes autonomy and a more equal partnership in the working alliance. Fundamentally, the client's experience is one of the therapist pulling back gradually to open a space that clients learn to fill for themselves, ideally with coping skills; a new capacity for affect regulation; tolerance for solitude; and, ultimately, growing self-efficacy and personal agency.

In contrast, the T-GRAF model posits that the direction of change for clients with deactivating tendencies is from Cell B to Cell C—that is, from Relief to Anxiety—as the therapist seeks to close the initially wide gap of therapeutic distance by increasing the emotional immediacy of sessions. Increasing tolerance for the anxiety of allowing themselves to become more vulnerable with the therapist is one marker that the working phase of therapy is now possible. For these clients, the experienced therapists interviewed by Daly and Mallinckrodt (2009) identified a number of other markers whose emergence indicates a shift is now possible from the engagement to the working phase of therapy. These markers include increased willingness to talk about relationships in specific rather than abstract terms and growing willingness to examine feelings toward relationship partners.

Of course, not only experienced therapists but also those just beginning their careers must work with clients who have attachment insecurities. Relatively novice therapists are quite understandably reluctant to provoke anxiety in their clients with deactivating tendencies by moving from Cell B to C and insisting on more disclosure and introspection in the sessions. Therapists (novice or not) are also understandably reluctant to risk their hyperactivating clients' ire by moving from Cell A to Cell D in their sessions—that is, by increasingly withholding what clients want by frustrating some of their dependency needs. It may help these therapists to see themselves not as withholding support but instead as providing continuing support of a different character that will, ultimately, be more beneficial for their clients.

It is beyond the scope of this chapter to delve into the rich literature focused on how therapist attachment styles might influence the psychotherapy process. However, one conclusion from this body of research might be that therapists' own attachment insecurities can set an upper bound on their capacity to pursue interventions they recognize will cause anxiety for clients with deactivating tendencies and frustration for clients with hyperactivating tendencies. For example, Marmarosh et al. (2014) found that, although therapist attachment style was not significantly directly correlated to client perceptions of the alliance, there were significant interactions between therapist and client attachment anxiety. Client-rated alliance early in treatment was most favorable when client and therapist attachment anxiety were opposite in valence—that is, high-anxiety clients worked best with low-anxiety therapists, and low-anxiety clients worked best with therapists higher in attachment anxiety than their peers. The therapists in this study were all graduate students in training. Some evidence suggests that novice therapists with high attachment anxiety, relative to their peers, may experience more difficulty successful repairing ruptures to the working alliance (Marmarosh et al., 2015).

Corrective Emotional Experiences

A *corrective emotional experience* (CEE) involves interactions in the here and now of the therapy relationship characterized by a new and more satisfactory response to clients' long-standing relationship difficulties (Teyber & Teyber, 2017). Clients' negative expectations formed through long experience in other relationships influence their initial impression of the therapist. Patterns that commonly occur with others are reenacted in the therapy relationship. Ideally, the therapist responds in a new way that provides insight and a healing resolution to these familiar painful patterns (Castonguay & Hill, 2012; Teyber & Teyber, 2017). Thus, the CEE represents a beginning much like the same old painful story experienced repeatedly by a client but concludes with a new, much more satisfying resolution in the therapeutic relationship. When clients' maladaptive patterns are rooted in childhood attachment disappointments and trauma, and are maintained by adult hyperactivating or deactivating tendencies, the CEE necessarily involves elements of establishing a new healthy, secure attachment to the therapist.

A final point from Daly and Mallinckrodt's (2009) interviews with expert therapists should be highlighted. Many noted that for both hyperactivating and deactivating clients, a significant marker of improvement is their willingness to examine the therapy relationship in the here and now. The difficult work of recalibrating the five key elements of attachment—down-regulation for hyperactivating clients and renewed engagement for deactivating clients—must be first performed in clients' relationship with their therapist (see also Teyber & Teyber, 2017). Generalization to other close relationships is only possible after this process has begun. From this perspective, some ruptures in the alliance are inevitable (Muran et al., 2009), perhaps especially when the therapist misjudges the hyperactivating client's tolerance for frustration or the deactivating client's tolerance for anxiety. These ruptures can be repaired if the therapist nondefensively validates the client's feelings, acknowledges the therapist's role in damaging the relationship, and works to resolve the misunderstanding (Safran et al., 2011). Thus, the therapist can respond in ways quite different than previous attachment figures and thereby contribute a new element to the client's corrective emotional experience.

Assessing Clients' Experience of Changing Therapeutic Distance

Mallinckrodt et al. (2015) developed the Therapeutic Distance Scale (TDS) to measure change processes described in the previous section. The instrument is intended to capture four aspects of clients' qualitative experience, each represented by a TDS subscale. In the initial sessions, many clients with hyperactivating tendencies may experience their therapist as (a) Too Distant ("I often feel disappointed with how little help I get from my therapist"). A core feature of the corrective emotional experience for these clients is a sense of (b) Growing Autonomy ("My therapist is helping me to face more challenges on my own"). Clients with deactivating tendencies in the early sessions may experience their therapist as (c) Too Close ("My therapist wants me to reveal too much personal information"). The corrective emotional experience for these clients is a sense of (d) Growing Engagement ("I have formed a much closer connection with my therapist than I expected at the start of therapy"). Appendix 5.2 shows the 36 items of modified the TDS Version 2, organized by subscales intended to capture these four aspects of clients' experience.

Growing Autonomy and Growing Engagement are both signs of significant progress in therapy for clients with hyperactivating or deactivating tendencies, respectively. Specific examples of each type of change are described later in this chapter.

To provide a comprehensive label, this chapter refers to the models developed by Daly and Mallinckrodt (2009) and Mallinckrodt (2010) together as *strategic regulation of therapeutic distance* (SRTD). To test SRTD as a model of change, Mallinckrodt et al. (2017) collected data from 47 clients at a university counseling center who completed the ECR and TDS after the fifth session and from the 34 clients in this sample who terminated after nine to 11 sessions. The first two columns of Table 5.2 show pairs of variables and the nature of

TABLE 5.2. Correlations Between Pretherapy Attachment and In-Session Client Perceptions of Therapeutic Distance and Corrective Emotional Experience

Variable pair	Expected association	Findings $r =$	Hypothesis supported?
All clients at midstage ($N = 47$)			
ECR Avoidance, TDS Too Close	Positive	.31*	yes
ECR Anxiety, TDS Too Distant	Positive	.36*	yes
(ECR Avoidance, TDS Too Distant)	Not significant	(.06)	yes
(ECR Anxiety, TDS Too Close)	Not significant	(.20)	yes
Only clients securely attached to therapist ($n = 17$, above CATS median Secure subscale)			
ECR Avoidance, TDS Growing Engagement	Positive	.60*	yes
ECR Anxiety, TDS Growing Autonomy	Positive	.15*	no
(ECR Avoidance, TDS Growing Autonomy)	Not significant	(–.21)	yes
(ECR Anxiety, TDS Growing Engagement)	Not significant	(.07)	yes

Note. Correlation coefficients in parentheses were not expected to be significant in the strategic regulation of therapeutic distance model. ECR = Experiences in Close Relationship scale; TDS = Therapeutic Distance Scale; CATS = Client Attachment to Therapist Scale. From "Pilot Test of a Measure to Assess Therapeutic Distance and its Association With Client Attachment and Corrective Experience in Therapy," by B. Mallinckrodt, G. Choi, and K. D. Daly, 2015, *Psychotherapy Research, 25*(5), p. 513 (https://doi.org/10.1080/10503307.2014.928755). Copyright 2015 by Taylor & Francis. Adapted with permission.
*$p < .05$.

the association expected if clients experience regulation of therapeutic distance as the SRTD model predicts. Note that for half of these pairings, the model predicts there will *not* be a significant association. These are shown enclosed in parentheses. Table 5.2 shows, as expected, ECR avoidance (a proxy for deactivating attachment tendencies) was significantly associated with client perceptions of their counselor as Too Close but not Too Distant. Also as expected, ECR anxiety (a proxy for hyperactivating attachment tendencies) was significantly associated with client perceptions of their counselor as Too Distant, but not Too Close, as assessed by TDS subscales.

Mallinckrodt et al. (2017) reasoned that only clients above the median in CATS Secure attachment to therapist at termination were likely to have experienced a meaningful corrective emotional experience. As expected, among 17 clients at termination, ECR Avoidance before therapy was significantly associated with the experience of Growing Engagement at termination, but—also as expected—Avoidance was not associated with Growing Autonomy. Contrary to expectations, among the 17 clients most securely attached to their therapist at termination, ECR Anxiety was not significantly associated with Growing Autonomy. Among the full sample of 34 clients remaining at termination regardless of secure attachment to therapist, none of these correlations were significant. Thus, the SRTD model has received some tentative support. Specifically, clients with generalized adult attachment anxiety before therapy do tend to experience their therapist as too distant in the early sessions, whereas clients with generalized adult attachment avoidance tend to experience their therapists initially as too close (Mallinckrodt et al., 2015). These results must be interpreted with a great deal of caution due to the small sample size. However, results of this pilot test support the retest reliability, internal reliability, and preliminary validity of the TDS subscales. Please note that both the CATS and TDS only yield valid data if clients are assured their therapists will never have access to these ratings of the psychotherapy relationship.

An observer-rated version of the Therapeutic Distance Scale (TDS-O; Egozi et al., 2021b) was developed using a sample of 66 university counseling center clients seen weekly for psychodynamic therapy that lasted a median of 14 months. These clients and their 29 therapists completed Relational Anecdote Paradigm (RAP) narratives after the fifth, 15th, and 28th sessions. Each 1-hour RAP interview asked participants to recount 10 "meaningful interactions" with target people (Wiseman & Tishby, 2017). Three of the 10 RAP narratives collected from clients targeted their therapist, and three therapist RAP narratives targeted their clients. Only these RAP data were used to develop the TDS-O. To assess reliability, a pair of raters evaluated 40% of the data in common. Interrater reliability was excellent for each of the four TDS-O subscales.

Because Egozi et al. (2021b) examined both client and therapist perspectives at three time points for four dimensions of therapeutic distance, their results are rich and complex. However, in keeping with the theme of this chapter, only analyses of client perceptions are reported here. Client attachment anxiety at 28 weeks was not related to RAP narratives coded with themes of the therapist being Too Distant at either the fifth or 15th session. Client attachment avoidance at 28 weeks was significantly associated with TDS-O coding of the therapist as Too Close after the fifth and 15th sessions. These findings were based on ECR scores collected, not at intake, but instead at 28 weeks. However, other researchers who used the same data (Wiseman & Tishby, 2014) reported that in a subset of 53% of clients who provided both intake and 28-week ECR data, there were no significant differences in attachment at the two timepoints. Therefore, Egozi et al. (2021b) interpreted 28-week ratings as a proxy for pretreatment levels of attachment. Subsequent analyses of these data (Egozi et al., 2021a) applied growth curve analyses but did not examine client attachment as a covariate. Results suggest that clients, regardless of general attachment insecurity, over the three time points were coded as having decreasing perceptions of their therapist as too distant and increasing perceptions of growing engagement. However, there was no significant change over time in perceptions of therapists as being too close, nor in growing autonomy. In another publication based on these data, Wiseman and Egozi (2021) presented excerpts from RAP interviews that provide richly detailed client narrative accounts of therapists perceived as too close, too distant, and appropriately responsive. Although quite interesting in their own right, these results do not constitute a direct test of the SRTD model because Egozi et al. (2021a) did not directly consider pretherapy client adult attachment and because neither analysis of these data (Egozi et al., 2021a, 2021b) considered secure attachment to the therapist. The SRTD model predicts significant change in Growing Autonomy and Growing Engagement only for clients who manage to establish a secure attachment to their therapist. Nevertheless, the TDS-O proved to be a valuable assessment tool for the data analyzed in these two studies (Egozi et al., 2021a, 2021b). Further research is needed to evaluate the congruence of observer and client ratings of therapeutic distance.

Earned Secure Attachment to the Therapist

Mallinckrodt et al. (2017) suggested the hard work of change for both hyper-activating and deactivating clients involves establishing an "earned secure attachment to therapist." The term "earned secure" has been previously used to describe individuals who manage to develop secure attachments later in life after overcoming early experiences of trauma, unresponsive parenting, or childhood attachment insecurity (Roisman et al., 2002). Many clients begin therapy with difficulties forming healthy secure attachments to others. These difficulties are soon manifested in early attempts to form productive working alliance bonds (Teyber & Teyber, 2017). As clients and their therapists work together to form a secure therapeutic attachment, they must overcome the same challenges the client faces in forming any close attachment; in other words, the client "earns" a more secure attachment to the therapist through this hard work. Such gains can be expected to result eventually in generalized reduction in distress, especially the distress that stems from interpersonal problems.

Before reporting empirical findings, it is necessary to unpack the rather complex concept of earned secure attachment to therapist from a research perspective. As we have seen, individuated–secure attachment at the conclusion of therapy can be assessed by the CATS Secure subscale scores, using multiple regression to partial out variance accounted for by CATS Preoccupied scores. By also partialing out pretherapy generalized attachment insecurity (using separate analyses for ECR Anxiety and ECR Avoidance) two residual gain earned secure scores result, one each representing individuated secure attachment to therapist gained at termination despite pretherapy adult attachment (a) anxiety and (b) avoidance. Mallinckrodt et al. (2017) calculated these indices for the 34 clients who provided termination data in the Mallinckrodt et al. (2015) study. For improvement in symptoms tracked by the Outcome Questionnaire (OQ), neither earned secure attachment coefficient reached significance (Avoidance, $r_{.part} = -.31$, $p = .053$; Anxiety, $r_{.part} = -.24$, $p = .131$). However, with a focus only on improvement in OQ interpersonal relationship symptoms, earned secure attachment despite Avoidance was significant ($r_{.part} = -.36$, $p = .021$) but not earned secure attachment despite Anxiety ($r_{.part} = .04$, $p = .082$). Essentially, these partial regression coefficients track the degree that the client's capacity to form a secure attachment to the therapist by the end of therapy, despite pretherapy attachment insecurity, parallels a reduction in psychological symptoms over the course of treatment.

Although it is possible for clients to improve in general adult attachment security during therapy, many clients may not be able to achieve this result. Taylor et al. (2015) conducted a systematic review of research published through 2012. Of the 14 studies that conducted pre- and posttest assessment of attachment for clients in treatment, 11 indicated some level of client improvement in attachment, and three did not. However, among these 11 studies that indicated improvement, there were subgroups of clients who did not improve significantly in attachment. Despite the daunting challenges these empirical findings suggest, an approach taken in the popular press (e.g., Levine & Heller, 2011) offers considerable hope and encouragement for individuals struggling with the impact of attachment insecurity on their relationships. The gist of this approach is to embrace one's attachment style and realize that it is not necessary to change this fundamental aspect of personality to enjoy satisfying, secure, and enduring relationships. Instead, readers are advised to view their avoidant or anxious attachment as a combination of unique vulnerabilities that can be successfully countered through changes in choices and attitudes but also unique skills that can be leveraged for advantage. For example, the heightened vigilance and exquisite interpersonal perception of persons with anxious tendencies can serve as a protective warning against toxic relationships if the individual also learns to manage maladaptive aspects of their anxiety and need for approval. Similarly, persons with avoidant tendencies have a strong sense of personal agency and self-reliance that can serve them well under stress—but could serve them even better if they also develop a capacity for connection, intimacy, and healthy reliance on others (Levine & Heller, 2011). The key to this hopeful, strengths-based approach seems to be developing an understanding of the vulnerabilities and unique strengths conferred by an attachment style, together with self-acceptance, affect regulation, and adaptation in one's interpersonal world, based on this new knowledge. Empirical evaluation of Levine and Heller's advice would be extremely valuable.

Research is also needed to shed more light on how improvement in attachment security to the therapist, that is, clients' Earned Secure Attachment to Therapist, corresponds to general improvement in emotional and interpersonal functioning and more secure attachment with others (Marmarosh, 2015). Qualitative studies are needed to examine clients' experience of developing a more secure attachment to their therapist, especially for clients with high pretherapy attachment insecurity. Clients with initial attachment insecurity may experience more intense and more frequent alliance ruptures than more securely attached clients—which is also an important empirical question. Qualitative research is needed to reveal whether the fundamental character of the rupture/repair cycle is different for clients with hyperactivating versus deactivation tendencies—especially because these two types of clients differ in holding a positive versus negative working model of others, respectively. Successful repair of these attachment insecurity mediated ruptures may prove to be a key factor for earned secure attachment with the therapist.

CONCLUSION AND FUTURE DIRECTIONS

Fuertes and Williams (2017) called for an increased research focus on the client's experience of therapy. They suggested an analogy to physical fitness, with the therapist likened to a personal trainer and the psychotherapy process to a "psychological gym where the client works out" (p. 370). An actual gym contains equipment for stretching, lifting against resistance, and learning new patterns of movement with the direction and encouragement of the personal trainer. Yet it is the client who must exert effort, endure discomfort, and commit to the regimen. In this analogy, although the therapist plays a vital role, clients' experiences matter more because they do the bulk of the work. Consequently, Fuertes and Williams argued that the power of clients to bring about successful therapy outcomes has been underestimated and is not sufficiently understood. They called for client-focused research to better understand elements of the "psychological workout that clients engage in during therapy" (p. 371).

Viewed through this lens, I hope this chapter has provided a glimpse into the metaphorical "workout gym" for clients who begin therapy with adult attachment insecurities. Specifically, for clients with hyperactivating tendencies, the essential work involves developing new self-management capacities that allow gradual downregulation of all five of the essential features of attachment to more normative levels of activation. For example, clients develop (a) a growing sense of personal agency and capacity to function more autonomously that replaces maladaptive proximity-seeking; (b) an increasing ability to self-soothe, which balances a continuing (but more appropriate) reliance on the therapist as a safe haven; (c) new affect regulation skills that provide a sufficient sense of comfort to permit secure base exploration; (d) confidence that they are in fact far "stronger and wiser" than they previously believed possible; and, finally, (e) an increased capacity to manage the anxiety of termination with new confidence in one's own abilities. Ultimately, the corrective emotional experience for many clients who enter therapy with strong hyperactivating tendencies is the SRTD model concept of Growing Autonomy through a new empowering attachment partnership—first with the therapist and then generalizing to others.

In Fuertes and Williams's (2017) terms, "workouts" for clients with deactivating tendencies involve strengthening underdeveloped capacities in each of the five attachment key components in the psychotherapy relationship. For example, clients must work to develop (a) gradually greater tolerance for proximity and disclosure of here-and-now feelings; (b) increasing willingness to risk vulnerability by soliciting safe haven comfort, first from the therapist and, eventually, with others; (c) growing openness to introspect through secure base exploration of painful experiences and threatening material; (d) relinquishing a need to always be stronger and wiser, while growing in acceptance of a collaborative partnership with the therapist; and (e) allowing the therapist to become a sufficiently meaningful figure so that, when the relationship inevitably ends, there will be a loss to grieve. These changes are the essential features of the SRTD model concept of Growing Engagement.

The therapist's role is similar to that of the personal trainer who does not insist the client use specific workout equipment but instead collaboratively suggests an overall fitness goal and listens carefully to the client's ideas about the best means to achieve the goal. After all, the "Verdict of the Dodo Bird" (Luborsky et al., 2002) applies to the psychotherapy workout gym as well. However, recognizing that all approaches are equally capable of achieving desired goals for clients in general does not eliminate the need to match a particular treatment to the needs of a specific client. Wampold and Imel (2015) pointed out that although the working alliance predicts more variance in treatment outcome than the choice of a particular technique, the alliance consists of tasks and goals as well as bonds. Thus, clients will ideally experience having their therapist explain the importance of developing more secure attachments, first by developing a secure attachment in the here and now of the ongoing therapy relationship and then generalizing these new skills to develop more secure attachments to others. Having agreed on these goals for attachment security, the next phase in the client's experience is developing an agreement with the therapist on the tasks (i.e., the particular workout plan) that is congruent with the client's cultural beliefs and mental health worldview (Grandbois, 2005).

When I share the concepts outlined in this chapter with practicum students, they often ask questions along these lines:

> I will have at most 15 hours of contact with my client before we terminate. On the other hand, the client has experienced thousands—maybe tens of thousands—of hours of contact with unreliable, unresponsive, and often traumatizing attachment figures. How can I possibly hope to counteract the weight of all that negative experience with anything corrective in our relationship?

I close this chapter by relating an allegory I share with these students to suggest something about the client's corrective emotional experience of secure attachment.

Imagine your client exists in a room that contains dozens of small black cloth bags. Somehow, the client understands that their continued survival depends on periodically reaching into a bag and drawing out one of the many egg-sized stones inside. Each stone is colored bone-white and covered with razor sharp spines. Thus, on every occasion, it is quite painful to pull out a stone, and yet survival depends on continuing this process every few hours. There are many such black bags in the room, so in dread of reaching for the next stone, the client begins to try other bags. But the result is always the same—a sharp white stone and a wounding experience repeated over years for hundreds of trials. Under these circumstances, it would be understandable if the client eventually gave up any hope of escaping this dilemma. Then, suddenly, one day, seemingly at random, the client tries yet another bag for the first time and now pulls out a beautiful, smooth, gleaming green stone. In an instant, despite all the weight of previous experience, the client's entire conception of stones, the bag, and perhaps the room itself are profoundly changed by this single counterexample. What the client previously believed with certainty is now, at the least, called into question. Let us further suppose that, over the next few days, this particular black bag yields almost all pleasing green stones and, only very occasionally, a painful white one. Not long afterward, it also yields the key to unlock the room itself. The client scoops up a handful of green stones and, drawing a deep breath, exits into the great unknown beyond the room.

After sharing this allegory, I remind students that they have heard clients make monolithic, all-inclusive statements such as "I can't trust anyone," "I will never be loved," "Only the fittest survive in this cruel world," "Everyone is out to get me," and "I'm a worthless piece of . . ." These all-or-nothing statements are the client's white stones—and, yes, they do accumulate a great weight over many hundreds of trials. But, as a therapist, *you* can prove yourself to be trustworthy for the client, *you* can demonstrate unconditional positive regard, and clients can learn to rely on you as a safe haven and a secure base—no matter what they have experienced from others. And, just to take the pressure off, you do not even need to be consistent. In fact, no counselor could ever maintain a consistently positive therapeutic relationship. Just do your best and trust that good intentions usually count for a very great deal with clients and that you will be able to repair the inevitable relationship ruptures. You can be a green stone, and that will make all the difference.

APPENDIX 5.1
CLIENT ATTACHMENT TO THERAPIST SCALE ITEMS REFLECTING THE SUBJECTIVE EXPERIENCE OF FELT SECURITY, HYPERACTIVATION, OR DEACTIVATION IN THE PSYCHOTHERAPY RELATIONSHIP

Primary secure strategy (13 items)

2. My counselor is sensitive to my needs. (S)
5. My counselor is dependable. (S)
17. I don't know how to expect my counselor to react from session to session. *(S)
34. I feel sure that my counselor will be there if I really need her/him. (S)
27. I feel safe with my counselor. (A)
14. When I show my feelings, my counselor responds in a helpful way. (S)
32. I know my counselor will understand the things that bother me. (S)
8. I feel that somehow things will work out OK for me when I am with my counselor. (S)
29. My counselor is a comforting presence to me when I am upset. (S)
26. My counselor helps me to look closely at the frightening or troubling things that have happened to me. (S)
9. I know I could tell my counselor anything and s/he would not reject me. (A)
20. I can tell that my counselor enjoys working with me. (S)
36. When I'm with my counselor, I feel I am his/her highest priority. (S)

Hyperactivation secondary strategy (15 items)

1. I don't get enough emotional support from my counselor. (S)
11. My counselor isn't giving me enough attention. (S)
10. I would like my counselor to feel closer to me. (P)
22. I wish there were a way I could spend more time with my counselor. (P)

7. I wish my counselor could be with me on a daily basis.   (P)

4. I yearn to be "at one" with my counselor.   (P)

23. I resent having to handle problems on my own when my counselor could be more helpful.   (S)

18. Sometimes I'm afraid that if I don't please my counselor, s/he will reject me.   (A)

3. I think my counselor disapproves of me.   (A)

13. I'd like to know more about my counselor as a person.   (P)

16. I think about calling my counselor at home.   (P)

19. I think about being my counselor's favorite client.   (P)

31. I often wonder about my counselor's other clients.   (P)

25. I wish I could do something for my counselor too.   (P)

28. I wish my counselor were not my counselor so that we could be friends.   (P)

Deactivation secondary strategy (eight items)

6. Talking over my problems with my counselor makes me feel ashamed or foolish.   (A)

12. I don't like to share my feelings with my counselor.   (A)

15. I feel humiliated in my counseling sessions.   (A)

24. My counselor wants to know more about me than I am comfortable talking about.   (A)

30. My counselor treats me more like a child than an adult.   (A)

33. It's hard for me to trust my counselor.   (A)

21. I suspect my counselor probably isn't honest with me.   (A)

35. I'm not certain that my counselor is all that concerned about me.   (A)

Note. S = CATS Secure subscale item, A = CATS Avoidant subscale item, P = CATS Preoccupied subscale item.
* Reverse keyed

APPENDIX 5.2
THERAPEUTIC DISTANCE SCALE VERSION 2.0

Too Distant

2. My therapist is not nearly as helpful as she/he could be.

6. I need a lot more from my therapist than I am getting.

10. There are times when my therapist seems cold and personally distant.

14. I sometimes feel frustrated with my therapist.

*18. My therapist has been very helpful so far.

22. I often feel disappointed with how little help I get from my therapist.

26. I don't have the sense of connection with my therapist that I need.

30. I have felt abandoned by my therapist when I needed help the most.

32. I wish my therapist had a closer relationship with me.

Growing Autonomy

3. As a result of therapy, I am able to handle situations more often without help from others.

7. My therapist is helping me to face more challenges on my own.

11. I realize that sometimes my therapist withholds something I want from her/him because it would be better for me to learn to do it for myself.

15. My therapist helps me to generate my own solutions instead of telling me what I should do.

19. My therapist is helping me to become a more independent and self-reliant person.

23. My therapist encourages my autonomy.

*27. Much of the time in the past 2 weeks I have felt overwhelmed or helpless.

*31. My therapist has done little to help me gain confidence in my own abilities.

*35. Much of the time in the past 2 weeks I wanted someone stronger and wiser to tell me how to solve my problems.

Too Close

1. My therapist is pushing me way too hard.

*5. My therapist respects my need to keep some things private.

9. I need to take things at a slower pace, but my therapist does not understand this.

13. Before a session starts, I often worry very much about what is about to happen.

17. My therapist wants me to reveal too much personal information.

*21. My therapist does not insist on pursuing a topic if I don't want to go there.

25. I would prefer a therapist who works without insisting on such a close relationship with me.

29. My therapist insists on talking about topics I do not feel safe discussing.

33. In some sessions I feel as though my therapist insists on invading my privacy.

Growing Engagement

4. My therapy sessions are not as stressful as I thought they would be.

8. My therapist provides a safe place for me to discuss some upsetting topics.

12. I have been able to put aside most of the worries I had at first about what therapy would be like.

16. My therapist has helped me feel more relaxed and comfortable to talk about very personal topics.

20. Sometimes I am surprised by how much I have learned to trust my therapist.

24. I am relieved that most of my worries about what might happen in therapy have not come true.

28. As time passes in therapy, I have grown quite a bit more comfortable talking about things that I rarely, if ever, discuss with others.

32. I have formed a much closer connection with my therapist than I expected at the start of therapy.

36. There are not many people I trust as much as I have grown to trust my therapist.

Note. *reverse keyed

REFERENCES

Ainsworth, M. D. S., Blehar, M. C., Waters, E., & Wall, S. (1978). *Patterns of attachment: A psychological study of the strange situation*. Erlbaum.

Bartholomew, K., & Horowitz, L. M. (1991). Attachment styles among young adults: A test of a four-category model. *Journal of Personality and Social Psychology, 61*(2), 226–244. https://doi.org/10.1037/0022-3514.61.2.226

Bernecker, S. L., Levy, K. N., & Ellison, W. D. (2014). A meta-analysis of the relation between patient adult attachment style and the working alliance. *Psychotherapy Research, 24*(1), 12–24.

Bowlby, J. (1973). *Attachment and loss: Vol. 2. Separation: Anxiety and anger*. Basic Books.

Bowlby, J. (1982). *Attachment and loss: Vol. 1. Attachment* (2nd ed.). Basic Books. (Original work published 1969)

Bowlby, J. (1988). *A secure base: Parent-child attachment and healthy human development*. Routledge.

Brennan, K. A., Clark, C. L., & Shaver, P. R. (1988). Self-report measurement of adult attachment: An integrative overview. In J. A. Simpson & W. S. Rholes (Eds.), *Attachment theory and close relationships* (pp. 46–76). Guilford Press.

Castonguay, L. G., & Hill, C. E. (Eds.). (2012). *Transformation in psychotherapy: Corrective experiences across cognitive behavioral, humanistic, and psychodynamic approaches*. American Psychological Association. https://doi.org/10.1037/13747-000

Daly, K. D., & Mallinckrodt, B. (2009). Expert therapists' approaches to psychotherapy with adult clients who present with attachment avoidance or anxiety. *Journal of Counseling Psychology, 56*(4), 549–563. https://doi.org/10.1037/a0016695

Daniel, S. I. F. (2006). Adult attachment patterns and individual psychotherapy: A review. *Clinical Psychology Review, 26*(8), 968–984. https://doi.org/10.1016/j.cpr.2006.02.001

Diener, M. J., & Monroe, J. M. (2011). The relationship between adult attachment style and therapeutic alliance in individual psychotherapy: A meta-analytic review. *Psychotherapy, 48*(3), 237–248. https://doi.org/10.1037/a0022425

Egozi, S., Tishby, O., & Wiseman, H. (2021a). Changes in clients' and therapists' experiences of therapeutic distance during psychodynamic therapy. *Journal of Clinical Psychology, 77*(4), 910–926. https://doi.org/10.1002/jclp.23077

Egozi, S., Tishby, O., & Wiseman, H. (2021b). Therapeutic distance in client–therapist narratives: Client attachment, therapist attachment, and dyadic effects. *Psychotherapy Research, 31*(8), 963–976. Advance online publication. https://doi.org/10.1080/10503307.2021.1874069

Fraley, R. C., & Waller, N. G. (1998). Adult attachment patterns: A test of the typological model. In J. A. Simpson & W. S. Rholes (Eds.), *Attachment theory and close relationships* (pp. 77–114). Guilford Press.

Franke, G. (1995). SCL-90-R. Die symptom checkliste von Derogatis. [SCL-90-R. The symptom-checklist by Derogatis]. *Zeitschrift für Klinische Psychologie, 26*, 77–79.

Fuertes, J. N., Mislowack, A., Brown, S., Gur-Arie, S., Wilkinson, S., & Gelso, C. J. (2007). Correlates of the real relationship in psychotherapy: A study of dyads. *Psychotherapy Research, 17*(4), 423–430. https://doi.org/10.1080/10503300600789189

Fuertes, J. N., & Williams, E. N. (2017). Client-focused psychotherapy research. *Journal of Counseling Psychology, 64*(4), 369–375. https://doi.org/10.1037/cou0000214

Gelso, C. J. (2004, June). *A theory of the real relationship in psychotherapy.* [Paper presentation]. International Conference of the Society for Psychotherapy Research, Rome, Italy.

Grandbois, D. (2005). Stigma of mental illness among American Indian and Alaska Native nations: Historical and contemporary perspectives. *Issues in Mental Health Nursing, 26*(10), 1001–1024. https://doi.org/10.1080/01612840500280661

Horowitz, L. M., Dryer, D. C., & Krasnoperova, E. N. (1997). The circumplex structure of interpersonal problems. In R. Plutchik & H. R. Conte (Eds.), *Circumplex models of personality and emotions* (pp. 347–384). American Psychological Association. https://doi.org/10.1037/10261-015

Horowitz, L. M., Rosenberg, S. E., Baer, B. A., Ureño, G., & Villaseñor, V. S. (1988). Inventory of interpersonal problems: Psychometric properties and clinical applications. *Journal of Consulting and Clinical Psychology, 56*(6), 885–892. https://doi.org/10.1037/0022-006X.56.6.885

Horowitz, L. M., Rosenberg, S. E., & Bartholomew, K. (1993). Interpersonal problems, attachment styles, and outcome in brief dynamic psychotherapy. *Journal of Consulting and Clinical Psychology, 61*(4), 549–560. https://doi.org/10.1037/0022-006X.61.4.549

Jeong, J.-S., Mallinckrodt, B., & Baldwin, D. R. (2021). *Attachment hyperactivation and deactivation: Emotional intelligence, affect regulation, and divergence between self-reported distress and salivary cortisol* [Manuscript submitted for publication].

Joyce, A. S., Piper, W. E., Ogrodniczuk, J. S., & Klein, R. H. (2007). Patient characteristics and variations in termination processes and outcomes. In A. S. Joyce, W. E. Piper, J. S. Ogrodniczuk, & R. H. Klein, *Termination in psychotherapy: A psychodynamic model of processes and outcomes* (pp. 109–131). American Psychological Association. https://doi.org/10.1037/11545-006

Kenny, D. A. (2019). *Interpersonal perception* (2nd ed.). Guilford Press.

Kiesler, D. J. (1983). The 1982 Interpersonal Circle: A taxonomy for complementarity in human transactions. *Psychological Review, 90*(3), 185–214. https://doi.org/10.1037/0033-295X.90.3.185

Kiesler, D. J., & Schmidt, J. A. (1991). *Octant scale version of the Impact Message Inventory: Form IIA.* Mind Garden.

Kinsler, P. J., Courtois, C. A., & Frankel, A. S. (2009). Therapeutic alliance and risk management. In C. A. Courtois & J. D. Ford (Eds.), *Treating complex traumatic stress disorders: An evidence-based guide* (pp. 183–201). Guilford Press.

Lambert, M. J., Hansen, N. B., Umpress, V., Lunnen, K., Okiishi, J., & Burlingame, G. M. (1996). *Administration and scoring manual for the OQ-45.2.* American Processional Credentialing Services LLC.

Levine, A., & Heller, R. (2011). *Attached: The new science of adult attachment and how it can help you find—and keep—love.* Penguin Random House.

Levy, K. N., Beeney, J. E., Wasserman, R. H., & Clarkin, J. F. (2010). Conflict begets conflict: Executive control, mental state vacillations, and the therapeutic alliance in treatment of borderline personality disorder. *Psychotherapy Research, 20*(4), 413–422. https://doi.org/10.1080/10503301003636696

Levy, K. N., Johnson, B. N., Gooch, C. V., & Kivity, Y. (2019). Attachment style. In J. C. Norcross & B. E. Wampold (Eds.), *Psychotherapy relationships that work: Vol. 2. Evidence-based therapist responsiveness* (3rd ed., pp. 15–55). Oxford University Press.

Levy, K. N., Kivity, Y., Johnson, B. N., & Gooch, C. V. (2018). Adult attachment as a predictor and moderator of psychotherapy outcome: A meta-analysis. *Journal of Clinical Psychology, 74*(11), 1996–2013. https://doi.org/10.1002/jclp.22685

Levy, K. N., Meehan, K. B., Kelly, K. M., Reynoso, J. S., Weber, M., Clarkin, J. F., & Kernberg, O. F. (2006). Change in attachment patterns and reflective function in a randomized control trial of transference-focused psychotherapy for borderline personality disorder. *Journal of Consulting and Clinical Psychology, 74*(6), 1027–1040. https://doi.org/10.1037/0022-006X.74.6.1027

Luborsky, L., Rosenthal, R., Diguer, L., Andrusyna, T. P., Berman, J. S., Levit, J. T., Seligman, D. A., & Drause, E. D. (2002). The dodo bird verdict is alive and well— mostly. *Clinical Psychology: Science and Practice, 9*(1), 2–12. https://doi.org/10.1093/clipsy.9.1.2

Main, M., & Hesse, E. (1990). Parents' unresolved traumatic experiences are related to infant disorganized attachment status: Is frightened and/or frightening parental behavior the linking mechanism? In M. T. Greenberg, D. Cicchetti, & E. M. Cummings (Eds.), *Attachment in the preschool years: Theory, research and intervention* (pp. 161–182). University of Chicago Press.

Main, M., Kaplan, N., & Cassidy, J. (1985). Security in infancy, childhood, and adult- hood: A move to the level of representation. *Monographs of the Society for Research in Child Development, 50*(1/2), 66–104. https://doi.org/10.2307/3333827

Mallinckrodt, B. (2010). The psychotherapy relationship as attachment: Evidence and implications. *Journal of Social and Personal Relationships, 27*(2), 262–270. https://doi.org/10.1177/0265407509360905

Mallinckrodt, B., Anderson, M. Z., Choi, G., Levy, K. N., Petrowski, K., Sauer, E. M., Tishby, O., & Wiseman, H. (2017). Pseudosecure vs. individuated-secure client attach- ment to therapist: Implications for therapy process and outcome. *Psychotherapy Research, 27*(6), 677–691. https://doi.org/10.1080/10503307.2016.1152411

Mallinckrodt, B., & Chen, E. C. (2004). Attachment and interpersonal impact percep- tions of group members: A Social Relations Model analysis of transference. *Psycho- therapy Research, 14*(2), 210–230. https://doi.org/10.1093/ptr/kph018

Mallinckrodt, B., Choi, G., & Daly, K. D. (2015). Pilot test of a measure to assess therapeutic distance and its association with client attachment and corrective expe- rience in therapy. *Psychotherapy Research, 25*(5), 505–517. https://doi.org/10.1080/10503307.2014.928755

Mallinckrodt, B., Gantt, D. L., & Coble, H. M. (1995). Attachment patterns in the psychotherapy relationship: Development of the Client Attachment to Therapist Scale. *Journal of Counseling Psychology, 42*(3), 307–317. https://doi.org/10.1037/0022-0167.42.3.307

Mallinckrodt, B., & Jeong, J. (2015). Meta-analysis of client attachment to therapist: Associations with working alliance and client pretherapy attachment. *Psychotherapy, 52*(1), 134–139. https://doi.org/10.1037/a0036890

Mallinckrodt, B., Porter, M. J., & Kivlighan, D. M., Jr. (2005). Client attachment to therapist, depth of in-session exploration, and object relations in brief psychother- apy. *Psychotherapy: Theory, Research, & Practice, 42*(1), 85–100. https://doi.org/10.1037/0033-3204.42.1.85

Marmarosh, C. L. (2015). Emphasizing the complexity of the relationship: The next decade of attachment-based psychotherapy research. *Psychotherapy, 52*(1), 12–18. https://doi.org/10.1037/a0036504

Marmarosh, C. L., Gelso, C. J., Markin, R. D., Majors, R., Mallery, C., & Choi, J. (2009). The real relationship in psychotherapy: Relationships to adult attachments, working alliance, transference, and therapy outcome. *Journal of Counseling Psychology, 56*(3), 337–350. https://doi.org/10.1037/a0015169

Marmarosh, C. L., Kivlighan, D. M., Jr., Bieri, K., LaFauci Schutt, J. M., Barone, C., & Choi, J. (2014). The insecure psychotherapy base: Using client and therapist attach- ment styles to understand the early alliance. *Psychotherapy, 51*(3), 404–412. https://doi.org/10.1037/a0031989

Marmarosh, C. L., Schmidt, E., Pembleton, J., Rotbart, E., Muzyk, N., Liner, A., Reid, L., Margolies, A., Joseph, M., & Salmen, K. (2015). Novice therapist attachment and perceived ruptures and repairs: A pilot study. *Psychotherapy, 52*(1), 140–144. https://doi.org/10.1037/a0036129

Mikulincer, M., & Shaver, P. R. (2016). *Attachment in adulthood: Structure, dynamics, and change* (2nd ed.). Guilford Press.

Mikulincer, M., & Shaver, P. R. (2019). Attachment orientations and emotion regulation. *Current Opinion in Psychology, 25*(1), 6–10. https://doi.org/10.1016/j.copsyc.2018.02.006

Muran, J. C., Safran, J. D., Gorman, B. S., Samstag, L. W., Eubanks-Carter, C., & Winston, A. (2009). The relationship of early alliance ruptures and their resolution to process and outcome in three time-limited psychotherapies for personality disorders. *Psychotherapy, 46*(2), 233–248. https://doi.org/10.1037/a0016085

Obegi, J. H., & Berant, E. (Eds.). (2009). *Attachment theory and research in clinical work with adults*. Guilford Press.

Petrowski, K., Pokorny, D., Nowacki, K., & Buchheim, A. (2013). The therapist's attachment representation and the patient's attachment to the therapist. *Psychotherapy Research, 23*(1), 25–34. https://doi.org/10.1080/10503307.2012.717307

Roisman, G. L., Padrón, E., Sroufe, L. A., & Egeland, B. (2002). Earned-secure attachment status in retrospect and prospect. *Child Development, 73*(4), 1204–1219. https://doi.org/10.1111/1467-8624.00467

Romano, V., Fitzpatrick, M., & Janzen, J. (2008). The secure-base hypothesis: Global attachment, attachment to counselor, and session exploration in psychotherapy. *Journal of Counseling Psychology, 55*(4), 495–504. https://doi.org/10.1037/a0013721

Safran, J. D., Muran, J. C., & Eubanks-Carter, C. (2011). Repairing alliance ruptures. *Psychotherapy, 48*(1), 80–87. https://doi.org/10.1037/a0022140

Sauer, E. M., Anderson, M. Z., Gormley, B., Richmond, C. J., & Preacco, L. (2010). Client attachment orientations, working alliances, and responses to therapy: A psychology training clinic study. *Psychotherapy Research, 20*(6), 702–711. https://doi.org/10.1080/10503307.2010.518635

Soldz, S., Budman, S., Demby, A., & Merry, J. (1995). A short form of the Inventory of Interpersonal Problems Circumplex scales. *Assessment, 2*(1), 53–63. https://doi.org/10.1177/1073191195002001006

Taylor, P., Rietzschel, J., Danquah, A., & Berry, K. (2015). Changes in attachment representations during psychological therapy. *Psychotherapy Research, 25*(2), 222–238. https://doi.org/10.1080/10503307.2014.886791

Teyber, E., & Teyber, F. H. (2017). *Interpersonal process in therapy: An integrative model* (7th ed.). Cengage Learning.

Tracey, T. J. (1993). An interpersonal stage model of the therapeutic process. *Journal of Counseling Psychology, 40*(4), 396–409. https://doi.org/10.1037/0022-0167.40.4.396

Tracey, T. J. G. (2005). Interpersonal rigidity and complementarity. *Journal of Research in Personality, 39*(6), 592–614. https://doi.org/10.1016/j.jrp.2004.12.001

Tracey, T. J. G., & Rohlfing, J. E. (2010). Variations in the understanding of interpersonal behavior: Adherence to the interpersonal circle as a moderator of the rigidity-psychological well-being relation. *Journal of Personality, 78*(2), 711–746. https://doi.org/10.1111/j.1467-6494.2010.00631.x

Vogel, D. L., & Wei, M. (2005). Adult attachment and help-seeking intent: The mediating roles of psychological distress and perceived social support. *Journal of Counseling Psychology, 52*(3), 347–357. https://doi.org/10.1037/0022-0167.52.3.347

Wampold, B. E., & Imel, Z. E. (2015). *The great psychotherapy debate: The research evidence for what works in psychotherapy* (2nd ed.). Routledge. https://doi.org/10.4324/9780203582015

Wei, M., Mallinckrodt, B., Arterberry, B. J., Liu, S., & Wang, K. T. (2021). Latent profile analysis of interpersonal problems: Attachment, basic psychological need frustration, and psychological outcomes. *Journal of Counseling Psychology, 68*(4), 467–488. https://doi.org/10.1037/cou0000551

Wiseman, H., & Egozi, S. (2021). Attachment theory as a framework for responsiveness in psychotherapy. In J. C. Watson & H. Wiseman (Eds.), *The responsive psychotherapist:*

Attuning to clients in the moment (pp. 59–82). American Psychological Association. https://doi.org/10.1037/0000240-004

Wiseman, H., & Tishby, O. (2014). Client attachment, attachment to the therapist and client–therapist attachment match: How do they relate to change in psychodynamic psychotherapy? *Psychotherapy Research, 24*(3), 392–406. https://doi.org/10.1080/10503307.2014.892646

Wiseman, H., & Tishby, O. (2017). Applying relationship anecdotes paradigm interviews to study client–therapist relationship narratives: Core conflictual relationship theme analyses. *Psychotherapy Research, 27*(3), 283–299. https://doi.org/10.1080/10503307.2016.1271958

Woodhouse, S. S., Schlosser, L. Z., Crook, R. E., Ligiéro, D. P., & Gelso, C. J. (2003). Client attachment to therapist: Relations to transference and client recollections of parental caregiving. *Journal of Counseling Psychology, 50*(4), 395–408. https://doi.org/10.1037/0022-0167.50.4.395

6

Clients' Agentic and Self-Healing Activities in Psychotherapy

Amy Greaves

The work being done on your marriage, are you having it done, or are you doing it yourselves?
—MICHAEL MASLIN, CARTOON PUBLISHED IN *THE NEW YORKER*, JUNE 19, 1989

Years ago, a radical new treatment for cancer was introduced, chemotherapy, which somewhat indiscriminately targets cancer cells (along with other fast-growing cells) in hopes that the cancer will die quicker than the patient. Another treatment, a bone marrow transplant, relies on the body's ability to replace its own destroyed marrow with healthy stem cells from carefully matched donors; these stem cells revitalize the body as they reproduce and grow into healthy blood cells, allowing doctors to administer heavier doses of chemotherapy. The donor stem cells may also have T cells that are more suited to attack the cancer. In more recent years, a new cancer treatment was introduced, immunotherapy, which utilizes a person's innate immune system to better fight cancer. For instance, one type of immunotherapy targets checkpoint receptors on the T cell (which can falsely identify a cancer cell as being healthy and thus attenuate the immune response). By blocking these molecules on the T cell, the immune system can unleash a much stronger response to cancer. In another

Portions of this chapter are from *The Active Client: A Qualitative Analysis of Thirteen Clients' Contribution to the Psychotherapeutic Process* [Unpublished doctoral dissertation], by A. L. Greaves, 2006, University of Southern California. Copyright 2006 by A. L. Greaves. Reprinted with permission.

https://doi.org/10.1037/0000303-007
The Other Side of Psychotherapy: Understanding Clients' Experiences and Contributions in Treatment, J. N. Fuertes (Editor)

immunotherapy, the patient's T cells are removed, genetically reprogrammed in the laboratory to better enable the T cell to recognize cancer cells, and then the T cells are infused back into the body and attack the cancer more efficiently (see American Society of Clinical Oncology, 2016).

In all these cases, the body's wisdom is harnessed to discover and implement the treatment at a cellular and systemic level. The parallels to psychotherapy are interesting in terms of potent interventions, foreign donors, and co-opting, retraining, blocking, and magnifying innate processes that result in healthier individuals. Tailored interventions based on an intricate understanding of a person's superpowers and vulnerabilities will result in more virile and fertile treatments with the least deleterious side effects. While comparing cancer treatment with psychotherapy may have its limitations, there are corollaries in the idea that the most revolutionary treatments will honor humans' salutary ability to heal.

We know that therapy works, but as Bohart and Tallman (Chapter 1, this volume) assert, the client works as well. To bolster their thesis that clients are heroes, too, we need only to look to some of our own researchers. We have many mental health scientist–practitioners to thank who advanced the field because of their insight into what works—insight they derived as survivors of mental health issues. Francine Shapiro (2013), the creator of eye movement desensitization and reprocessing therapy (EMDR), was walking in the park in 1987 and, while worrying about a particular issue in her life, noticed that her eyes were darting side to side in quick succession. This behavior was not something she intended to do, yet when she returned to thinking about that same issue, she noticed that the topic did not have the same intensity as before the eye phenomenon. She recounted, "Luckily, I'd been using my own mind and body as a 'laboratory' for the previous ten years after a bout with cancer" (Shapiro, 2013, p. 24). Marsha Linehan (2020) spent years in an inpatient facility and created dialectical behavior therapy (DBT) as an outgrowth from her experiences of what worked for her. She wrote that she was once asked by her clients, "Are you one of us?" She responded, "You mean have I suffered?" The response was, "No, Marsha . . . I mean one of us. Like us. Because if you were, it would give all of us so much hope." The answer is yes: Marsha was one of them, and in that fact lies quite a bit of hope for therapist and client alike!

Clients are uniquely attuned to their problems and just might have the ingenuity to create a befitting cure, just as Dr. Linehan did. Now, we can say that Dr. Shapiro and Dr. Linehan are extraordinary, but it does make one wonder what extraordinary processes are at work inside our own clients. Carl Rogers (1964) talked about an organismic valuing process that grounded his work with clients, counting on the fact that there was a mental health corollary to the body's innate healing processes just described. What could happen if psychotherapy practitioners, researchers, and consumers accounted for the healing capacities and unique contributions of psychotherapy clients? What if clients' self-healing tendencies were catered to as the fuel source of psychotherapy? Co-opting this ability of clients to heal may be key in reducing treatment duration, reaching different populations, and increasing the breadth of treatment success.

In this chapter, I present a four-dimensional model of client self-healing that highlights the processes and activities that clients engage in during therapy, which are often invisible to therapists and even to the clients themselves. The hope is that therapists can better recognize these self-healing capabilities and help clients notice them and capitalize on them as well.

TURNING THE PARADIGM ON ITS HEAD

If a client spends 1 hour a week in therapy, that is less than 1% of a client's healing time that week. This percentage puts into perspective the extraordinarily limited amount of time the client will be interacting directly with the therapist during a course of treatment and highlights the idea that clients put to use all sorts of people and activities in their quest to feel relief and experience more fulfillment in their lives. For much of the world, psychotherapy remains out of reach as a resource for healing due to the cost of therapy, access to trained professionals in rural or underdeveloped nations, or the constraints of the cultural taboo of turning to a therapist (Cohen Veterans Network & National Council for Behavioral Health, 2018). For those who do access psychotherapy, the average course of therapy is about nine hourly sessions and only 15 to 20 sessions to see clinically significant gains (Lambert, 2013).

When clients are not sitting across from a therapist, they are using a vast array of other modalities. Some are using a socially situated healing practice (Wampold & Imel, 2015) where family and friends help them resolve a problem. Others consult with a spiritual or indigenous healer (Wampold, 2017), attend peer-support groups (Kelly & Yeterian, 2012), consult with a deity (Puchalska-Wasyl & Zarzycka, 2020), or use social media to learn from others but also create content themselves to share how they are conquering mental health struggles (Sangeorzan et al., 2019).

I have had clients volunteer for projects, serving people in similar predicaments (see Biggs et al., 2019). They leave friend groups and form new ones, move to get a fresh start, apply for a new job, go back to college, develop a new hobby, form a single mother's group, sign up for a dating website, adopt a pet, reconnect with their religion, visit a parent's grave, start a nonprofit to address issues they are passionate about, and so on—all socially derived healing adjuncts that I never thought to recommend to them. I have seen my clients derive healing from participating in creative endeavors like making art, writing an autobiography, singing their theme song, rapping about their pain, writing comedy scripts, and acting professionally in ways that transfigured their rocky past. Other creative self-healing activities tap into the body's healing movement like yoga, martial arts, or dancing spontaneously (see van der Kolk, 2014). Even without invoking conscious thought, the body can unlock potentiated energy in the vagal system through means such as yawning, sighing, smelling pleasant aromas, or petting a cat (see Porges, 2011).

My clients have taken up reflective activities such as meditation and gratitude practices and adventurous activities such as ascending heights through ambulatory or aeronautical means to gain expansive perspectives. They have also engaged in confrontational practices such as facing and forgiving a loved one, filing a harassment lawsuit, or leaning into a fear of needles to get vaccinated to fulfill a dream of volunteering in Africa—all examples of ways my clients have endeavored to heal in ways unprompted by therapy. All of this is important to hold in mind as we research the psychotherapy process and client–therapist interplay. If we as researchers, producers, and even consumers of psychotherapy don't attend to the 99% of what clients are doing when they are not in the room with us, we will surely miss out on opportunities to discover, tap into, piggyback onto, reinforce, or amplify people's agentic activities that are extensions of the innate yearning for wholeness.

OVERVIEW OF CLIENT SELF-HEALING IN THERAPY

There is a call for psychotherapy research to include more process-oriented research (Crits-Christoph et al., 2013). Emphasis on tracking the client's contribution to the change process has been underwhelming compared with the attention that has been given to therapist participation (Bohart & Wade, 2013). Various reasons, including training needs and the advancement of the counseling profession, might account for this imbalance in the body of research. Several significant limitations apply to the current body of literature on client process variables. First, there is a disparity of attention paid to client processes that represent their views and contributions to therapy. Second, there is a reactive quality in how many categories are framed, suggesting that the presumed causality is unidirectional and initiates with the therapist. Third, client process measurements vary significantly in their design to capture intentionality or active versus just receptive client processes (see Gaston, 1991; Hill et al., 2001; Honos-Webb et al., 2003; Klein et al., 1986; Rice & Kerr, 1986; Stiles, 1986; Suh et al., 1989; Toukmanian, 1986). While intentionality may be hard to deduce, the trade-off in using these measures comes at the price of providing data about the meaning-filled process of psychotherapy. Finally, process measures generally attempt to represent the full range of client activities with relatively few categories, and thus rich content is collapsed into a more generic taxonomy. This may make the process measure easier to use by external raters, but the descriptive thinness of the categories impacts the epistemological breadth that can be obtained by such categorical collapsing of the phenomena under investigation.

This chapter represents the subject and findings from my dissertation, which I have advanced and refined over the years of full-time clinical practice and part-time research activities. I studied and created a taxonomy of four main categories to describe the microprocesses of clients in psychotherapy (Greaves, 2006). The qualitative analysis involved 13 clients who ranged in age from 18 to 63 and only one of whom identified their ethnicity (as Mexican American). There were seven therapists, all in graduate training, who engaged in supportive therapy and insight-oriented therapy, implementing gestalt and cognitive-behavioral techniques. Only two of the therapists gave their ages, 39 and 43 years old. I also used my own client records and reflection memos to expand my empathy for the phenomenon under study, an advisable practice in qualitative analysis (Rhodes et al., 1994). As I reviewed the notes and the 70 transcripts, I focused solely on how the clients were active and agentic in ways that seemed to promote their healing. I asked the following questions:

1. How do these clients' activities contribute to the nature and quality of the therapeutic relationship?

2. How do these clients' creativity or agency evidence itself in the therapeutic process?

3. How do these clients assert themselves despite power differences in their prescribed roles?

4. How do these clients collaborate with therapists in pursuing the process of change? (Greaves, 2006, p. 89)

I used an ethnographic approach like the one used by Bohart and Brock (2003); I put myself in the position of the client, curious about how their words and actions aligned with stated goals and how the client's activities might culminate in healing outcomes. I also put myself in the role of the therapist, imagining the effect certain dialogue would have on my own internal process. From the textual analysis, I created 767 codes, organizing these into hierarchies of superordinate and subordinate themes based on hypothesized conceptual relationships. The result is a taxonomy composed of four global client dimensions of self-healing, and within each are related therapy processes (a total of 21) and 66 activities that the client engages in that promote healing. The four dimensions and their related self-healing processes are listed in Table 6.1. All the clinical examples are actual statements from the clients and therapists and are included to highlight each identified dimension, process, or activity.[1]

In framing the taxonomy, four dimensions emerged from the data. Two dimensions involved how the client used therapy to problem solve and reconstruct the self, and two dimensions highlighted ways clients used the therapist for healing ends. The dimensions, Self-Directed Problem Solving and Reconstruction and Remoralization of the Self, include processes and activities that could potentially be prompted by the therapist as well, but in the analysis of whole transcripts, these processes and activities were also initiated by the client. This does not seem to discount the important role the therapist plays in problem solving or in remoralization of the client, but instead, it highlights activities that clients intuitively engaged in that were not as a direct response

---

[1]The identities of the individuals in this chapter's case examples have been properly disguised to protect client confidentiality.

TABLE 6.1. Dimensions of Client Self-Healing Capacities

Client self-healing dimensions	Self-healing processes
Self-directed problem solving	• formulates and clarifies problems • defines goals • implements meaning-making heuristics • consolidates and expresses insight • generates and evaluates plan • enacts and reports on change
Reconstruction and remoralization of self	• defines and redefines self • affirms and accepts self • experiences emotional renewal • assumes and assigns responsibility • protects and advocates for self • fortifies motivation and commitment to change
Mobilization and application of the therapist's expertise	• elicits interventions • contextually prepares therapist • complies with interventions • customizes interventions • coordinates therapeutic attunement
Nurturance and use of the therapeutic relationship	• builds rapport and strengthens bond with therapist • tests interpersonal assumptions • repairs ruptures in relationship • qualifies trustworthiness of therapist

Note. From *The Active Client: A Qualitative Analysis of Thirteen Clients' Contribution to the Psychotherapeutic Process* [Unpublished doctoral dissertation] (p. 109), by A. L. Greaves, 2006, University of Southern California. Copyright 2006 by A. L. Greaves. Reprinted with permission.

to therapist intervention. The other two dimensions, Mobilization and Application of the Therapist Expertise and Nurturance and Utilization of the Therapeutic Relationship, capture when the client worked more dialogically with the therapist. In the analysis, I kept an attentive eye on how clients were contributing to and digesting the synergistic partnership and how therapists seemed to respond to clients' influence. Although therapy is dialogic in nature and therefore bidirectional in its influence, by attempting to parse out clients' singular contributions to therapeutic processes, we can gain a better understanding of how clients manifest in session the organismic valuing process that Rogers (1964) theorized about and the self-healing that Bohart and Tallman (1999) discussed in their writings.

SELF-DIRECTED PROBLEM SOLVING

The first dimension of self-healing involves problem-solving processes and their related activities, which are reviewed in this section (see Table 6.2 for a summary).

TABLE 6.2. Self-Directed Problem-Solving Dimension

Self-healing processes	Self-healing activities
Formulate and clarify the problems	• identify problems • describe problems • organize problems • reexperience problems
Define goals	• define ideal outcome • declare goal • negotiate relationship among needs, desires, values, and goals
Implement meaning-making heuristics	• compare and contrast • uncover and examine assumptions • symbolize experience with metaphors, similes, and imagery • search for and analyze new or incongruent information • craft a narrative • reframe experience
Consolidate and express insight	• express insight • evaluate insight • integrate insight • absorb insight
Generate and evaluate plan	• devise possible plan • evaluate plan • propose and confirm plan • revise plan
Enact and report on change	• practice new behavior • evidence new attitude • report on progress

Note. From *The Active Client: A Qualitative Analysis of Thirteen Clients' Contribution to the Psychotherapeutic Process* [Unpublished doctoral dissertation] (p. 114), by A. L. Greaves, 2006, University of Southern California. Copyright 2006 by A. L. Greaves. Reprinted with permission.

Formulate and Clarify the Problems

Identify the Problems

Clients seem to have a good idea about the issues necessitating counseling and engage in a process of identifying a cluster of concern (e.g., enumerating character flaws, ineffective coping strategies, or overwhelming emotions).

Describe the Problems

Clients appear to "have notes" about their lives, presenting evidence about their problems at the commencement of therapy. The therapists help to guide the process with questions, but clients seem to notice details that the therapists would miss or not ask about. They elaborate on the details of their problems: the who, what, where, when, and how. For instance, some clients noticed who was the recipient of their angry outbursts, what quantities of food were consumed during a typical binge–purge episode, where they were likely to have a panic attack, when they would have more nightmares, or how often they drank to excess. My observation is that while both therapist and client have questions, it is the clients who are in-the-field fact gatherers and reporters, providing important pieces for the team to solve the puzzle.

Organize the Problems

Clients impose order and structure on their presenting concerns. This takes the form of mapping the relationship among the problems (i.e., positioning the whole among its parts, identifying overlap between the problems, etc.) as well as ranking the importance and order of concerns based on personal criteria, such as the severity of the pain one particular problem is causing, how much a problem interferes with an important desire, or how one problem compounds all the others. Some choose an "easy" problem for a particular session because they seem to want a quick win early on. Whereas therapists have ideas about the "main problem," clients seem to recognize that if a smaller problem were cleared, they would feel better equipped to face the more difficult problem. For instance, one client pushed to resolve her childcare problem, knowing if she didn't do that first, efforts to have more work–life balance and reduce anxiety would be somewhat futile.

Reexperience the Problems

Some clients reexperience their symptoms or dysfunction in session. For example, one client defined her core complaint as anxiety stemming from over-analysis. Later, while discussing a different problem, the client reenacted the confusion and obsession that characterized her analytic process. She stated,

> I've done things like that. I don't know why. I remember thinking, "What am I doing?" I do that with something. I want to think of an example but I can't right now. Things that are really important to me . . .
>
> [*Two exchanges later*] I wish I could think of something . . .
>
> [*Four exchanges later*] I'm stuck on—I keep trying to find an example. Let it go—you can't find an example right now. Let it go. You can't find an example right now. It will bother me . . .
>
> [*Eight exchanges later*] Okay, a perfect example—I came up with one. My mom wrote me. (Greaves, 2006, p. 116)

This type of experiential knowing of the problem seemed to allow the client to go beyond the cognitive descriptors and make contact with the problem in a safe environment.

Define Goals

Define the Ideal Outcome

The act of setting a course and following through on plans to change demonstrates the purposive aspect of the client's agentic capacity. Clients can envision how their ideal outcome will look. As a personal endeavor, clients tap into their drive and creativity to envision a blueprint of their healing and growth.

This defining of their ideal is characterized by statements such as "I want," "I need," "I hope," or "if only" or, conversely, stating the antithesis of their desired outcome. One client stated, "I'm trying really hard to figure out how to turn this around to where I'm not always the scapegoat, the walking man, the whatever" (Greaves, 2006, p. 117).

Declare Goals

This category refers to an informal way clients state their intention to behave, feel, or think differently. It may take the form of an explicit and measurable goal, such as when a client states, "I'm going to be nicer to myself and try to hire outside help to care for my mom," or "I'm going to see if I can take a month off from drinking." Clients declare goals for the entire treatment or a goal for just that session. One client remarked, "That's what I want to work on in the counseling. How to change my thinking. . . . How I think people perceive me" (Greaves, 2006, p. 118).

Negotiate Goals

Embracing a goal can be complicated if desires and values conflict. For instance, one client desperately wanted to feel more included in her sorority and set a goal to attend all the functions to effect that change. She also believed this goal would interfere with her goal to maintain a 3.5 grade point average so she could keep her scholarship. In this case, the client engaged in a negotiating process where goals, values, and desires were weighed and prioritized. The client reasoned through the competing intentions, finding trade-offs she could live with.

Implement Meaning-Making Heuristics

Compare and Contrast

One way clients wrestle with material is to attend to the similarities and differences of the subject matter. This takes the form of comparing themselves with others, two alternative explanations, comparing a current problem with how a past problem was resolved, and so forth. For instance, one client compared her relationship with a roommate with her relationship with her father, illuminating the difference in relationship styles:

> I feel like, for the first time in my life, I stood up to my dad last year. It was one of the hardest things I had to do in my life, and it felt good. Everything [good came] of it. But my roommate—I don't know what it is about him that scares me to death to stand up to him. I just don't know. It bothers me so much that I can't do it to him because my dad was much scarier than him, so I don't understand why he would freak me out more. I'm mad at myself that I won't stand up to him. It really frustrates me. (Greaves, 2006, p. 119)

Uncover and Examine Assumptions

Challenging their assumptions, clients look at the origin of their beliefs, the consequences of those beliefs, and the motivation to hang onto the status quo. For instance, one client responded to her therapist's suggestion to ask for a colleague's help by uncovering an assumption that had previously blocked her from asking for help. She described growing up in a family where asking for help meant you were a wimp or trying to get attention, and she had learned to associate being trustworthy with never asking for help.

Symbolize Experience

The use of symbolic language—metaphors, similes, and imagery—is another heuristic clients use to grasp complex inner material. One client created a simile to better circumscribe a challenging part of her personality: "No, I mean the personality, [my inner critic is] like, kind of like speed and alcohol is a superior being. It doesn't care about anything else" (Greaves, 2006, p. 122). Similarly, clients' dreams and other imagery drill down into an issue. One client told of a dream in which she was building a house, but it was too close to the waves. Her interpretation was that she feared building her life anew with a partner who had not fully dealt with his addiction. By using metaphors, clients are able to access and express a problem or issue in a way that makes it available to the therapist for their joint cognitive problem solving.

Search for and Analyze New or Incongruent Information

Some clients seem to search at the periphery of their cognitive awareness—feeling after what is almost known. Indicators of this process are when clients used phrases such as "I don't know, but maybe," "It's on the tip of my tongue," or "I'm not exactly sure why this memory fits with what we're talking about, but it seems to be related." Another way clients introduce a new puzzle piece is to delve into the hypothetical. One client who was trying to make a good decision about her son's custody arrangement asked a series of "what if" questions, allowing her to imagine multiple scenarios:

> If he was a teenager, he doesn't need me as much. I don't feel like he needs me as much once he gets older, but he's a little boy. And then I think, well, if I have him live down there, then he has his dad like he wanted, but what if he isn't happy, and he's stuck down there, and he's trapped? And I don't want him to ever feel like I can't help him, you know. (Greaves, 2006, p. 120)

In their analysis, clients also identify "the exception"—when something was out of the ordinary, adding discrepant information to the way they were making sense of things. This client looked at the exception to make sense of her anxiety:

> [I'm] anxious all the time. Yeah, anxious when I'm home. When my roommates aren't there I feel so good, but once they come home, I lock myself in my room, and I don't come out. I don't know. There's just lots of fear that I hate because in other instances, like when I do extreme sports, I'm fearless, but like with people there's something about it I don't know how to shake, I don't know how to get rid of. (Greaves, 2006, p. 120)

Clients also grapple with paradoxes. For instance, after finally discovering the truth about her husband's affairs, one client explored the strength it would take to leave him while also exploring the strength it would take to forgive him and stay.

Craft a Narrative

Organizing their experience into a narrative format allows some clients the opportunity to try on different meanings based on the way they narrate their story. One client examined the details surrounding her mother's death, portraying the characters in a way that created some sense to her:

CLIENT: I don't really blame my dad . . . I find myself blaming her—that maybe if she wasn't drinking this wouldn't happen. Why did she have to drink? Did she kill herself because she wouldn't put her seatbelt on? I remember that; I was in there, so I remember the fighting, and she wouldn't put her seatbelt on. But still my dad was yelling at her. If he had known, why didn't he stop the vehicle and put the seatbelt on her.

THERAPIST: It's hard and confusing.

CLIENT: I know I would have. I don't go anywhere until I know everyone has their seatbelt on.

THERAPIST: Now that you talk about it, seatbelts were not commonly used back then.

CLIENT: In my family they were.

THERAPIST: They were?

CLIENT: Yes. My family is very—have always been—overly safe, overly protective.

THERAPIST: Do you think that was before your mother died? . . .

CLIENT: Yes. I remember we would go to Disneyland, and we always had to get in our seatbelts. . . .

CLIENT: That sounds good. She didn't want to go. She wanted another beer.

THERAPIST: She was not happy.

CLIENT: But she didn't act like an alcoholic. People think of an alcoholic as a skid row bum, but that's not always the case.

THERAPIST: So your mom was made to leave an occasion before she wanted to.

CLIENT: I think so. I'm not sure. I just know that they were over at other people's house, and they were drinking. And drinking makes— I know how it makes me to where I don't want to go somewhere, but when you're drinking, you don't want to go home.

CLIENT: So she didn't put her seatbelt on. . . . She killed herself to control the whole family. (Greaves, 2006, pp. 123–124)

Reframe Experiences

One client began to consider what he had termed "negative" emotions in a new light. He attempted an activity, hoping to be more like his mother, who did not seem to fear anything. Later, he wondered aloud whether he was even braver than she was because, when he followed in her footsteps, he did so trembling all the while with fear. In this instance, he tried on a new perspective on anxiety by including the possibility that anxiety could bring to light redeeming qualities as well.

Consolidate and Express Insight

Express Insight

The dialogue with the therapist is often what helps a client arrive at insights, although clients do express insights that they arrived at outside of counseling. At times, the expression of insight is solid and established, and other times the client is hesitant as if "trying something on for size." To illustrate this, one client explained one contributing factor for his poor relationship with his father:

> CLIENT: My dad still doesn't get along with my mom; he hasn't forgiven her.
>
> THERAPIST: So he's still mad at her.
>
> CLIENT: For 15 years.
>
> THERAPIST: You think he blamed you for that.
>
> CLIENT: He doesn't blame me but it's like I . . .
>
> THERAPIST: You had to hear about it.
>
> CLIENT: It's like my personality is just like my mom's, where my sister's is just like his. So he sees my mom every time I talk or have an idea. (Greaves, 2006, pp. 124–125)

When clients arrive at insights outside of session, they relate them to their therapist in a way that is more conclusive, a product of what had already been discovered. The following is an example of this "relating the insight" process versus discovering it in real time:

> I just discovered last week—you know what? I'm not sick. I'm not the one who's sick. And I am definitely not going to let myself get there. But on anything that I can control, I'm going to do that. But I still don't know who I am. (Greaves, 2006, p. 125)

Sometimes clients relay to the therapist others' insights about the situation, one they can adopt whole or mix with their own interpretation, as in the following example:

> I don't know. My mom was telling me I'm never happy unless I have a girlfriend. Which is true. It's the only time I feel real happy. . . . Yeah, I guess [it's] the feeling of being wanted. I don't know. (Greaves, 2006, p. 125)

Evaluate Insight

Clients scrutinize the validity of an insight and measure how valuable the insight is on the basis of the impact it has on their lives. For instance, one client recognized that her disinterest in sex came from her irrational fear of dying during childbirth, should she ever get pregnant. She wrestled with the explanatory power of this one explanation and revised it to include her fear of pain, having her clothes not fit anymore, and losing some control over her day-to-day life should she accidentally get pregnant. She believed if she was purposefully trying to get pregnant, though, these fears could simply be chalked up as fears she was bravely trying to confront, and then her interest in sex would return.

Absorb Insight

Some clients repeat the same insight in separate sessions as if it is new, possibly as if it is gaining marinating concentration. For instance, after many weeks of making the connection between his bingeing and his "relational" feelings, one client no longer referred to his addiction temptation as simply an urge to get high. Instead, his "languaging" around addiction incorporated the idea that it was a way to medicate the emptiness he felt in his marriage.

Integrate Insight

Newly acquired self-understanding seemed to find its relationship with the rest of the clients' wisdom bank. They revise and process new ideas and beliefs until these become integrated with previously held understanding. One client who had been raised in a shaming environment always had to solve problems to avoid the next blowup. As she got in touch with how exhausting it is to serve herself up on a platter, she learned to accept her limitations and let go of some perfectionism. She hoped that in the future, she could say something like, "Whoops! I made a simple mistake. Now I know."

Generate and Evaluate Plan

Devise a Plan

Making a plan involves executive functioning processes that allow clients to anticipate how they might get from Point A to Point B. One key activity involved in devising possible plans is the quality of brainstorming. Clients engage in planning and strategizing on the fly. This monologue demonstrates this free-form planning about how to replace compulsive study behavior with more socializing:

> I've been thinking about getting involved, but I feel like I'm so stuck that I can't do anything else [besides watch TV]. I could go out and not do a team thing, but go shoot around or play volleyball without a commitment. . . . That's like why I want to volunteer—but my parents say no—like at the animal shelter. . . . I know I have time—like once a week maybe I can just go there. . . . I need to find something that I can do when I want to . . . but not commit. Like not having to be there [at a] certain time, certain place. (Greaves, 2006, p. 127)

Evaluate the Plan

Clients evaluate their plans by contrasting two or more options, identifying the pros and cons, or predicting possible impediments to implementing the plan. Clients are the ones implementing the plan and know the intricacies of their life and are thus uniquely qualified to evaluate the plan. One client, whose parents had serious health concerns, considered her options of how to care for her younger siblings should her parents die while she was still in college:

> I think any day they can die. They can smoke too much coke, and they can die. Just drink too much beer and die. And what do I do? I'd take the kids, and what do I do? How would I care for the kids? I have a two-bedroom apartment. I think it would be a good thing because I could mold them and help them. But it would be a bad thing because I don't know if I want that responsibility. I want more kids but with my husband. Not have two—you know what I mean? It would be a burden—we have to have more people in our home and less money. I don't want to do that . . . [but] I don't want to not be able to do it if something happened to them. I wouldn't allow them to go anywhere else. I'm stuck in a hard place. (Greaves, 2006, p. 127)

Propose and Confirm the Plan

Clients articulate firm plans about how to go about accomplishing a desired goal. The detail that clients put into their plan varies in the level of precision, but the plan is spoken with an air of decisiveness, as in the example of a client with an eating disorder who determined how she would begin eating breakfast at her dorm cafeteria. She elaborately mapped out what time she would arrive, what table to be seated at, what direction to face, and what foods she would eat. Clients also firm up their plans as they speak. The following client conveyed her determination to start her own business, thus becoming financially independent and no longer needing to live with her daughter:

> So I would start with that, and I would do covered wagon rides and have people contact me for birthday rides and take them up on Table Mountain or whatever and see the spring flowers to get started. . . . Oh, yeah, and I've already figured out what the chuck wagon would have to have with it and how much it would have to be for whatever meal you have. . . . I think I could do it a lot of times. The thing that I can't do—you just said that—it made me think that I don't have to be the wagon driver. I could arrange it, couldn't I? (Greaves, 2006, p. 128)

Revise Plan

Often, plans did not go off as expected, and clients reflect on these failed attempts. This activity consists of appraising the details of the plan: What went wrong? What could be improved? What worked well and perhaps just needs to be fine-tuned? In some cases, an extension of this evaluative process results in a revision to the original plan.

Enact and Report on Change

Practice a New Behavior

The safety of the therapy space can become a "testing ground," with clients experimenting with a new behavior before venturing out and trying their new way of being with family, friends, or foe. One client, who feared if she took note of any of her positive traits, she would then become too vain, began noticing aloud in session qualities that she valued in herself. Another client, who was usually on the receiving end of a breakup, practiced his newfound autonomy in therapy: He announced that while he appreciated his therapist, he no longer felt the sessions beneficial enough to continue.

Evidence a New Attitude

The therapy hour can be an "incubator" for revised attitudes and hypothesis testing. One client, who received the family message to never show "unpleasant" emotions in public, dared not cry, raise her voice, or show fear unless she was completely alone. In her shame, she kept tight control of these emotions, not even displaying them in front of her fiancé. As therapy progressed, she permitted herself to weep in her therapist's presence. At first, she expressed her embarrassment about being unable to hold back the tears. But then she began to see these emotions in a new light—feeling proud that she was sensitive enough to experience a range of emotions, prizing the tenderness of sharing her emotions with another person.

Report on Progress

A common activity is the reporting of progress—or lack thereof. This activity serves the purpose of both a self-diagnostic check as well as holding themselves accountable to another person. Clients report when they have success with a difficult conversation, reducing their drinking, detaching from the outcome of a fertility procedure, and so forth.

RECONSTRUCTION AND REMORALIZATION OF SELF

The second dimension is like the first in that it involves creative, executive, and emotional functioning activities that happen to be driven by the client, although they can be therapist driven as well. However, this dimension differs in that it is less focused on how clients address concrete problems and more on the way clients fortify themselves as a whole person. Table 6.3 summarizes the self-healing processes and the associated activities that fall under this dimension.

Define and Redefine Self

Name and Own Characteristics

The therapy experience provides a safe opportunity for clients to explore who they are. They identify and claim their strengths. Such is the case with the client who stated, "I know that I've always been stubborn so I knew that I could always muster through things" (Greaves, 2006, p. 133). In having a safe place to talk about their weaknesses, clients make room for all aspects of their being and can come out of hiding. This facilitates the change process as weaknesses are put into context and the implications are examined. In this example, a client looked at what makes communication difficult for him:

> I have a way of saying things just as I'm thinking them. I don't think through things before I say them. I have a habit of just blurting things out. So, it would

TABLE 6.3. Reconstruction and Remoralization of Self Dimension

Self-healing processes	Self-healing activities
Define and redefine self	• name and own characteristics • define values, beliefs, needs, and desires • give and revise self-narrative
Affirm and accept self	• validate self • appreciate self
Experience emotional renewal	• identify emotions • experience emotions • integrate emotional experience
Assume and assign responsibility	• assume responsibility • assign responsibility
Protect and advocate for self	• defend self • set pace of therapy process • negotiate structure of therapy
Fortify motivation and commitment to change	• inspire hope • declare a commitment to change • challenge own resistance

Note. From *The Active Client: A Qualitative Analysis of Thirteen Clients' Contribution to the Psychotherapeutic Process* [Unpublished doctoral dissertation] (p. 133), by A. L. Greaves, 2006, University of Southern California. Copyright 2006 by A. L. Greaves. Reprinted with permission.

be hard for me, I would have to really sit down and go through my mind, really reword things so that they don't come off as—I don't want to say "rude" but uncensored, if that makes any sense. (Greaves, 2006, p. 133)

Define Values, Beliefs, Needs, and Desires

In defining their values and beliefs, clients lay out what constitutes their version of health or sickness, what their worldview is, what their moral code is, and so on. One client shared her perspective on the importance of friendship: "But I still think it's important to meet new people. It's good to have the same group of friends your whole life, but it's good to incorporate more" (Greaves, 2006, p. 134). Clients also define themselves in relation to other people, cultural influences, and those in their social milieu. One client began to describe her level of acculturation as a second-generation Asian American, noting how she is similar to and different from her Filipino mother and European American father. As therapists listen, they will hear clients spell out their own moral code—which therapists can draw on as needed. The following is one small example of a client defining expectations for himself: "I can't get mad because they aren't the way that I want them to be" (Greaves, 2006, p. 134).

When clients explore their authentic preferences, they give their therapist guideposts for future reference. In this vignette, one client confidently expressed what gives her life force energy:

It's something that I like to do; I love nature, and I like being alone, just walking and wandering around and listening to sounds. I don't like to go alone or be away from people but to just enjoy nature—I feel better. (Greaves, 2006, p. 142)

Give and Revise a Self-Narrative

The act of narrating one's story goes beyond solving a particular problem and is an essential part of constructing a coherent sense of self. Through this self-narrative, with its leading characters, plot twists, and "moral of the story" reminders, clients understand themselves as historical beings with a rich past that differentiates them from others. One client depicted how she came to embody self-reliance and bravery:

CLIENT: I don't know. You just come from something, and you make yourself totally different. There's no limitation. I don't know, you can't . . .

THERAPIST: You were able to overcome your circumstances, and that's gratifying to you. That's . . . because I remember you said you could've gone the exact opposite.

CLIENT: Yeah. Which a lot of people do.

THERAPIST: Uh-huh. And yet somehow you were able to—

CLIENT: Whatever that was. Something I was born with, I guess. I don't really know. 'Cause, like, I am the one that at 4 years old told the cops that my mom did drugs. And I am the one that got taken away from that situation. And if I didn't say that then, it wouldn't have happened that way. So at 4 years old I made the choice.

THERAPIST: At four, you were able to—

CLIENT: Four or five.

THERAPIST: Be cognizant enough to say . . .

CLIENT: Yeah because I knew what drugs were and everything like that. I knew what, I knew what was going on around me for some reason, and I knew I wasn't supposed to say anything to anybody about it because it was bad, and bad things would happen to me if I said that she was doing drugs or anything like that. So when the police came to the door, they asked if they could talk to me out in the hallway. And I said yeah and everything and I went out there and they asked me if my mom was doing marijuana or whatever and I said yeah she does a little marijuana but she also does drugs and all that stuff. And I knew I wasn't supposed to say anything like even though I said something.

THERAPIST: Was it an unspoken message? You weren't supposed to—

CLIENT: No.

THERAPIST: She had outright told you?

CLIENT: Yeah. And we had talked about it like, don't tell anybody. You know you're not supposed to say anything, even before they had come to the door. Because, my mom and the guy that she was living with were asleep on the bed and I heard them coming so, it's like I was kind of trying to clean up the room because you could hear the footsteps down the hallway, and so I like cleaned up the room and threw any drugs like laying around because I cleaned it up, and I woke her up, and they knocked on the door and everything—

THERAPIST: At five years old you did all these things?

CLIENT: Yeah.

THERAPIST: Wow.

CLIENT: Yeah it was like around five years old. So I made a decision at that point not to be there. So I don't know how I made that decision, whether it was God or if it was, like I didn't know who God was at that point in my life, but something told me to say what I needed to say, so. And then when I moved in with my grandparents, I lived there for a little while and then they asked me if I wanted to stay and I wanted to stay. And then we had to go to court and I had to tell the court that I wanted to stay. Those were some pretty big changes in my life, but I kind of made them on my own for whatever reason. (Greaves, 2006, pp. 143–144)

Affirm and Accept Self

Validate Self

Clients seek validation from their therapists, but in doing so, they also provide validation for themselves. This may take the form of self-sympathy by using objective information. One client validated the severity of her history as an abuse survivor by declaring that she wouldn't wish that treatment on her worst enemy.

Appreciate Self

As a natural termination approaches, clients will occupy time in therapy recounting more and more successes while therapists celebrate their progress. But throughout therapy, clients remark on their good qualities, take pride in reaching a goal, or savor the satisfaction of making a difficult choice. For example, one client believed others saw her as rotten to the core, but she knew she was genuine, empathetic, nonjudgmental, and funny. She held on to these qualities even though certain situations necessitated having her guard up.

Experience Emotional Renewal

Experience Emotions

Therapy allows clients the opportunity to give fuller expression to their feelings. This emotional catharsis takes many forms, ranging from paralinguistic gestures of emotion (e.g., crying, laughing, speaking softly, hand wringing, pounding a fist, wincing, sighing) to verbal gestures such as the use of particularly vivid language.

Identify Emotions

Clients label the emotion (e.g., mad, sad, scared) or elaborate with metaphor (e.g., a crazy fog, unlit bomb), making it a part of them or possibly more separate from them. One client did her own "parts work," identifying cutoff emotions and stating that her "[inner critic] wants to cry" (Greaves, 2006, p. 140).

Integrate Emotional Experience

Just as the etymology of "emotion" comes from the root *e* (outward) and *motion* (movement), when clients experience a variety of emotions and integrate each one as parts of a whole, they can move through their stuck point. The following dialogue highlights three emotion-related activities: experiencing, identifying, and integrating emotions. In this example, the client gained a fuller understanding of the range of emotions that she experienced when she was around children. She was able to identify and sift through a variety of emotions and begin to make sense of each one.

CLIENT: I didn't apply for [the job]. . . . I felt really strange when I walked into the place. I think I would like to work with kids.

THERAPIST: I can see you really meshing well with kids.

CLIENT: I'm at that age when my mother had me. I don't want to have kids. I'm way too young to handle a kid. I can't even handle myself; how could I handle a kid? I think that would be really good. It's so hot in here.

THERAPIST: You get real emotional talking about kids.

CLIENT: Yeah, 'cause I like kids. They make me sad.

THERAPIST: How come?

CLIENT: I don't know. I guess 'cause they are so cute and not unhappy. That's not unfair [*tearing up*]. It doesn't make me sad 'cause I'm not jealous of them, but I'm just sad. I remember how it was. It was sad.

THERAPIST: Do you feel like you were gypped?

CLIENT: Uh-huh, kind of.

THERAPIST: Do you wish you could do it over again?

CLIENT: No. I really liked my childhood. I really had a lot of fun. I think I miss the feeling inside.

THERAPIST: Of being a child?

CLIENT: Yeah. The way it feels and stuff. I think I miss that. I wouldn't want a different stuff. I remember a lot of stuff that was really fun, like butterflies. I think that's why I want to work with kids: They put that feeling back. Like, I remember I went over to this house, and there were all these—he has this daughter that's like 7, and they all come running up to me. And they try telling me all this stuff. It was like this wave of energy come into me, and it was crazy feeling. And I tried talking to them, and they were pulling me here and there. Even after I left, I still felt all their energy and stuff. It was so cool. It was so weird. It's like oh, my God, that's what we were talking about. I think I like that feeling. I like all that energy that they give you.

THERAPIST: It's exhilarating, isn't it?

CLIENT:	It is. It's kind of like when I perform on stage, and you're filled with energy. They are like curious, and they are like that. It's the same feeling. I think that's why I like it.
THERAPIST:	It's nonjudgmental.
CLIENT:	Yeah.
THERAPIST:	It's a pure thing from a child.
CLIENT:	Yeah, like the things that they are into. You can see how much they are into it; they just glow with it. They find so many things pretty. It's really calming. A lot of stuff is really ugly in the world, and it's really nice being with a kid and stuff.
THERAPIST:	What kinds of emotions is this stirring up for you?
CLIENT:	I don't know. I'd say sadness, but not really. I'm not really sad, kind of like. I don't know. Like ummmm . . .
THERAPIST:	Mixed emotions?
CLIENT:	Yeah, kind of mixed. I'm really happy, and I'm kind of sad, but it's like it feels good when I talk about how cute they are.
THERAPIST:	Like you told me a little bit about your childhood. Like with your father, there were some tough times in there and that whole situation.
CLIENT:	I think that brings up a lot of that when I talk about it. It kind of brings back that unhappy, sad feeling. I think that's where it comes from.
THERAPIST:	It reminds you of your childhood?
CLIENT:	Yeah I think it does when I talk about it and stuff. It was really awful, but it also had some really nice moments.
THERAPIST:	Your childhood?
CLIENT:	Yeah, so it made it really worth it. I like the little moments. (Greaves, 2006, pp. 140–141)

Assume and Assign Responsibility

Assume Responsibility

Another aspect of clients' remoralization process is holding themselves accountable according to their own standards. By honestly evaluating the appropriateness of their behaviors and attitudes, clients demonstrate and potentially fortify their integrity and capacity to manage imperfection. One wife acknowledged the impact her behaviors had in the relationship:

> And I know he's not here to give his side of the story. And he could very well have his own issues with me. . . . And I know that there's my temper. I've got a temper when it comes to him. I do; I have a short fuse. I know that a lot of times all I have to do is hear his voice, and I put my guard up. And I'm sure it changes the tone in my voice and puts him on defense. So little things like that I would like to have brought to my attention, just so I can work on my part of it. (Greaves, 2006, pp. 137–138)

Assign Responsibility

As clients took the time to explore their sense of responsibility, they became more aware about the limits of their responsibility. One client illustrated this and how she came to terms with the imbalance of expectations within her family structure:

> Sometimes I think that it's not my responsibility because I'm doing—sometimes I think that I'm doing more than they're doing because they are just going either to school . . . or they're going to work, and they're not doing anything in the afternoon. And I do—go to school, I work. Sometimes I work full time. . . . And I go to school full time too. . . . About the house—sometimes I feel that it's not my responsibility because I do a lot of things. But you know, our culture, where the girls have to do, you know. . . . Since I'm the only girl . . . so, like, it's my responsibility because my mom is not here. (Greaves, 2006, p. 138)

Five sessions later, this client demonstrated the refinement of assuming and assigning responsibility with her siblings:

> I feel good. I don't feel like before I told you I feel guilty or bad because I didn't cook or anything. I'm getting over that feeling. I don't feel bad no more. I know that there's food from the day before. I know they can do something; they can buy something. (Greaves, 2006, p. 139)

Fortify Motivation and Commitment to Change

Inspire Hope

Peppered throughout many clients' dialogue were what could be considered "hope boosters." Clients seem to inspire hope in their change process by reminding themselves of past successes—bringing into the forefront of their minds evidence that they are capable of overcoming the illusion of insurmountable barriers. The following illustrates a client's motivational monologue:

> Just 'cause, like, I would know what I'd be doing instead of wasting my time trying to relax or something, but if I plan something out where I know I will have fun and get my mind off it 'cause I planned ahead. That would help a lot. That would be a good break for once, and then I would be, like, maybe it would be a reward in a way too. Like if I study this long and take a break I would have something fun to do and then go back and maybe another thing. I could focus on the good of that, too. (Greaves, 2006, p. 143)

Declare a Commitment to Change

The language of resolve is the hallmark feature of the process of declaring a commitment to change. Rather than a more logical-sounding declaration of goals, clients adopt the *language of resolve*, a declaration with an emotional tone that belies the client's move from merely wishing to sincere intention. The following client exhibited her resolve to take some time to know herself rather than hopping from one relationship to another:

> Yeah, like, I did that with [Ricardo] and [Miguel]. I made myself sick over it. How am I going to go on without them? Yeah, I can be with other people. Right now, my biggest fear is oh, my God, I'm going to be alone. Not that I can't live without him;

it's just—can I live without somebody? I know I can, but I haven't done it for the longest time. Now I want to. For the first time in my life there's a part of me that wants to. There still is a little part of me that still wants someone, but then there's such a bigger part that I don't want anyone right now. . . . Yeah, yeah, like, I'm scared, "Oh, my God, I'm going to do this." But at the same time, I know that I'm going to learn so much and get so much out of it. . . . I think I'm a person that's aware of things, but it takes me a long time to do something about it—to be strong enough and willing enough to do it. I think, for once, I'm so fed up with—like in a good way. . . . [Like, with] him coming up here, it's like, yeah, I don't want to be with anybody. I can't have anyone come into my life and pick up all my pieces for me. I have to do it myself, and who can do it better than me. (Greaves, 2006, p. 144)

Challenge Their Own Resistance

Clients are at times aware something is blocking them from moving forward in the therapy and confess it outright. They seem to challenge their resistance by enumerating the consequences of inaction or addressing how the problem affects them. The following example illustrates how a client began to address his resistance to giving up smoking, growing, and selling marijuana:

CLIENT: Yeah, I just feel like it's the only life. I make my money by it; I smoke it. I want to get away from it. I want to learn something else.

THERAPIST: You don't think you can do that on your own.

CLIENT: No, I'm tired of the life.

THERAPIST: You don't think you can just cut it out?

CLIENT: Yeah, if I end up in jail.

THERAPIST: Otherwise you don't think you could?

CLIENT: No.

THERAPIST: Huh.

CLIENT: That's my income; that's how I get my money. I'm tired of that life. It's been a while now—well, not that long, but it's "paranoia-ing." My dad doesn't know. (Greaves, 2006, pp. 144–145)

Protect and Advocate for Self

Defend the Self

Although the word "defend" usually has poor connotations, clients' healthy protection mechanisms are activated as clients defend themselves against mistreatment. Clients describe the offending behavior and artfully formulate their defense and practice with the therapist. This includes boundary setting, including with the therapist. One client, who was considering joining the military, listened to his therapist sharply criticize the military and frowned on the client's decision to enlist. The client defended his intentions and sent a message to the therapist, in subtle ways, that he resented the therapist's unsolicited opinion about his career choice.

Set the Pace of the Therapy Process

Clients manage what and when they disclose and at times retreat into a somewhat superficial level of conversing. Other times, they speed the pace by shifting to a more vulnerable topic or letting the therapist know they have already grasped the therapist's message. Silences, detaching from intense processes, or noncompliance with in-session activities are ways clients control the level of immersion. One client who was grieving over losing custody of her son managed the intensity of the therapy as follows:

CLIENT: I don't think I want to talk about this anymore; it's just going to keep me going.

THERAPIST: Okay.

CLIENT: I can't do this right now—you know?

THERAPIST: Okay, okay, sure.

CLIENT: I just feel like once it starts, I could just sit here for hours and cry, and it's not going to do any good right now.

THERAPIST: Okay, we will back off then. Okay? One thing I do want to show you though before you go today: It's a little breathing technique. And it might help you, if you can keep it in your head in the moment; it might help you to breathe through the anxiety, breathe through the sadness until you can get to a place where you can take care of yourself. [*Explains breathing technique*]

CLIENT: Uh-huh.

THERAPIST: So that might be something, and maybe we'll try a couple of things of that before you go today, just to help you get grounded and centered before you go back out. But that might be something that could be useful to you in the moment if you feel overwhelmed. Just try something as simple—just try a couple of minutes of [*breathes in and out*] and see how that—see where that takes you. How does that sound to you? Does that seem like something you could possibly?

CLIENT: Yeah, yeah.

THERAPIST: Okay. [*Pause. Client is crying*] I can see so much pain, and I just want you to know how much I empathize with you. . . . Do you want to try a couple of deep breathing relaxations?

CLIENT: No.

THERAPIST: No?

CLIENT: No, I mean I can sort of get the idea, and I'll practice it, but I don't think I can really do that now.

THERAPIST: Okay, okay. So, do you feel like you just want to close right now or what? How can I help you right now?

CLIENT: I don't think anything can help me right now. (Greaves, 2006, p. 147)

Negotiate the Structure of Therapy

At times, clients and therapists negotiate when therapy will begin, how often they meet, and how many sessions before termination. Even though there may be external guidelines for session frequency, clients may push for what they feel they need. One client asked to come more than once a week, explaining that it seemed to her a better alternative than to be hospitalized—having already been hospitalized—and she did not want to go back again. Another client asked to stretch her covered sessions out over a longer period by coming to therapy biweekly. Clients exert their influence over which day of the week and what time of day sessions occur. One client requested to come Friday afternoons so he could access certain painful material but still have the weekends to recover before going back to work.

MOBILIZATION AND APPLICATION OF THE THERAPIST'S EXPERTISE

When clients come to therapy, it is often because they have exhausted the resources available to them and are looking for professional help. The expertise of a professional therapist may be sought to fill in the knowledge gaps of the client's understanding to provide an objective viewpoint, provide outside support and encouragement, or direct the client's attention to areas unfamiliar and unexplored. While therapists have their own unique set of skills and wisdom, the implementation and timing of this expertise may be subtly or overtly influenced by the client. Once the therapist's interventions are "delivered," it is left up to clients to use that expertise in a manner they see fit—and that may not be exactly the way the therapist originally intended. Furthermore, clients pull for therapists to take certain stances with them, possibly indicating the client's intuitive sense of what would be the most healing at that time. This section reviews the processes and associated activities that are part of this third dimension of client self-healing (see Table 6.4 for a summary of these processes and activities).

Elicit Interventions

Elicit an Authoritative Stance

When clients yearn for more structure, they may send a signal—"advise me, confront me, evaluate me." One client asked her therapist, "I know you haven't known me very long, but what do you think of me going to the abbey in Nova Scotia?" (Greaves, 2006, p. 150). Clients also send signals that they are stuck and need direction in what topic to explore or how to deepen their emotional process. Clients also use their therapist as an accountability person. Without solicitation, one client brought in a food journal each week, tracking her progress in overcoming binge eating, eliciting her therapist's evaluative stance on progress or setbacks. Another client related how powerful it was to hear Robin Williams's character in the movie *Good Will Hunting* (1997) repeatedly

TABLE 6.4. Mobilization and Application of the Therapist's Expertise Dimension

Self-healing processes	Self-healing activities
Elicits interventions	• elicit authoritative stance • elicit supportive stance • elicit informative stance
Contextually prepares therapist	• display the problem • imbue vicarious knowledge • provide historical, cultural, and situational context • encourage outside learning
Cooperates with interventions	• defer to therapist's lead • accept suggestions and reports on compliance
Customizes interventions	• interpret and develop therapist's direction • individualize therapist's assignments
Coordinates therapeutic attunement	• direct focus • ensure understanding of therapist • keep therapist on track

Note. From *The Active Client: A Qualitative Analysis of Thirteen Clients' Contribution to the Psychotherapeutic Process* [Unpublished doctoral dissertation] (p. 149), by A. L. Greaves, 2006, University of Southern California. Copyright 2006 by A. L. Greaves. Reprinted with permission.

tell his client that his mother's death was in no way his fault. It was as if the client was hinting to his therapist, "I also need someone of authority to convince me that my own mother's death is not my fault." Clients may elicit an authoritative stance as they ask for constructive criticism as follows:

> I want—if there's something that you see that I don't see in myself; maybe I'm too judgmental. I want to know because I want to work on it. I don't want somebody to agree with me—that's why I don't go to my dad or boyfriend because they're one-sided. I want an outsider's point of view to see things that I don't see about myself because maybe I'm doing something that sets him off. Something I can do to change. I want constructive criticism about what I can do differently, about what I'm doing that could be causing or adding to the problem. I think that's what I want more than anything. (Greaves, 2006, p. 151)

Elicit a Supportive Stance

Clients seem to know when they need more encouragement or empathy from their therapist and draw out a more supportive stance than their therapist usually provides. One client asked his therapist if he could try to understand what it is like to be him. Clients may ask directly, use more dramatic language, or become more emotional to elicit this more supportive stance. One client elicited supportive empathy in the following way:

> CLIENT: It's always something, you know. It doesn't seem like we're ever— it's been a long 6 years, you know?
>
> THERAPIST: I can see that you're really just kind of tired and worn out with this whole thing. (Greaves, 2006, p. 151)

Elicit an Informative Stance

Clients tap into therapists' training and knowledge bank about a variety of topics. These clients drew on their therapist's book learning, asking about such things as sleep hygiene, side effects of abusing a particular drug, or the stages of the coming out process. Clients also solicit insight about themselves, as in the case of one client who posed the question "How does one [adopt] a savior complex?" (Greaves, 2006, p. 152).

Contextually Prepare the Therapist

Display the Problem

One way for the therapist to become attuned to their client is to witness the problem in action. Personality disorders, couples' fight patterns, compulsions, delusions, depression, and so on can all be evident in the room. If clients only talked about their problem rather than displaying it, therapists would have less information and possibly be less helpful. One client reported a conflict between her family's wish that she remains submissive and her fledgling attempt to embrace a more assertive personality. Several sessions later, her therapist began the session by asking if he could read a parable to her and then followed that with a visualization exercise, never asking what her goal or agenda for the session might be. The therapist summed up his main point and then announced, "That's all the time we have for today" (Greaves, 2006, p. 153). The client provided the therapist with an experiential example of how she could remain quiet instead of interjecting when the session was not going in the direction she had intended.

Imbue Vicarious Knowledge

Another useful way clients prepare their therapist is by creating an experience that allows the therapist to feel what it's like to be them. A client who feels hopeless and pessimistic seems to begin to impact the therapist's hope regarding the client's treatment. One client, who reported that his father rarely credited him for his success, attributed all his improvements to a recent antidepressant trial, possibly transferring the feeling of devaluation that he often received from his father onto his therapist. When clients imbue vicarious knowledge of what the client feels, it allows therapists to gain an accurate and empathic frame of reference to better help the client.

Provide Historical, Cultural, and Situational Context

The client's provision of background information turns "run of the mill" depression into a vivid and idiosyncratic picture for the therapist. While clients are "telling their stories," they are clueing the therapist into their values, relationship dynamics, the impact of their problems on everyday life, past attempts at managing a problem, and so forth. For instance, a client who was adjusting to conflicts between gender roles in her old and new culture gave her therapist insight into how this plays out in daily life:

> I also live with five of my brothers. So, my parents are in Mexico, and I have kind of, you know, we have Mexican traditions, so I have to do all the things at home like clean, wash the clothes, and cook everyday for them and all that. And that's basically what I do. (Greaves, 2006, p. 155)

By contextualizing a problem within a historical, cultural, and value-laden backdrop, clients better equip their therapists to choose what type of response might be most effective.

Encourage Outside Learning

Clients can overtly or subtly encourage therapists to do outside homework to better understand and help them. For instance, a recent immigrant was surprised that the therapist was unaware of his country's civil war, which had a profound impact on him, so by the next session, the therapist had learned more about that country's political history. Clients refer to movies or books with characters or story lines that are relatable to clients, like the client who wanted his therapist to watch *The Godfather* (1972) because it paralleled his relationship with his father.

Cooperate With Interventions

Defer to the Therapist's Lead

There is often a back-and-forth process as client and therapist determine how the session unfolds. Clients may defer to the therapists' expertise in deciding what the focus should be, answering the therapist's questions or elaborating on topics that seem a priority to the therapist. For instance, when one therapist was symptom focused, clients would begin sessions by reporting on symptoms. When one therapist showed enthusiasm for dream interpretation, the clients brought in dreams to work on.

Accept Suggestions and Report on Compliance

As therapists prescribe in-session and homework activities and even informal suggestions, clients choose to comply with these suggestions—and if it happens outside of session, they report back. Even if they do not accept the challenge right away, they may deliberate and follow through at some later point. For instance, one client who was shy about doing an empty-chair exercise declared in a later session that she wanted to give it a try.

Customizes Interventions

Interpret and Develop Therapist's Direction

Even when clients are compliant with therapists' interventions, it is evident that a fair amount of interpretation takes place. For example, a client will report that they "did what the therapist suggested," but in reality, it is somewhat different from what the therapist mentioned in the previous session. During in-session exercises, clients must interpret therapists' instructions and carry out the prompts in ways that make sense to them. This takes the form of using their imagination to heighten the effect in an imaginal exposure exercise, constructing the dialogue in two-chair work, creating a mantra to challenge a negative belief, and tuning into the unfinished action in somatic experiencing work.

In some cases, clients do not wait for the therapist to finish a thought before jumping in to complete a sentence, assuming they know where the therapist is going and building on the therapist's insightful offering. The following illustrates fruitful results that can stem from a client interrupting her therapist:

CLIENT: I never got along with my mom; we couldn't have a conversation without fighting—really bad and stuff.

THERAPIST: Was it because of . . .

CLIENT: Yeah, she didn't trust me. She didn't trust me for a while. It was a huge trust issue. (Greaves, 2006, p. 158)

The client used the partial question as a prompt so she could expound on the root of the conflict—a line of thinking that may not have otherwise been explored. This type of assumption extends to the client "hearing" the kinds of interpretations and advice the client may intuitively need to hear. An example of this involves a client who was meeting up with strangers in hotel rooms and asked her therapist for her opinion regarding the matter. Although the therapist did not advise and instead reflected and asked questions, in the following session, the client reported she had done just as the therapist recommended by stopping the practice. Perhaps the client was looking for a particular kind of support, hearing what she needed to hear.

Individualize the Therapist's Assignments
A therapist's idea of how to proceed can inspire a client to reshape that same idea into a variation that fits more perfectly with what the client needs. This is another way that clients and therapists blend their expertise. For example, one client tailored the therapist's homework assignment to write a letter detailing her unexpressed anger to her boss. When the client returned, she not only had written a letter to her boss but also her mother, brother, and one of her close friends and proceeded to read all four letters aloud. Clients may also use an in-session intervention as a springboard for their own homegrown interventions. The following exchange illustrates how a client refashioned an exercise her therapist had initiated:

THERAPIST: Let's switch places for a minute: you are me. What would you tell me to do?

CLIENT: I would tell you to get over it. I have had friends—not really friends, but I know her—who have had boyfriends that have been

> cheating. She knew it, and everyone knew it, but she still talked to him. I was sitting here telling her—well, the thing is, my first boyfriend cheated on me about four times, and at the fourth time he admitted [it] to me, and so we broke up. So I tell her you have to forget about him; it is not that big of deal. Then I look back at what I did and well. I kept taking him back when I knew it was true. Okay, I went with it. So I would tell you: You can't be with someone like that—who cheated on you. You don't do that. (Greaves, 2006, p. 159)

The client did what the therapist asked but then piggybacked on it her own intervention—that of relating the advice she had given to a friend in a similar predicament.

Coordinate Therapeutic Attunement

Direct Focus

Some therapists offer their clients the lead in determining the focus of the current session. But even when this is not the case, clients can seize an opportunity to shift the focus to what would be most suitable to their goals. They may do this subtly or simply announce it more directly, as in the following case: "Yeah . . . I don't even want to talk about [my ex-girlfriend] anymore. There's more deep root to my problems than her" (Greaves, 2006, p. 160).

Ensure Understanding of the Therapist

To properly use the expertise of the therapist, clients make efforts to understand what the therapist is communicating. They listen and check in with restatements and summaries or express confusion (verbally or nonverbally), thus allowing the therapist to make an adjustment. The following demonstrates how a client attempts to clarify what a therapist is wanting to convey:

> THERAPIST: One thing that popped out of my intuition, one thing that came to me is you might ask your intuition what its interacting with in maybe a kind of journal writing experiment or exercise, where you would sit down and just try and work through—give it a little time, as awkward sometimes experiments are to start with; just say, intuition, who are you interacting with?
>
> CLIENT: Fear, that's what came to mind when you said that, but I'm not sure if that's what you meant by interacting. (Greaves, 2006, p. 161)

Keep the Therapist on Track

Clients keep their therapists on track, making sure their therapist understands the meaning of what was conveyed and encouraging their therapist to work toward the same immediate or long-term goals. They may say, "You know what I mean?" to ensure the two are in sync or give positive affirmations indicating that the current direction is useful. Sometimes, clients give negative feedback to calibrate the therapist's attunement, rephrasing until they feel understood or highlighting the dissonance by using more impassioned language. One therapist was steering the client toward having more empathy for his father, who was roping the client into divorce squabbles, but the client countersteered, possibly hoping the therapist would support the client's resistance to feeling enmeshed with his dad:

> THERAPIST: Can you put yourself in his shoes and understand how he might have felt? I'm not saying what he did was right . . .
>
> CLIENT: I understand how he felt, but I mean, he could have gone to a damn counselor and said all those things. (Greaves, 2006, p. 162)

NURTURANCE AND UTILIZATION OF THE THERAPEUTIC RELATIONSHIP

Just as therapists' expertise is co-opted by clients' healing endeavors, the sustenance of the interpersonal relationship with the therapist is also metabolized by clients as they heal relationally. While the literature tends to focus on what therapists do to create a relationship with "medicinal power," my research showed that clients engage in similar and complementary practices to create a "medicinal compound." Beyond that, the clients I studied seemed to care about the quality of the relationship; it mattered who their travel companion was on their healing journey. Therapists and clients alike can be motivated to invest in creating a strong therapeutic bond because it has major implications for their satisfaction and wellness outcomes, respectively. The clients' contributions to a healing therapeutic relationship are reviewed in this fourth dimension of self-healing activities, as outlined in Table 6.5.

TABLE 6.5. Nurturance and Utilization of the Therapeutic Relationship Dimension

Self-healing processes	Self-healing activities
Build rapport and strengthen bond with therapist	• attend to etiquette • foster healing qualities in the therapist • create mutuality
Test interpersonal assumptions	• directly process relationship • enact role of others • recreate own role
Qualify trustworthiness of therapist	• check compatibility with therapist • determine therapist's competence • test therapist's commitment
Repair ruptures in the relationship	• address therapist's mistakes • explore solutions to rupture • make amends with therapist

Note. From *The Active Client: A Qualitative Analysis of Thirteen Clients' Contribution to the Psychotherapeutic Process* [Unpublished doctoral dissertation] (p. 164), by A. L. Greaves, 2006, University of Southern California. Copyright 2006 by A. L. Greaves. Reprinted with permission.

Build Rapport and Strengthen the Bond With the Therapist

Attend to Etiquette

Prosocial behaviors can help build rapport, and therapy relationships are no exception. Clients engage with their therapist in ways that convey respect and courtesy. Examples include laughing at the therapist's jokes, maintaining eye contact, being on time, waiting for their turn to speak, or accommodating therapists' schedule changes. They show respect for their therapist in a variety of ways, including asking permission to call them by their first name, giving credence to their experience and ideas, and not intruding on the therapist's personal life. When clients engage in these types of prosocial behaviors, it may facilitate their therapist in being more mentally and emotionally available as a working partner. For instance, one client apologized for cutting the therapist off but then shared an important detail that took the conversation in a new and fruitful direction.

Foster Healing Qualities in the Therapist

The way clients treat their therapists seems to impact their therapists' motivation levels as well as draw out interpersonal qualities that are conducive to healing. Clients seem to earn the respect of their therapists by working hard in therapy, revealing and developing strengths, showing good judgment, and so forth. Some clients command the attention of their therapist through their engaging presence or by casting their problems in an interesting light or a compelling way. When clients embody genuineness, it seems to inspire their therapists to do the same. When clients are more obviously vulnerable in their emotions or use vivid and descriptive language, it seems to enhance their therapists' empathic language. Clients seem to motivate their therapist to work hard in and out of session by showing appreciation or, alternatively, their desperation. Clients also give therapists a reason to hope by reporting progress to the therapist or reminding their therapist of previous therapeutic successes. For example, after one client revealed a series of unscrupulous choices, he then told the therapist how much it meant to him that he felt safe enough with her to open up. I imagine that would even further reinforce the therapist's nonjudgmental stance with the client.

Create Mutuality

Therapist and client come together in a particular way to create a unique union or mutuality. As clients invest in this relationship, they stand to glean fortification if the relationship is healthy. Many clients choose to trust their therapist, telling them things they have "never told anyone." Another way clients create mutuality with their therapist is by introducing language that then becomes a common language as well as a shared history. Clients refer in a short-hand way to stories previously shared with the therapist or the shared stories created in the therapy room over the course of the therapy. Comments such as "You remember when . . ." or "You know me" hint at the realness and importance of their connection. Other ways this mutuality is formed is by cocreating their shared sense of humor, communicating about their relationship, or conveying the sense that they simply enjoy one another. For example, after one client shared his latest obsession, the therapist began speaking, but the client cut her off, saying he knew what she was going to say next—he guessed she wanted him to do yet another exposure exercise—and they both started laughing.

Test Interpersonal Assumptions

Directly Process the Relationship

The therapy relationship is often referred to as a test tube for later experimentation in the outside world. Clients test out their perceptions of the relationship and compare notes with the therapists' perceptions. For instance, one client experienced anxiety in situations where she feared she was imposing on others (meeting with her thesis advisor or making phone calls to donors). At times in the therapy, she would experience this same anxiety if she hesitated about what to talk about in therapy or reported feeling better. She directly asked whether her therapist thought she was wasting the therapist's time. She queried if she bored or annoyed the therapist, taking up valuable resources because she was not in the direst of circumstances. At times, clients initiate processing of their relationship with the therapist and then transfer what they learn to other relationships.

Recreate the Other's Role

Clients seem to learn how to respond differently in a troubled relationship by watching how the therapist responds when posed with a similar challenge. Although it may be unconscious, clients may set up a situation where the therapist is in a similar position as the client and could thus model how to handle the situation. An example of this happened when a client set up an oppositional relationship with the therapist like the one he had with his father. In this situation, the client challenged much of what the therapist said or did, just as his father challenged him. The therapist's responses to this opposition provided alternative methods for dealing with his oppositional father.

Recreate Their Own Role

In a similar vein, clients also recreate with their therapist their part in a conflicted relationship. For instance, one client was late to therapy on a regular basis and had mentioned that her lack of punctuality was also a source of contention with her husband. At one point, the therapist processed how it felt to wait for the client to show, wondering if she valued therapy or wanted to avoid the full amount of time with the therapist. The client wondered aloud whether her husband might be having a similar reaction to her tardiness.

Qualify the Therapist's Trustworthiness

Check Compatibility With the Therapist

Before investing so much into what could be a highly influential therapy relationship, clients vet their therapist. They ask about background, looking for commonalities or, conversely, important sought-after differences. Clients test to see if their therapist has similar values, worldviews, and so forth. For instance, one client made a derogatory comment about a particular ethnic group, seemingly wanting to see if the therapist would agree with the stereotype. A few sessions later, the client shared her fears that professors were silently prejudiced, and she wondered how she could detect which ones held biases before choosing her thesis advisor. These types of compatibility checks help the client invest resources into a potentially healing relationship.

Determine the Therapist's Competence

Clients ask questions about training to determine competency—for example, they ask about the therapist's degree, license, alma mater, number of years of experience, and areas of expertise. They test for cultural competency, querying to see if the therapist is culturally literate and aware. Clients also garner information about their therapist's personal life to vet for relevant experiences. For instance, one curious client asked whether her therapist was married and had children—because her primary concerns involved her role as wife and mother, she wanted guidance from someone who had some sense of what it was like to be in a similar situation.

Test the Therapist's Commitment

Some clients seem to want to know they are not "just another client" for the therapist. They engage in experiments of sorts to see whether their therapist has a genuine concern for them. One client tested the memory of his therapist, loosely referring to an issue but wanting to see how thoroughly the therapist recollected the details of a trauma. Another client wrote provocative things in her written intake questionnaire, and when the therapist delved further in person, the client admitted she was just checking to see if the therapist was actually paying attention. It seemed important to one client to know that his therapist would be able to join him for the long haul, inquiring how long she would be at that clinic.

Repair Ruptures in the Relationship

Address Therapist's Mistakes

Inevitably, therapists make mistakes, which run the gamut of inconsequential to irreparable. In graduate school, therapists' mistakes are referred to as "grist for the therapeutic mill"—and clients operate the mill! Clients confront the therapist directly, allowing the therapist the opportunity to work on the relationship. At times, it seems that clients more subtly address the therapist's mistake. One client, who had experienced multiple losses (the deaths of her mother, father, and son) seemed to have difficulty getting her therapist to attend to her grief. At the end of the first session, the client began to cry and mentioned how her needs tended to be neglected in the family. At the same moment, the therapist abruptly ended the session. The dialogue went as follows:

CLIENT: My mother died when I was 4, and everyone else was kind of focused on that, and my grandfather died and everyone focused on that. I was always—it wasn't their fault, but things happened in my life that made them pay no attention.

THERAPIST: I have to run. I so enjoyed our time together. (Greaves, 2006, p. 171)

The ill-timed ending was not mentioned at the beginning of the second session. However, partway through the second session, the client readdressed her pain over losing her mother.

CLIENT: Like with my mother's death, and I was wondering why. . . . Lately, I've been mourning for her. Something broke loose, and I was able to cry. *I don't know if it was something that I talked to you about* [emphasis added], but whatever happened, it did something about my mother, which I never knew, which is maybe underneath the problem, all the problems. . . . So, maybe if I stay there—like this week with my mother and think how I feel about her leaving me. (Greaves, 2006, pp. 171–172)

The client continued to talk about her mother for two exchanges when the therapist switched topics. The client complied. At the end of the second session, the therapist asked if she was interested in coming back the following week, something the therapist had not said to other clients in the study. Again, the client took this question in stride and responded that she would. The beginning of the next session went as follows:

THERAPIST: Did you have anything on your mind?

CLIENT: Oh a lot. I keep going back to when I was a little child and my mother died. (Greaves, 2006, p. 172)

Finally, the majority of the third session was spent processing the loss of her mother, and it appeared the client had forgiven the therapist for seemingly avoiding the painful subject.

Explore Solutions to Rupture

When clients have invested a lot into a therapy relationship, it makes sense they would want to look for ways to resolve the rupture so as not to have to start over with a new therapist. For example, one client was hurt by the therapist's word choices when talking about past abuse, feeling the therapist was not being sensitive enough. She suggested the therapist talk in a less pointed way, leaving out names and not referring to exact details of the abuse.

Make Amends With the Therapist

At times, clients can offend or wear down a therapist, which can also have deleterious effects on the alliance and consequently the fruitfulness of therapy. Clients may ask if the therapist is offended by certain actions or comments. Some offer an apology or try to set things straight. For example, one client who repeatedly went over time even after it was announced that time was up eventually acknowledged the difficulty of knowing therapy was over, and she would again be alone with her problems. After admitting the pattern, she followed through on her plan to manage the endings of the session more respectfully.

IMPLICATIONS FOR THERAPISTS

Noting the client's words and behavior is part of the therapist's natural domain. However, the lens through which therapists see their clients' words and behavior can have a dramatic effect on how therapists respond and coordinate synergistically with their clients. The implications given here are just a sampling of ideas of how a new pair of lenses may reveal how to partner with clients' inherent strengths.

Client-Directed Problem Solving

This dimension highlights what clients can do as therapists assist them with what is described as the organization of the problem and the hermeneutical understanding of the problem. Therapists are equipped with diagnostic tools and specialized problem-solving skills, but determining which problem the client wants to solve is key. Paying attention to subtleties, even word choices (Lacan, 1968), reveals the idiosyncratic manifestation and meaning of the problem for that specific person. Besides, clients may have different priorities and ideas about what is changeable, what problems can be lived with, and what they can afford to fix at the moment. If therapists align with the motivation that the client has to solve a particular problem (see Prochaska et al., 1992), they will have gained "capital" with the client, opening the way to help alleviate other problems the client is reluctant to address or has grown accustomed to.

The client's identification of a problem and their impromptu intentions of how to address it are like crafting a "work order." Even if clients are not completely aware of their plans (Rennie, 1990), this work order can be a crucial guide to therapists. Intention is a hallmark of agency at work, and when clients identify a problem or direction, therapists can lend their curiosity, remind them of their plans, or cater interventions to what the client is already gravitating toward. Similarly, when clients are reporting on progress, the therapist may be an accountability partner, a cheerleader (Rennie, 2004), and a revering admirer who may inspire the client to do more of the same.

Therapists must recognize and yield to client meaning-making processes. For instance, most metaphors have roots in the lived bodily experience (Lakoff & Johnson, 2003), so by using their own metaphors, clients are able to access their internal felt sense of a problem and map it to something more tangible and more available for cognitive problem solving. Therapists may also feel inclined to finish clients' thoughts; however, if therapists patiently sync with their clients who are searching at the periphery of their awareness (Gendlin, 1998) or the periphery of what they have felt comfortable sharing thus far, they may be surprised at the rewards of yielding to that hesitancy and what the client is able to convey next. When therapists assume insight and healing activities are happening all week long and take the time to inquire about and highlight these, it reinforces to clients that their intuitive problem-solving processes are valuable, and they themselves should pay attention to them.

Reconstruction and Remoralization of the Self

Frank and Frank (1991) asserted that clients often seek out therapy after years of struggle when they are demoralized and that the most important goal of therapy is to regain hope. By noticing and encouraging when clients talk positively about their own qualities, ideas, and even partially successful attempts at change, therapists can fan the flame of hope that starts from within (Blundo et al., 2014). Gradually, the self is reconstructed as clients risk being their true selves, accessing cutoff emotions that they "don't usually let themselves show," and doing so in the context of a supportive relationship is a key to remoralization.

Rennie (1998) proposed that the main goal of therapy is to increase the degree to which clients act in purposeful or agentic ways. Therapists can be sensitive to the remoralization process by recognizing when clients increase their exercise of agency, and sometimes that means allowing the client to have more control of the session, as Rennie (2000) found some clients desired. Sometimes that means clients "do our job" as they assert themselves by structuring the session, setting the pace, interrupting to get "back on" their topic, challenging their own resistances, and so forth. This is a time to pivot, where therapists can see their role as cotherapist. When therapists make room for silence, it sends a message that not all the work will be done in a dialogic way and allows clients the space to drop into their bodies and into an emotional experience or take the space for insight incubation. Researchers have discovered that shortly before an "aha" moment, brain scans show a quieting down in one area of the brain taking in stimuli and a burst of activity in the right superior temporal gyrus, a part of the brain associated with new learning (Kounios & Beeman, 2014).

There may also be a moral component to the concept of clients maximizing their agentic capacity. R. N. Williams (1992) noted that "whether a person is free is to ask *how* he or she is 'in the world' depends on whether or not he or she is involved in the world truthfully" (p. 757). As clients create safe spaces to explore the truth, their agency is enhanced. R. N. Williams (1994) further elaborated that if "the very essence of our humanity is our obligation to the other" (p. 38), to live in the world truthfully and thus exercise agency, one must take on this ethical obligation. When clients are working on moral concerns such as defining their beliefs and values or assuming responsibility for their actions, therapists may want to defer to the client's reasoning and instead marvel at their agentic growth, which in and of itself is a morale boost! At times, clients' maturation advances beyond the level of the therapist, as Yalom (2003) described:

> Karen Horney's view of the self-actualizing drive . . . is relevant: if the therapist removes obstacles, patients will naturally mature and realize their potential, even attaining a level of integration beyond that of the facilitating therapist. . . . Indeed, I have often had patients whose change and whose courage have left me gaping in admiration. (pp. 104–105)

Mobilization and Application of the Therapist's Expertise

This dimension includes those activities that are readily mentioned in the process literature: deferring to the therapist's expertise and complying with interventions. After all, many clients are looking for a directive approach to psychotherapy (Cooper et al., 2019), and psychology as a science has much specialized knowledge to offer (E. N. Williams, 2020). However, as Bohart and Tallman (Chapter 1, this volume) note, even in compliance, clients engage in the active process of "adopting" the therapist's way. Furthermore, some techniques require more of the client's interpretation and development than others. Psychodrama, two-chair work, guided imagery, and the like require the client's linguistic or visual creativity to work at all. During an EMDR protocol, there are long stretches where the therapist does not even know what is happening as the client quietly, and possibly nonlinguistically, processes and integrates memories.

Clients may implement the directive as expected by the therapist, but clients often customize these interventions, using them as a "prosthesis" (Bohart & Tallman, 1999). When clients start customizing the in-session activity or homework, therapists could look for cues about what special thing the client gleaned from making the modification. Even when clients comply with suggestions, which intervention the therapist chooses can be influenced by the subtle pull of the client (see Chapter 12, this volume). Therapists notice those things that surprise them (clients' tangents or objections or even the therapist's own feelings and behavior) and appraise these as possible indicators that clients have contextually prepared them to be the most helpful. On rare occasions, clients might be the ones giving the homework to therapists or subtly inspiring them to get consultation or learn a new method when treatment failure seems inevitable.

Polkinghorne (2004) drew on the work of philosopher de Certeau, comparing the power differential between client and therapist with that of institutional marginalization. He noted that while therapists employ formal strategies, clients claim their power through the use of tactics that can be "ordinary . . . hidden . . . less structured, and less precise" (p. 67). These tactics can balance the power and are used a lot more often than meets the eye, as I have attempted to demonstrate. Not only can therapists strive for an egalitarian relationship that, if successful, might make clients' self-healing tactics less hidden, but they can also keep their eyes peeled for the ways clients are agentically showing up and explicitly defer to their lead.

Some models address how therapists can intricately draw on their own empathic, experiential, and scholarly understanding in responding to clients' clues about what approach is needed. Constantino et al. (2020) demonstrated the value of context-responsive psychotherapy integration methods through the following example: A therapist administering an evidence-based therapy pivots to another treatment method, recognizing the adaptive quality (not resistance) of a typically unassertive client who stands up to defend the value of her worry. Because of the therapist's flexibility, an emotionally corrective experience is possible as the therapist defers to the client. With the post-traumatic growth model, Tedeschi and Moore (2020) developed the idea of an *expert companion*, where a therapist "accompanies the trauma survivor by assuming a stance as a learner of their experience and its personal meaning, and is a sharp listener for signs of growth that become an emphasis in therapy beyond symptomatic improvement" (p. 7). Expert companions implement trauma-based strategies from various theoretical orientations at appropriate times based on what they are reading from their "companion."

Nurturance and Utilization of the Therapeutic Relationship

Therapists recognize that each relationship they form with clients has its own unique qualities; no two are alike. Why are these relationships so distinct? Therapists are virtually the same one hour to the next (unless the previous hour, the client changed them, which is possible). I think back to the things I learned in graduate school about forming a therapeutic bond with my clients—being respectful, empathic, attentive, competent, reliable, genuine, trustworthy, nonjudgmental, and humorous—and I wonder, "Why wouldn't clients do the same?" In spite of their problems, they want the therapist to like them! And, in fact, treatment outcomes improve if the therapist likes the client (Gelso, 2019). Clients must balance how to interact with their therapist so as to not bore them asleep, irritate them into reactivity, or scare them off—yet still not dilute the potency of the relationship to fix the very problems that may make them boring, annoying, or overwhelming. This aspect of the bond, or the real relationship (Gelso, 2019) that clients help create, is separate from efforts to simply be socially desirable, the working alliance, or transference–countertransference effects.

Genuineness is a crucial component of the real relationship (Gelso, 2019). Rennie (1992) found that clients "[appraise] . . . whether or not [they are] in 'good hands' with the person of the therapist [and] . . . sense . . . whether or not [the] therapist has clients' interest at heart" (p. 20). When clients perceive therapists to be "agents of the establishment," they may perform credibility tests to see whether gender, cultural differences, or other differences are disruptive enough to halt therapy (Sue & Sue, 1999, p. 46). Put into their proper perspective, therapists can honor these trustworthiness tests as signs of healthy functioning, paving the way for the safety to do deeper therapeutic work.

And what about when the therapist does blow it? Owen et al. (2014) found that when racial microaggressions occurred, if they were discussed, the overall alliance ratings were similar to those where no rupture occurred. Thankfully, clients are sometimes the ones to initiate those repair ruptures. When clients were interviewed about ruptures, it was found that clients intentionally weighed the need to either have the trust repaired through direct confrontation versus covert toleration of the therapist's mistake (Rennie, 1994). Ironically, even when therapists are not being helpful, they are supplying the client with "grist for the therapeutic mill" as clients recognize that no matter how much the therapist may care, ultimately, the client must find their own grounding because therapists are not fully dependable. However, if therapists are willing participants and allow the client to practice working successfully through the ruptures with them, this too can be a corrective emotional experience as they practice forgiving and being forgiven. If the rupture cannot be adequately mended, clients can also have a corrective emotional experience by terminating the therapy, an often-overlooked aspect of healthy agentic functioning.

IMPLICATIONS FOR FUTURE RESEARCH

In our meta-analytic review of client-focused research, Bohart and I noted that there was a paucity of research looking at the neurobiological, psychological, and social underpinnings of clients' participation (not client traits) and how clients act on the therapy (Bohart & Wade, 2013). Exploratory qualitative studies that use recordings (see Elliott, 1986; Rennie, 2012) to capture more nuanced phenomena, followed by well-timed interviews that capture covert processes, paired with quantitative measures of change, have the potential to culminate in complex theories of interdependent change in psychotherapy. Naturally, clients, therapists, observers, and quantitative measures will reveal different aspects of the story. However, if the questions and observations are not specifically attuned to how clients contribute to the change process, we will fill the annals with more technique and therapist-centric research.

Even with complex modeling, the models can only work as well as the measures that capture client phenomena. With the use of observational research like that presented here, process measures could be adapted to include categories that account for active and agentic client contributions, along with measures that capture the mutual influence process. Empirically supported principles or practices (Bohart, 2000), as opposed to empirically supported protocols or manuals, are valuable in that they allow for a coconstructive change process where therapists and clients are free to react to the agentic flow of the moment. This bidirectional influence is real life, and as Kazdin (2008) noted, "We are letting knowledge from practice drip through the holes of a colander" (p. 155).

Research on *role induction* (the term used to describe the formal education of clients about what is expected of them in therapy) highlights that it can attenuate early termination (Swift et al., 2012). However, role induction can also take place informally in therapists' paracommunication and metacommunication with clients (Beitman & Viamontes, 2007). Experimenting with formal or informal role induction protocols that debunk myths of passive participation and highlight instead clients' unique contributions and the bidirectional influence model could prove fruitful in enhancing treatment outcome. Indeed, the general public is curious about psychotherapy from the client's perspective, as evidenced by the fact that the 2019 number one Audible nonfiction book of the year gave a peek into psychotherapist Lori Gottlieb (2019) taking her turn on the other side of psychotherapy, as a client. I wonder then what could happen if consumers of psychotherapy saw this paradigm shift of psychotherapy, away from being expert driven and toward a relationship that is truly a collaborative meeting of the minds.

CONCLUSION

The matter of agency is intricate, and therapists and clients alike have varying adeptness at embodying their agency in various circumstances (see R. N. Williams, 1992). But I am excited to think that the field is shifting to a serious investigation of the bidirectional influence process of psychotherapy, honoring therapist and client alike as healers and agents of change. The resulting research will create a repository of dynamic duos, human feats of strength, and people overcoming odds and blossoming despite the pain, disappointments, and even torture of this life. What a boon to therapists, clients, and laypeople alike! While I draw on several theoretical orientations as a psychologist, I am grateful that early on, my practice was shaped by Bohart and Tallman's (1999) theory of the meeting of the minds—and I would add the word "hearts" as well. Last, I am grateful to my clients who allow me to partner with them, sometimes riding in their "slipstream," and rewarding me with lasting memories of the beautiful lives they have fashioned in the throes of the inevitable problems of living. I hope their stories—our stories—are told more fully in the years to come.

REFERENCES

American Society of Clinical Oncology. (2016). *Clinical cancer advances 2016: Annual report on progress against cancer.* https://www.asco.org/research-progress/reports-studies/clinical-cancer-advances

Beitman, B. D., & Viamontes, G. I. (2007). Unconscious role-induction: Implications for psychotherapy. *Psychiatric Annals, 37*(4), 259–268.

Biggs, L. J., McLachlan, H. L., Shafiei, T., Small, R., & Forster, D. A. (2019). Peer supporters' experiences on an Australian perinatal mental health helpline. *Health Promotion International, 34*(3), 479–489. https://doi.org/10.1093/heapro/dax097

Blundo, R. G., Bolton, K. W., & Hall, J. C. (2014). Hope: Research and theory in relation to solution-focused practice and training. *International Journal of Solution-Focused Practices, 2*(2), 52–62. https://doi.org/10.14335/ijsfp.v2i2.22

Bohart, A. C. (2000). Paradigm clash: Empirically supported treatments versus empirically supported psychotherapy practice. *Psychotherapy Research, 10*(4), 488–493. https://doi.org/10.1080/713663783

Bohart, A. C., & Brock, G. (2003, July 6–11). *How does empathy facilitate?* Paper presented at the meeting of the World Conference for Person-Centered and Experiential Psychotherapy and Counseling, Egmond aan Zee, The Netherlands.

Bohart, A. C., & Tallman, K. (1999). *How clients make therapy work: The process of active self-healing.* American Psychological Association. https://doi.org/10.1037/10323-000

Bohart, A. C., & Wade, A. G. (2013). The client in psychotherapy. In M. J. Lambert (Ed.), *Bergin and Garfield's handbook of psychotherapy and behavior change* (6th ed., pp. 219–257). Wiley.

Cohen Veterans Network & National Council for Behavioral Health. (2018). *America's mental health 2018.* https://www.cohenveteransnetwork.org/wp-content/uploads/2018/10/Research-Summary-10-10-2018.pdf

Constantino, M. J., Coyne, A. E., & Muir, H. J. (2020). Evidence-based therapist responsivity to disruptive clinical process. *Cognitive and Behavioral Practice, 27*(4), 405–416. https://doi.org/10.1016/j.cbpra.2020.01.003

Cooper, M., Norcross, J. C., Raymond-Barker, B., & Hogan, T. P. (2019). Psychotherapy preferences of laypersons and mental health professionals: Whose therapy is it? *Psychotherapy, 56*(2), 205–216. https://doi.org/10.1037/pst0000226

Coppola, F. F. (1972). *The Godfather* [Film]. Paramount Pictures.

Crits-Christoph, P., Gibbons, M. B. C., & Mukherjee, D. (2013). Process-outcome research. In M. J. Lambert (Ed.), *Bergin and Garfield's handbook of psychotherapy and behavior change* (6th ed., pp. 298–340). Wiley.

Elliott, R. (1986). Interpersonal process recall as a psychotherapy research method. In L. S. Greenberg & W. M. Pinsof (Eds.), *The psychotherapeutic process: A research handbook* (pp. 503–527). Guilford Press.

Frank, J. D., & Frank, J. B. (1991). *Persuasion and healing: A comparative study of psychotherapy* (3rd ed.). The Johns Hopkins University Press.

Gaston, L. (1991). Reliability and criterion-related validity of the California Psychotherapy Alliance Scales—Patient version. *Psychological Assessment, 3*(1), 68–74. https://doi.org/10.1037/1040-3590.3.1.68

Gelso, C. J. (2019). *The therapeutic relationships in psychotherapy practice: An integrative perspective*. Routledge.

Gendlin, E. T. (1998). *Focusing-oriented psychotherapy: A manual of the experiential method.* Guilford Press.

Gottlieb, L. (2019). *Maybe you should talk to someone: A therapist, her therapist, and our lives revealed.* Houghton Mifflin Harcourt.

Greaves, A. L. (2006). *The active client: A qualitative analysis of thirteen clients' contribution to the psychotherapeutic process* [Unpublished doctoral dissertation]. University of Southern California.

Hill, C. E., Corbett, M. M., Kanitz, B., Rios, P., Lightsey, R., & Gomez, M. (2001). Client behavior in counseling and therapy sessions: Development of a pantheoretical measure. In C. E. Hill (Ed.), *Helping skills: The empirical foundation* (pp. 21–40). American Psychological Association. https://doi.org/10.1037/10412-002

Honos-Webb, L., Stiles, W. B., & Greenberg, L. S. (2003). A method of rating assimilation in psychotherapy based on markers of change. *Journal of Counseling Psychology, 50*(2), 189–198. https://doi.org/10.1037/0022-0167.50.2.189

Kazdin, A. E. (2008). Evidence-based treatment and practice: New opportunities to bridge clinical research and practice, enhance the knowledge base, and improve patient care. *American Psychologist, 63*(3), 146–159. https://doi.org/10.1037/0003-066X.63.3.146

Kelly, J. F., & Yeterian, J. D. (2012). Empirical awakening: The new science on mutual help and implications for cost containment under health care reform. *Substance Abuse, 33*(2), 85–91. https://doi.org/10.1080/08897077.2011.634965

Klein, M. H., Mathieu-Coughlan, P., & Kiesler, D. J. (1986). The experiencing scales. In L. S. Greenberg & W. M. Pinsof (Eds.), *The psychotherapeutic process: A research handbook* (pp. 21–71). Guilford Press.

Kounios, J., & Beeman, M. (2014). The cognitive neuroscience of insight. *Annual Review of Psychology, 65*(1), 71–93. https://doi.org/10.1146/annurev-psych-010213-115154

Lacan, J. (1968). *Speech and language in psychoanalysis*. The John Hopkins University Press.

Lakoff, G., & Johnson, M. (2003). *Metaphors we live by*. University of Chicago Press. https://doi.org/10.7208/chicago/9780226470993.001.0001

Lambert, M. J. (2013). The efficacy and effectiveness of psychotherapy. In M. J. Lambert (Ed.), *Bergin and Garfield's handbook of psychotherapy and behavior change* (6th ed., pp. 169–218). Wiley.

Linehan, M. (2020). *Building a life worth living: A memoir*. Random House.

Owen, J., Tao, K. W., Imel, Z. E., Wampold, B. E., & Rodolfa, E. (2014). Addressing racial and ethnic microaggressions in therapy. *Professional Psychology, Research and Practice, 45*(4), 283–290. https://doi.org/10.1037/a0037420

Polkinghorne, D. E. (2004). *Practice and the human sciences: The case for a judgment-based practice of care*. SUNY Press.

Porges, S. W. (2011). *The polyvagal theory: Neurophysiological foundations of emotions, attachment, communication, and self-regulation*. Norton.

Prochaska, J. O., DiClemente, C. C., & Norcross, J. C. (1992). In search of how people change. Applications to addictive behaviors. *American Psychologist, 47*(9), 1102–1114. https://doi.org/10.1037/0003-066X.47.9.1102

Puchalska-Wasyl, M. M., & Zarzycka, B. (2020). Prayer and internal dialogical activity: How do they predict well-being? *Psychology of Religion and Spirituality, 12*(4), 417–427. https://doi.org/10.1037/rel0000255

Rennie, D. L. (1990). Toward a representation of the client's experience of the psychotherapy hour. In G. Lietaer, J. Rombauts, & R. Van Balen (Eds.), *Client-centered and experiential therapy in the nineties* (pp. 155–172). Leuven University Press.

Rennie, D. L. (1992). Qualitative analysis of the client's experience of psychotherapy: The unfolding of reflexivity. In S. G. Toukmanian & D. L. Rennie (Eds.), *Psychotherapy process research: Paradigmatic and narrative approaches* (pp. 211–233). SAGE.

Rennie, D. L. (1994). Clients' deference in psychotherapy. *Journal of Counseling Psychology, 41*(4), 427–437. https://doi.org/10.1037/0022-0167.41.4.427

Rennie, D. L. (1998). *Person-centered counseling: An experiential approach*. SAGE. https://doi.org/10.4135/9781446279854

Rennie, D. L. (2000). Aspects of the client's conscious control of the psychotherapy process. *Journal of Psychotherapy Integration, 10*(2), 151–167. https://link.springer.com/article/10.1023/A:1009496116174

Rennie, D. L. (2004). Reflexivity and person-centered counseling. *Journal of Humanistic Psychology, 44*(2), 182–203. https://doi.org/10.1177/0022167804263066

Rennie, D. L. (2012). Qualitative research as methodical hermeneutics. *Psychological Methods, 17*(3), 385–398. https://doi.org/10.1037/a0029250

Rhodes, R. H., Hill, C. E., Thompson, B. J., & Elliott, R. (1994). Client retrospective recall of resolved and unresolved misunderstanding events. *Journal of Counseling Psychology, 41*(4), 473–483. https://doi.org/10.1037/0022-0167.41.4.473

Rice, L. N., & Kerr, G. P. (1986). Measures of client and therapist vocal quality. In L. S. Greenberg & W. M. Pinsof (Eds.), *The psychotherapeutic process: A research handbook* (pp. 73–105). Guilford Press.

Rogers, C. R. (1964). Toward a modern approach to values: The valuing process in the mature person. *Journal of Abnormal and Social Psychology, 68*(2), 160–167. https://doi.org/10.1037/h0046419

Sangeorzan, I., Andriopoulou, P., & Livanou, M. (2019). Exploring the experiences of people vlogging about severe mental illness on YouTube: An interpretative phenomenological analysis. *Journal of Affective Disorders, 246*, 422–428. https://doi.org/10.1016/j.jad.2018.12.119

Shapiro, F. (2013). *Getting past your past: Take control of your life with self-help techniques from EMDR therapy*. Rodale Books.

Stiles, W. B. (1986). Development of a taxonomy of verbal response modes. In L. S. Greenberg & W. M. Pinsof (Eds.), *The psychotherapeutic process: A research handbook* (pp. 161–199). Guilford Press.

Sue, D. S., & Sue, D. (1999). *Counseling the culturally different: Theory and practice*. Wiley.

Suh, C. S., O'Malley, S. S., Strupp, H. H., & Johnson, M. E. (1989). The Vanderbilt Psychotherapy Process Scale (VPPS). *Journal of Cognitive Psychotherapy, 3*(2), 123–154. https://doi.org/10.1891/0889-8391.3.2.123

Swift, J. K., Greenberg, R. P., Whipple, J. L., & Kominiak, N. (2012). Practice recommendations for reducing premature termination in therapy. *Professional Psychology, Research and Practice, 43*(4), 379–387. https://doi.org/10.1037/a0028291

Tedeschi, R. G., & Moore, B. A. (2020). Posttraumatic growth as an integrative thera-peutic philosophy. *Journal of Psychotherapy Integration.* Advance online publication. https://doi.org/10.1037/int0000250

Toukmanian, S. G. (1986). A measure of client perceptual processing. In L. S. Greenberg & W. M. Pinsof (Eds.), *The psychotherapeutic process: A research handbook* (pp. 107–130). Guilford Press.

van der Kolk, B. A. (2014). *The body keeps the score: Brain, mind, and body in the healing of trauma.* Viking.

Van Sant, G. (Director). (1997). *Good Will Hunting* [Film]. Miramax.

Wampold, B. E. (2017). What should we practice? A contextual model for how psycho-therapy works. In T. Rousmaniere, R. K. Goodyear, S. D. Miller, & B. E. Wampold (Eds.), *The cycle of excellence: Using deliberate practice to improve supervision and training* (pp. 49–65). Wiley-Blackwell. https://doi.org/10.1002/9781119165590.ch3

Wampold, B. E., & Imel, Z. E. (2015). *The great psychotherapy debate: The research evi-dence for what works in psychotherapy* (2nd ed.). Routledge. https://doi.org/10.4324/9780203582015

Williams, E. N. (2020). Putting psychotherapy outcomes in context: The need for more exploratory and process research. *Journal of Psychotherapy Integration, 30*(4), 528–534. https://doi.org/10.1037/int0000237

Williams, R. N. (1992). The human context of agency. *American Psychologist, 47*(6), 752–760. https://doi.org/10.1037/0003-066X.47.6.752

Williams, R. N. (1994). The modern, the post-modern, and the question of truth: Perspec-tives on the problem of agency. *Journal of Theoretical and Philosophical Psychology, 14*(1), 25–39. https://doi.org/10.1037/h0091125

Yalom, I. (2003). *The gift of therapy.* HarperCollins.

II

CLIENT–THERAPIST INTERACTIONS

7

The Client's Function in the Psychotherapy Relationship

What Clients Experience and Contribute

Charles J. Gelso and Kathryn V. Kline

In any treatment situation (e.g., therapy, teaching, supervision), we can broadly consider three classes of factors: (a) input, (b) intervention, and (c) output. In therapy research, these three factors pertain to the client (input), the psychotherapy treatment (intervention), and the treatment outcome (output). Of the three, by far the greatest attention in theory and research has been given to the intervention factor, including the therapist's actions. However, in virtually all such situations, including psychotherapy, the evidence overwhelmingly favors the importance of the input factor (Norcross & Lambert, 2019), specifically the client's experience of and contribution to the therapy situation.

Similar to what we have said about the importance of the client factor, the therapy relationship that develops between the client and therapist has also been seen as a vital element of virtually all approaches to therapy. An abundance of empirical research supports this assertion (see Norcross & Lambert, 2019). In the present chapter, our focus is the therapy relationship, particularly on the client's experience of and contribution to the relationship that develops with the therapist.

THE THERAPY RELATIONSHIP AND ITS COMPONENTS

What is the *therapy relationship*? Despite decades of research and theory, surprisingly little effort has gone into defining the relationship. At times, researchers have equated the relationship (usually implicitly) to what Carl Rogers famously

https://doi.org/10.1037/0000303-008
The Other Side of Psychotherapy: Understanding Clients' Experiences and Contributions in Treatment, J. N. Fuertes (Editor)

viewed as the therapist-offered conditions for successful therapy: therapists' empathic understanding of the client, unconditional positive regard for the client, and congruence or genuineness with the client. Similarly, at times the relationship seems to be equated with what has been termed the *working alliance* that forms between the therapist and the client. Elsewhere, the first author (Gelso) has discussed why neither the therapist-offered conditions nor the working alliance is a satisfactory definition of the therapy relationship. Because the therapist-offered conditions pertain to only the therapist, they cannot define the relationship, which is inherently bipersonal. The working alliance is an insufficient definition of or proxy for the therapy relationship because, as we discuss subsequently, it pertains to only one element of the therapy relationship, albeit an important element.

A definition of the therapy relationship that gets at its bipersonal nature and also does not restrict it to a single element was offered by Gelso and Carter (1985, 1994). They defined the relationship as the feelings and attitudes that the client and therapist have toward one another and the manner in which these are expressed. This very general definition has been viewed as "concise, consensual, theoretically neutral, and sufficiently precise" (Norcross & Lambert, 2019, p. 3) and has often been adopted in recent years. As can be seen from this definition, both the client and the therapist contribute to the relationship, and their experiences in and of the relationship are vitally important. However, in this chapter, our focus is on the client's experience and contribution because that has been the neglected side of the psychotherapy relationship.

When discussing the therapy relationship, usually noted is the division between the relationship, on one hand, and therapist techniques, on the other. Although this division makes sense when researchers seek to understand the different elements of psychotherapy, in the reality of the clinical situation, the two are highly intertwined, as the first author has discussed (Gelso, 2019), with each pervasively influencing the other. Using the verbal technique of therapist interpretation as an example, the content, emotional tone, depth, specificity, length, timing, and accuracy of interpretations have much to do with the feelings and attitudes that therapy participants have toward one another and vice versa. Thus, "the qualities and subtleties of the relationship deeply affect all aspects of technique, and all aspects of the techniques that are used just as deeply affect the quality of the therapeutic relationship" (Gelso, 2019, p. 4). Subsequently, we have more to say about the interconnection between the therapy relationship and the therapist technique from the perspective of the client.

Finally, our emphasis in this chapter is on the client's role in what may be considered key elements or components of the psychotherapy relationship (real relationship, working alliance, and transference–countertransference) rather than on the client's experience of and contribution to the therapy relationship as a whole. Next, we define these elements of what may be termed a tripartite model of the relationship, and we then discuss the client's experience of and contributions to each element, combining research findings, clinical/ theoretical evidence, and case material.

A TRIPARTITE MODEL OF THE THERAPY RELATIONSHIP

Over a period of several decades, the first author and his collaborators have formulated and empirically investigated a model in which the therapy relationship is seen as consisting of three highly interrelated components: a real relationship, a working alliance, and a transference–countertransference configuration (Bhatia & Gelso, 2018; Gelso, 2014, 2019; Gelso & Carter, 1985, 1994; Gelso & Hayes, 1998; Gelso & Samstag, 2008). These elements are viewed as existing from the first moment of contact between therapists and clients and in some cases even before the participants make contact (e.g., the client's fantasies and images of the expected therapist). Each component exists in all theoretical persuasions of psychotherapy, although the components are likely to manifest themselves in different ways and to varying degrees in each persuasion. The three elements contribute importantly to the process of therapy and its outcomes for all theoretical orientations.

The Real Relationship: The Foundation

We begin by discussing the real relationship because this may be considered the most fundamental element of the therapy relationship (e.g., Gelso, 2011, 2019). The *real relationship* may be defined as the personal or person-to-person connection between therapist and client marked by the extent to which each is genuine with the other and perceives or experiences the other in ways that befit that person (Gelso, 2011). Thus, as Greenson (1967) formulated early on, the real relationship consists of two key constructs: *genuineness* and *realism*, or the extent to which each participant perceives/experiences the other realistically (vs. distorting the other due, for example, to transference; see subsequent sections on transference and countertransference). To understand the real relationship, two additional constructs are needed: magnitude and valence. *Magnitude* pertains to the extent or amount of real relationship that exists in any interaction, whereas *valence* reflects the degree of positivity versus negativity of the real relationship. Terms such as *caring, liking, appreciating*, and *respecting* get at the valence construct. Regarding valence, it is important to clarify that a relationship can be highly realistic and genuine but be mostly negative. In therapy as well as all relationships, people may not, for example, like, take to, or care for one another genuinely and realistically, and we cannot simply explain these reactions away on the basis of transference distortions. In any event, when we combine realism, genuineness, valence, and magnitude, we get a measure of the overall strength of the real relationship, with greater magnitudes and more positive valences of genuineness and realism indicating stronger real relationships. Virtually all measures to date of the real relationship have assessed its strength (e.g., Gelso et al., 2005; Kelley et al., 2010), and thus all studies have done so as well.

The real relationship is posited to exist within all relationships, all therapy sessions, and likely even all relational responses by therapists and clients (Gelso, 2011, 2014, 2019). It is very clearly bidirectional and is experienced and contributed to by both the client and the therapist. Furthermore, the main measures of it seek to tap three sources: the client, the therapist, and the relationship itself. Thus, both the client-rated and the therapist-rated real relationship measures ask the rater to evaluate items pertaining to the therapist, the client, and the relationship. Still, like so much of the therapy literature, the focus has been more on what the therapist contributes to the creation, maintenance, and development of the real relationship. But what of the client's role in this process? Next, we first discuss clinical/conceptual material on the client's experiences and contributions based on clinical experience and research, and we then follow with a summary of the relation of the client's experience and contribution of the real relationship to treatment outcome.

The Client's Experience of and Contribution to the Real Relationship
An important part of the client's role in psychotherapy is to say what is on their mind, explore difficult feelings and thoughts, share their thoughts and feelings about the therapist, and engage in the other tasks of therapy (e.g., homework). The extent to which the client shares and explores genuinely is a manifestation of the genuineness element of the real relationship. In addition, the client's sense of the therapist's genuineness is part of this real relationship. The concept of genuineness from the client's perspective may be understood through the items used to assess client-rated genuineness on the Real Relationship Inventory—Client Form (RRI-C; Kelley et al., 2010), the most commonly used measure of the real relationship from the client's perspective. A selection of these items presents a picture of the client's experience and expression of the real relationship. The following items from the RRI-C, reproduced from Kelley et al. (2010, Table 3), reflect genuineness:

- I was able to be myself with my therapist.
- I was holding back significant parts of myself.
- I was able to communicate my moment-to-moment inner experience to my therapist.
- My therapist seemed genuinely connected to me.
- My therapist was holding back his/her genuine self.
- My therapist and I were able to be authentic in our relationship.

Similarly, to the extent that the client perceives and experiences the therapist accurately and believes the therapist is accurately perceiving the client, the realism component of the real relationship is being enacted. Selected realism items of the RRI-C, also reproduced from Kelley et al. (2010, Table 3), are as follows:

- My therapist and I had a realistic perception of our relationship.
- My therapist liked the real me.
- My therapist's perceptions of me seem colored by his or her own issues.
- I had a realistic understanding of my therapist as a person.
- My therapist did not see me as I really am.
- My therapist's perceptions of me were accurate.

It should be reiterated that the valence of genuineness and realism is a key element of their strength. Thus, as the client experiences and expresses more genuineness and realism, and experiences greater liking, caring, and so forth, for and from the therapist, the real relationship becomes strengthened. Clients typically experience and express strong real relationships, according to their perceptions. For example, clients' overall ratings of the real relationship are typically 4 or above on a 5-point scale measuring the strength of the real relationship (Fuertes et al., 2007; Kelley et al., 2010). Furthermore, as treatment progresses, clients' ratings increase so that, for example, in the fourth quarter of therapy, their ratings are close to a 4.5 (Gelso et al., 2012).

How does the real relationship manifest in the client during the therapy hour? As noted earlier, the real relationship shows itself whenever clients express their thoughts and feelings genuinely and experience/perceive therapists and themselves realistically. One of the ways is the client's commenting honestly on some realistically perceived aspect of the therapist and their interaction. As an example, many years ago, the psychoanalyst Ralph Greenson (1967) beautifully described a somewhat painful manifestation of the real relationship with one of his analysands:

> A young man, in the terminal phase of his five-year analysis, hesitates after I have made an interpretation and then tells me that he has something to say which is very difficult for him. He was about to skip over it when he realized he had been doing just that for years. He takes a deep breath and says, "You always talk a little bit too much. You tend to exaggerate. It would be much easier for me to get mad at you and say you're cockeyed or wrong or off the point or just not answer. It's terribly hard to say what I mean because I know it will hurt your feelings."
> I believe the patient has correctly perceived some traits of mine and it was somewhat painful for me to have them pointed out. I told him he was right, but I wanted to know why it was harder for him to tell me simply and directly as he had just done than to become enraged. He answered that he knew from experience that I would not get upset by his temper. Telling me about my talking too much and exaggerating was a personal criticism and that would be hurtful. He knew I took pride in my skill as a therapist. In the past he would have been worried that I might retaliate, but he now knew it was not likely. Besides, it wouldn't kill him. (pp. 217–218)

This patient was experiencing the therapist accurately (realism element) and sharing his experience of the analyst very honestly (genuineness element). Greenson also responded genuinely, while also maintaining his analytic exploration. This is an example of one manifestation of the real relationship during a long treatment in which a more general, stronger, and more real relationship appears to have developed.

Often the client's expression of the real relationship is mixed with transference. One of the first author's (subsequently referred to in the first person) favorite examples of this is drawn from my long-term work with a client in which I ignored an expression of the real relationship, instead seeking the transference element.[1] The patient and I had worked together for 6 years; knew

---

[1]The identities of the individuals in this chapter's case examples have been properly disguised to protect client confidentiality.

each other well, as inevitably happens in work that has gone on for several years; and genuinely liked and cared for each other.

In the first session following a serious surgery I had undergone, the client, John, expressed concern by asking, "How are you doing, buddy?" I replied briefly, "I am doing well, thanks." I then began to pursue how his expression of concern was transferentially related to his need to please others and be pleasing to them. This need stemmed from a traumatic childhood in which his charm helped him avert great emotional and physical dangers within a deeply troubled family life. In a word, John knew how to be pleasing. However, in response to my seeking a connection of his concern for me and his defensive pattern, John replied, "Well, that may be so, but I was also just concerned about you as a person." Here I believe John was expressing caring within our real relationship, but my zeal to work with the transference got in the way of seeing the real relationship element. I told John that I appreciated his concern, and we proceeded to explore other relevant material.

Client Factors in the Real Relationship

What qualities in clients facilitate the strength of the real relationships they form with their therapists? The little research that has been done points clearly to a small but cohesive cluster of qualities: the tendency to form secure attachments to others, including their therapist (Marmarosh et al., 2009; Moore & Gelso, 2011); ego strength, including the capacity to observe themselves and others clearly (Kelley et al., 2010); insightfulness during the therapy hour; a tendency to attend to their inner feelings; and, negatively, a tendency to hide their true feelings and conform to others' expectations (Kelley et al., 2010).

One client factor that has been discussed clinically as mattering a great deal in the development of the real relationship is a client's sense of self or the cohesiveness of the sense of self (Gelso & Silberberg, 2016). This is why clients who have borderline or narcissistic disorders appear to experience great difficulties forming strong real relationships. As Gelso and Silberberg (2016) stated,

> The RR [real relationship] by definition is a genuine connection between two people, but it is contingent on having two people who are able to see each other as separate beings. If the client does not have a clear and strong sense of self for the psychotherapist to connect with, the RR will be extremely difficult to establish. Helping the client build his or her sense of self is a slow and deliberate process, which will ultimately allow the client to view his or herself as a separate person with permeable, yet clear boundaries with others. (p. 160)

In sum, clients who have a strong enough sense of self and self-cohesion; an ability to observe themselves and others; and a capacity to form sound attachments with others, including their therapist, are more inclined to develop strong real relationships with their therapists. Similarly, clients who seem to have a good capacity to look inward, understand their inner workings, and do not hide their feelings too much in order to look good tend to form strong real relationships. It follows that as these qualities strengthen during therapy, the real relationship should likewise change, and there is an abundance of clinical and empirical evidence that such changes do unfold during successful treatment (see Gelso, 2014, 2019; Gelso & Silberberg, 2016).

Does the Client's Experience of the Real Relationship Matter?

One way of assessing whether the client's experience of the real relationship matters is through its relation to session outcome, treatment progress, and treatment outcome. We can point to at least 16 studies of the relation of real relationship to these criteria. In a recent meta-analysis (Gelso et al., 2018), the overall correlation coefficient between the strength of the real relationship and the outcome was 0.37, representing a moderate effect size, which did not vary with the type of outcome (e.g., session vs. treatment) and is larger than is typically found for the association of the working alliance and the outcome. To the point of this chapter, the client rating of the real relationship was as strongly associated with outcome (regardless of whether client or therapist rated the outcome) as was therapist ratings of the real relationship. So, the client's experience of and contribution to the real relationship clearly matters in terms of its effect on the success or failure of psychotherapy. Unfortunately, we have no qualitative studies that examine clients' perceptions of the real relationship, how important it is to clients in their own words, and how it relates to the success or failure of treatment in clients' eyes. A small sample of potentially useful questions that could be explored in qualitative studies are as follows: What has helped you develop a person-to-person relationship with your therapist? What hinders this? In what ways has this personal relationship facilitated (or hindered) your work with your therapist? What can you or your therapist do to strengthen your person-to-person connection to each other?

The Working Alliance: The Catalyst

Although the real relationship may be the foundation of the overall therapy relationship, the work relationship, or working alliance, is necessary if the work of therapy is to be done successfully. Indeed, it is hard to imagine successful therapy in the absence of a sound working alliance. We may define this alliance as the alignment or joining together of the client's reasonable ego or self and the therapist's therapizing ego or self for the purpose of accomplishing the work of therapy (see Gelso & Carter, 1994). This joining together reflects a working bond between the participants and an implicit or explicit agreement on the goals of therapy and the tasks that are useful to accomplish those goals. The joining together both affects and is affected by these bonds and agreements. Conceptualization of working alliance in terms of a bond, an agreement of goals, and an agreement on tasks needed to attain the goals was first offered by Bordin (1979) and operationalized by the Working Alliance Inventory (WAI; Horvath & Greenberg, 1989). This measure has a client- and a therapist-completed version and now appears in several different forms. From its initial development, the WAI has been the dominant measure of the working alliance, due to its conceptual clarity and its ease of use. Similarly, Bordin's conception of the working alliance has been the dominant theory for many years (Fuertes et al., 2020).

It should be noted that we have conceptualized the bond element of the working alliance as related to but different from the real relationship (Gelso & Kline, 2019). The bond of the working alliance is a working bond and has to do with the participants' feelings toward one another as the client and the therapist. For example, the client's respect for the therapist as a professional is part of the working bond, as we view it. On the other hand, the bond in the real relationship is a personal or person-to-person bond, one that exists between two human beings with feelings toward one another as people.

Whereas the real relationship may be conceptualized as a part of all human relationships, the working alliance exists for the sole purpose of getting a piece of work done. In this sense, it may be seen as an artifact of the therapy relationship. Like the real relationship in psychotherapy, the working alliance is a bipersonal phenomenon, with its nature, strength, and effects being contributed to by both the therapist and the client. In this chapter, our focus is on the client's role in the alliance formation and its effects.

The Client's Experience of and Contribution to the Working Alliance

To exemplify clients' experience of and contribution to the working alliance, a few items from the WAI (Horvath & Greenberg, 1989, Table 2), probably the major measure of this concept, are presented next (the subscale the item comes from is in parentheses following the item):

- I believe the way we were working with my problem(s) was correct. (Agreement of tasks)
- My therapist and I were working toward mutually agreed upon goals. (Agreement on goals)
- I believe my therapist is genuinely concerned for my welfare. (Working bond)

A key client contribution to the working alliance is the willingness of the client to invest in the work. If the client does not invest, there is bound to be little collaboration and, ultimately, little bonding in the alliance. Or if clients begin to disinvest, the alliance will not have the sustenance to continue meaningful work. Such investment includes being willing to share what is on one's mind and make an effort to do the tasks of therapy. It also includes speaking up when part of the work does not seem useful to the client. Speaking up can help the client and therapist get on the same page about the therapeutic work. Conversely, if clients do not raise concerns, this is likely to lead to potentially unsolvable ruptures (discussed subsequently).

According to a theory developed by Fitzpatrick et al. (2006, 2009), alliance formation may begin with comments made by the therapist that communicate something positive to or about the client. But alliance formation is also fostered by the client's openness to exploration. For example, the client has a positive response to the therapist asking an insight-rendering question or making a comment that facilitates the client's feeling appreciated or understood. Then the client's positive responses to the therapist's actions and the client's openness to exploration lay the groundwork for the client's contribution to the formation of the working alliance.

When considering what makes for a strong working alliance in clients' eyes, it is important to understand the obvious: Clients differ! This fact was made clear by a now-classic qualitative study by Bachelor (1995) in which clients at a university consultation center were asked what they viewed as a good client–therapist working relationship. Their responses divided clients into three clusters or alliance types. Bachelor labeled the first as the *nurturant* type. The nurturant working relationship was characterized by the therapist being attentive, nonjudgmental, understanding, and respectful. This kind of alliance was similar to that of a close friend, as well as what Rogers considered the good relationship in his humanistic therapy. The second cluster of clients viewed the good working relationship as involving therapist-fostered *insight or self-understanding*. Therapist activities that facilitated this kind of alliance were interpretation, uncovering of underlying states, exploration, and integrating the past with the present in a way that had not previously been understood. For this insight cluster of clients, a more psychodynamic approach would likely foster a good working alliance. Finally, a third cluster of clients wanted a *collaborative relationship* in which the therapist and client worked together to set agendas and solve problems.

It is noteworthy that the collaborative cluster was by far the smallest in Bachelor's (1995) study. This is in contrast to most therapist-constructed alliance conceptions, where the collaborative aspect of the alliance is prominently featured. As Bedi and Hayes (2020) pointed out, clients typically place responsibility on therapists and their clinical contributions for the development and maintenance of the working alliance. Bedi and Hayes further remind us that "clinicians should not necessarily expect clients initially to be thinking about therapeutic collaboration as clients often enter treatment in great psychological distress, feeling incompetent in resolving their problems" (p. 126) and "unable to handle much responsibility" (Bedi, 2006, p. 32). This is one area in which it is highly important to be aware of the client's perspective. Bedi and Hayes's viewpoint is consistent with the meta-analytic results indicating that therapists typically contribute more to the alliance development than clients (Flückiger et al., 2019).

Another aspect of the Bachelor (1995) study is noteworthy. Despite the different clusters of clients in terms of what makes for a good work relationship, Bachelor also found that for nearly all clients, therapist qualities that we might summarize as empathy, caring, and affirmation were important (see Gelso, 2019). Thus, for the alliance to develop effectively, therapists need to offer these fundamental conditions to all clients, while, beyond that, they should also offer one or more of the three approaches Bachelor discovered, depending on the particular client's needs.

The qualities of empathy, caring, and affirmation are similar to what Bedi and Hayes (2020) referred to as *confirmation*. In clients' words, Bedi (2006) told us that confirmation means the therapist said "that my reactions were understandable and reasonable, that it is okay to feel this way" and that the therapist "normalized my experiences," "made encouraging comments," "made positive comments about me," and "agreed with what I said" (p. 31). Bedi noted that confirmations such as these play a highly significant role in alliance formation according to clients. At the same time, it seems to us that part of the art of effective psychotherapy is knowing or learning when and how to communicate these messages. For example, while the client may feel good when the therapist "agreed with what I said" or "normalized my experience," there are times when such communications are uncalled for and counterproductive in the long run.

The idea that the alliance involves a warm, supportive, caring response by the therapist was part of early conceptualizations of alliance development (Luborsky, 1976). However, for Luborsky, this represented the first phase of alliance development. The second phase involved a greater collaborative effort. Research is needed to determine whether this theoretically and clinically reasonable assertion holds up in terms of clients' experience.

We earlier pointed to the deep connection between therapist techniques and the therapy relationship. This connection is underscored when we consider what constitutes the working alliance in clients' eyes. For clients, it appears that therapy strategies and interventions are a key part of clients' experience of alliance formation (Bedi & Hayes, 2020). For example, Bedi et al. (2005) found that clients point to specific therapist techniques as influential in alliance formation. Similarly, it has been found that the techniques that were most influential in alliance formation were those that helped the client most (Fitzpatrick et al., 2006, 2009; Kivlighan, 1990). The take-home message in these consistent findings is that the effective use of techniques is perhaps the most potent determinant of the working alliance.

Clients typically evaluate the working alliance favorably, just as they do the real relationship. For example, Tryon et al. (2008) found that clients' ratings on several alliance measures tended to be in the upper fifth of the rating scale. And there tends to be a slight improvement in clients' alliance ratings across sessions (Falkenström et al., 2015). Clients' ratings of the alliance tend to be higher than therapists' ratings, and although the correlation between clients' and therapists' ratings are statistically significant, they tend not to be strong (in the 0.30–0.35 range). Therapists and clients, in other words, often have differences in how they see the working alliance.

Client Factors in the Working Alliance

Are there qualities in the client that foster or impede the working alliance? As we have indicated, therapists typically contribute more to the alliance formation than clients. Still, certain client factors are substantial and important. From a clinical perspective, it seems obvious that a key client factor in alliance formation and development is the ability to form sound attachments to others (e.g., the therapist). Similarly, the capacity for trusting others has been found to be important (Birkhäuer et al., 2017). If clients cannot form attachments and trust, it is hard to imagine a working alliance, and this connection has been empirically supported (e.g., Levy et al., 2018).

Although the empirical evidence is mixed, from a clinical perspective, personality disorders such as borderline personality, antisocial personality, and schizoid personality all likely affect the development of the working alliance in complex ways. For example, the high levels of aggression and negativity evidenced in most borderline patients can significantly impede alliance formation. These qualities make skillful therapeutic work (including management of countertransference; discussed in more detail later) essential if an effective alliance is to develop.

Does the Client's Experience of the Working Alliance Matter?

There have been several decades of research seeking to determine the association of the working alliance to therapy outcomes (e.g., session outcome, treatment outcome, treatment progress). The overall findings taken from several hundred studies is that the working alliance is indeed associated with outcome (see Flückiger et al., 2019). The magnitude of this relationship is statistically significant but modest, with alliance–outcome correlations being between 0.23 and 0.30. This magnitude is statistically seen as small to medium. Such a magnitude may seem rather trivial, but when considering the numerous potential variables and confounds that may suppress such an association, it is generally seen as clinically meaningful.

More to the point of this chapter, the client's ratings of the working alliance were related to treatment outcome at the same level statistically (correlation coefficients of 0.25) as the therapist's rating of alliance ($r = 0.29$). Thus, although the therapist may contribute more to alliance formation than the client, clients' and therapists' assessments of the alliance are about equally important to the success or failure of treatment.

Tear and Repair: The Impact of Alliance Ruptures

The concept of alliance ruptures was originated by Bordin (1979, 1994) and further refined and empirically investigated by Safran, Muran, and Eubanks (e.g., Eubanks et al., 2019; Safran & Muran, 2000). *Rupture* may be defined as a deterioration in the working alliance as manifested in a disagreement between client and therapist on the goals of therapy, lack of collaboration on the tasks needed to attain those goals, or a strain in the working bond (Eubanks et al., 2019; Gelso & Kline, 2019). It should be noted that although Safran and his collaborators referred to the bond as an emotional bond, we prefer the term *working bond* because this helps differentiate the working alliance and its ruptures from the real relationship. The idea behind tear and repair is that the process of experiencing ruptures and then there being a repairment by the client and therapist is common to therapy and ultimately helpful.

Naturally, the client's perspective is fundamentally important in identifying both ruptures and repairs. This is so because the rupture and repair ordinarily occur in the client's experience of the working relationship. As described by Eubanks et al. (2019, pp. 550–551), key items used to study clients' perceptions of alliance ruptures and repairs are as follows: Did you experience any tension or problem, misunderstanding, conflict, or disagreement in your relationship with your therapist during the session?

- If yes, please rate how tense or upset you felt during the session.
- To what extent did you find yourself and your therapist overly accommodating or overly protective of each other?
- To what extent was this problem addressed in this session?
- To what degree do you feel the problem was resolved by the end of the session?

As Eubanks et al. (2019) clarified, there are essentially two kinds of ruptures: withdrawal and confrontation. *Withdrawal* ruptures are marked by the client moving away from the therapist and the work, often hiding dissatisfaction with the therapist and the work. *Confrontation* ruptures, on the other hand, involve the client moving against the therapist, often by expressing anger or dissatisfaction with the therapist and therapy or with some aspect of the work. Confrontation ruptures require immediate attention from the therapist, whereas withdrawal ruptures more easily go unnoticed. It is, however, important that ruptures be both noticed and explored by therapists. As the first author has elsewhere noted,

> In sum, the therapist needs to be sensitive to the occurrence of ruptures, and s/he needs to sensitively explore what the rupture is about. Repairing the rupture may involve the therapist clarifying where s/he was coming from, apologizing, and exploring the patient's feelings around the rupture. When the time is right, it is also important to explore the relation of the rupture, as well as the patient's way of dealing with the rupture, to the patient's core issues. However, to the extent that the rupture is fundamentally the responsibility of the therapist, it is important that the therapist not simply place the root of the rupture on the patient and his/her conflicts. (Gelso, 2019, p. 66)

Although the therapist's attention to the rupture experienced by the client is a key step in the repair of the rupture, client factors in the repair process are also crucial. As Eubanks et al. (2019) pointed out, clients who are best suited to contribute to rupture resolutions are those who are highly motivated, experience a strong bond with the therapist to begin with, are committed to the therapy/therapist, and have qualities such as psychological mindedness and nondefensiveness. In addition, in a qualitative study of 19 therapy cases (Rhodes et al., 1994), it was found that clients' expression of negative feelings, rather than the therapist's examination, was the first step in the process of repairing ruptures. Here again, clients and therapists do not see things in the same way! A central finding of the Rhodes et al. (1994) study was that for misunderstandings or ruptures to be resolved, clients needed to feel the therapy relationship was good to begin with, which allowed them to bring up the misunderstanding. On the negative side, unresolved ruptures usually came from therapies in which the relationship was not sound to begin with, and when ruptures went unresolved, clients often quit therapy. An example is the client who stated that "we always had a rocky relationship. This was the icing on the cake, I distanced myself from her and eventually ended the relationship" (Rhodes et al., 1994, p. 478).

The effective tear-and-repair process is similar to, if not the same as, the idea that in successful therapy the working alliance is initially strong as the therapist concentrates on empathically understanding the client. Then, as the therapist begins to examine and point out the client's issues and defenses, tensions increase and the alliance weakens. These tensions signal alliance rupture. This is followed by a working-through process during which the alliance regains its strength. This high-low-high pattern in the alliance may repeat itself several times during treatment, depending on, among other things, how long the therapy lasts. Empirically speaking, it has been found that one or more high-low-high patterns during treatment is related to treatment success (Horvath et al., 2011; Stiles et al., 2004). Similarly, in a recent meta-analysis, the tear-and-repair or rupture-resolution process has been found to predict successful therapy (Eubanks et al., 2019). In sum, the occurrence of ruptures accompanied by the repair of these ruptures is indicative of effective psychotherapy. From the perspective of clinical experience, we add that it seems important that the initial alliance is strong, for if ruptures occur very early in treatment, before a sound alliance has formed, it seems likely that the therapy will be endangered.

Some potentially useful general questions that might be asked of clients (using language that is jargon free) in future research on both the working alliance and the tear–repair process are as follows: What therapist actions facilitated the development of a working relationship with you? What did you do or feel that may have hindered or helped your working relationship with your therapist? What did your therapist do that hindered alliance development? What actions caused misunderstanding or ruptures? What helped repair ruptures?

Transference: A Window Into the Client's Conflict

Of the relationship elements we discuss in this chapter, transference most clearly emerges from the client, given that its source is the client's early relational experiences and unresolved conflicts. Because transference offers insight into clients' early relationship history and internal conflict, psychoanalytic therapists, in particular, see it as crucial for understanding the client and guiding the treatment. Transference may be defined as

> the client's experience and perceptions of the therapist that are shaped by the client's psychological structures and past, involving carryover from earlier significant relationships and displacement onto the therapist of feelings, attitudes, and behaviors belonging rightfully to those earlier relationships. (Gelso & Hayes, 1998, p. 51)

Thus, as Freud (1888) discovered and articulated, clients view their therapist in distorted ways that reflect attributes of their early caregivers. Freud proposed that transference originated from unresolved issues during the Oedipal period, but different psychoanalytic schools of thought have extended upon and/or disagreed with this assertion. For example, Bowlby's (1982) attachment theory proposes that transference originates from clients' internal working models of their early caregivers' availability and responsiveness, which begin to crystallize much earlier in development. In addition, transference is not limited to the straightforward displacement of early figures and relational patterns onto the therapist but often represents a host of defenses, meanings, and motivations (McWilliams, 1999). For example, an erotic transference can symbolize anything from how a client gains attention and power to how they avoid fears of aging and death. Hence, like many aspects of the psychotherapy process, the origins and functions of transference are numerous and complex.

The degree of client distortion involved in transference is also a debated topic. Classical analysts believe that the distortion involved in transference emerges primarily from the client's psyche. By contrast, modern intersubjective/relational analysts believe transference is significantly coconstructed by the client and the therapist. Hence, in comparison to classical analysts, the intersubjective/relational camp pays more attention to how the client may be reacting to realistic parts of the therapist and how the therapist pulls for certain reactions from the client. In our view, the specifics of any transference reaction are coconstructed by the client and the therapist, although the general themes represent core conflicts of the client. One way core conflicts have been defined is by Luborsky and Crits-Christoph's (1990) core conflictual relationship theme (CCRT) method. This method allows research observers to assess similarities between clients' narratives of significant others and clients' narratives of their therapists. The CCRT is defined as the client's wishes and needs in relationships, perceived responses of other toward the client, and the subsequent responses of the client. Thus, this method highlights the client's role and projections in the transference.

Although psychoanalysis gave birth to the discovery and exploration of transference, research suggests it appears in nonanalytic treatments as well (Gelso & Bhatia, 2012). However, the extent to which it is attended to in the therapy may differ depending on the therapist's theoretical orientation. Researchers have examined transference using qualitative client interviews and client-rated object relations (e.g., Response of Others subscale of the Central Relationship Questionnaire; McCarthy et al., 2008), observer reports (e.g., core conflictual relationship theme method; Luborsky & Crits-Christoph, 1990), and therapist ratings (therapy session checklist-transference items; Graff & Luborsky, 1977). These different empirical vantage points and over a century of clinical theory provide insight into the complexity and richness of the client's experience of and contribution to transference.

The Client's Experience of and Contribution to Transference

The client's experience of transference—involving feelings, attitudes, and behaviors toward the therapist—is heavily influenced by their attachment history. Internal working models (IWMs) established from experiences with early caregivers influence a client's "forecasts" (predictions) of the therapist, including how the therapist will behave toward the client (Bowlby, 1988). In general, IWMs are either positive (the client believes that the therapist will be available and responsive to their needs) or negative (the client believes that the therapist will be unavailable and unresponsive to their needs). Of course, there is more nuance based on the type of unresponsiveness a client experienced early in life. For example, one can imagine a client who had an abusive early caregiver might experience their therapist as frightening or demeaning, whereas a client who had a withdrawn caregiver might experience their therapist as withholding or bored. It is important to note that a client's distortion, especially early in the treatment, is unconscious (i.e., a client does not recognize they are mis-attributing characteristics to the therapist that are true of earlier figures). Thus, it is imperative that therapists use good timing and sensitivity when pointing out this distortion to help clients understand the misattribution and eventually to alter their interpersonal expectations and ways of being with others.

Transference from the client's lens has been examined qualitatively and quantitatively, although the empirical research is relatively sparse. In a classic qualitative study examining clients' experiences in behavior therapy, Ryan and Gizynski (1971) found that—from the client's perspective—interpersonal feel-ings toward their therapist were more influential on treatment outcome than the behavior modifications their therapists employed. The interviews shed light on how early relationship dynamics unfolded in the therapy. For example, one client said her therapist "was the kind of mother for whom it could be worth being good" (Ryan & Gizynski, 1971, p. 7) and described how she missed this opportunity with her own mother, whom she found inadequate. Another client described her therapist, whom others found intellectual and cold, as "warm and sensitive underneath—just like her brother" (p. 7). She explained that she overcame her minor phobia to "show him she was a brave person" (p. 7). Hence, in these clients' own words, their experiences of the therapist were connected to dynamics of earlier relationships. Barber et al. (1998) developed a standardized measurement of clients' self-reported interactions with signif-icant others named the Central Relationship Questionnaire (CRQ), which is based on the observer-rated measure of transference (CCRT; Luborsky & Crits-Christoph, 1990) noted earlier. Clients' expected responses of others (e.g., "controls me," "loves me"), responses of self (e.g., "feels anxious," "feels valued"), and underlying wish in the relationship (e.g., "to be independent," "not to be abandoned") are assessed. Although the CRQ has demonstrated reliability and concurrent validity with scales assessing interpersonal func-tioning and symptomatology (Barber et al., 1998; Wiseman et al., 2002), it has yet to be used to assess clients' transference experiences. Although this mea-sure is unable to capture the unconscious elements of transference, it could still provide illuminating information about clients' perspectives on their inter-actions with therapists. There is a body of research indicating significant simi-larities in clients' narratives between significant others and therapists, a pattern that becomes stronger over time in therapy (e.g., Connolly et al., 2000; Tellides et al., 2008). However, these studies have used observer-rated methods, and clients' perspectives are sorely needed.

The client's experience of transference is also heavily influenced by unre-solved conflict, including maladaptive defenses and unconscious motivations (McWilliams, 1999). One client's experience indicative of a transference reaction in the Ryan and Gizynski (1971) study highlights a defensive projective mechanism. This client reported that she believed her therapist had many of the same problems as a fellow single woman and wanted to "chuck it all and get married" (p. 7) just like the client. The type of unresolved conflict that is projected onto the therapist has a major impact on the affective quality of the transference (McWilliams, 1999). For example, a client may experience intense feelings of love for the therapist, which may represent an unconscious wish to merge with the therapist to bolster the client's self-esteem. Alternatively, a client may not be able to shake sexual feelings toward the therapist, highlighting a sexualization defense that prevents the client from relating in other ways. Hence, clients' transferential experiences can range in emotional quality as well as intensity. At times, certain content may stir up a client's transferential feelings more strongly, to the extent that it cannot be ignored by the therapist. Other times, transference may be more akin to background music—the therapist need not explicitly address it but can use it to guide their conceptualization of the client and the treatment. One of the second author's cases, shared next, illustrates the different elements of a client's experience of transference.

The client and I worked together for 2 years with the primary goals of understanding why the client continually found herself in unfulfilling relationships and why she underperformed in her career despite her immense aptitude. As a child, the client had to navigate an extremely critical and demanding father who rarely, if ever, mirrored the good in her. I found the client to be funny, smart, and insightful in the therapy, which is why it came as a surprise during therapy moments when her whole body shifted into a defensive posture as if preparing to be ridiculed. During these times she expressed how stupid she felt talking to me. Upon exploration, the client felt that I looked down on her and deemed her hopeless and worthless. Hence, her history with a critical caregiver emerged in her feelings and attitudes toward me. Because she was unaware that she was seeing me through the lens in which she saw her father and because I did not want to make her feel more "stupid," I gently explored what made her feel this way. Over time, she began to see that these feelings and attitudes she carried in her relationships belonged rightfully to her father and that she had internalized and projected his critical voice. In addition to experiencing me as a critical caregiver, she at times had intense feelings of envy toward me and wished to be more like me. We came to understand that these envious feelings represented a belief that her father would be proud of someone like me (a PhD student at the time), highlighting an unhealed narcissistic injury that she unconsciously attempted to heal through idealizing me. The intensity of her transference reactions fluctuated throughout the treatment but grew during times when we discussed her career. We came to understand this phenomenon as partly emerging from her father being especially critical about the client's intellect and partly from my pursuit of a PhD (therapist contributions to transference are discussed later in the chapter). By the end of treatment, she gained insight into how she projected her internalized critical voice—which originated from her father's criticism of her—onto others (how attachment influenced the transference experience) and how her feelings of envy represented a wish to fix the parts of herself she felt were inadequate (how unresolved conflict influenced the transference experience). These insights improved her ability to engage in reality testing in her relationships and work. In addition, she was able to tone down her critical voice, thereby allowing her to feel more confident as an employee, a friend, and a romantic partner.

The client's experience of and contribution to the transference are intertwined. Specifically, the client's cognitive, affective, and physiological experience of the transference—rooted in early attachment history and unresolved conflict—is both what they experience and what they bring to the therapy relationship. How willing a client is to address and explore how they perceive their therapist is another client contributing factor affecting the nature and outcome of the treatment.

Client Factors in the Transference

What client factors underlie the nature and intensity of client transferential reactions? The research and clinical literature suggest two primary variables: a client's personality structure and their attachment style. Client personality structure has been written about extensively in how it appears in the therapy relationship/transference and how this influences treatment (McWilliams, 2011). One robust finding among clinicians is that clients with narcissistic personalities tend to develop particular kinds of transferences, the main ones of which may be referred to as idealizing or mirror transferences. Because the core feature of a narcissistic personality is an undeveloped sense of self, narcissistic clients often idealize their therapist or look to their therapist to reflect (i.e., mirror) their goodness back to them—both of which serve as a self-esteem maintenance function for the client. Arachtingi and Lichtenberg (1999) provided empirical evidence for the phenomenon. They found that clients with poorer self-esteem and weaker ego identities rated their therapists as more different from their parents on measures of empathy, positive regard, and genuineness, suggesting that these clients were more prone to positive or idealizing transferences. Although idealizing and mirror transferences, as well as other types of transference (e.g., erotic), are often discussed in the psychoanalytic literature, Bradley et al. (2005) empirically examined how therapists of different theoretical orientations (cognitive, psychodynamic, and eclectic) view the association between personality pathology and transference reactions. They found that dramatic/erratic personalities were positively associated with angry/entitled and sexualized transferences and anxious/fearful personalities were positively associated with anxious/preoccupied transferences. Results approached significance for a positive association between odd/eccentric personalities and avoidant/counterdependent transference. Hence, personality pathology appears correlated with the nature of transference (i.e., the types of transference feelings and attitudes expressed). In addition to personality organization, there is also evidence that the level of personality pathology plays a role in how transference unfolds. Specifically, the more severe the client's pathology, the more readily the client projects internalized object relations onto the therapist (Kernberg, 2004).

Another finding from empirical literature is the association of client attachment and transference. A small cluster of studies (Bradley et al., 2005; Marmarosh et al., 2009; Woodhouse et al., 2003) have found that client emotions associated with attachment anxiety and therapist-perceived amount of transference are positively associated. Client attachment anxiety experienced in the therapy relationship was positively associated with therapist-rated negative transference (Woodhouse et al., 2003), whereas client attachment anxiety as experienced in romantic relationships was positively associated with positive transference and negatively associated with negative transference as rated by the therapist (Marmarosh et al., 2009). Thus, it seems that attachment reactions in the therapy relationship versus romantic relationships have different associations to negative and positive transference. Interestingly, Woodhouse et al. also found that a client's secure attachment to the therapist was positively associated with negative transference. The authors speculated that feeling secure in the therapy relationship allows for negative transference to emerge so that it could be addressed and worked through. In sum, there is an emerging body of findings that client attachment underlies the amount and type of transference.

The Therapist Contributes to Transference

Although we have shown that transference involves core conflictual themes of the client, it is also influenced by the therapist. Therapist characteristics, style, and personal conflicts can strengthen or weaken particular transference reactions in the client. A host of social–cognitive research on transference in everyday interactions indicates that individuals apply their internalized object relations onto others, even when there is no similarity between past and present person (Andersen & Przybylinski, 2012). However, individuals transfer to a greater degree when new people resemble earlier figures in their lives (Levy & Scala, 2012). This suggests that a similar phenomenon would happen between clients and therapists. Zilcha-Mano et al. (2014) investigated how clients' pretreatment representations of others (ROs) were projected onto the therapist and how these projections were influenced by the therapist across treatment. They found that clients early in treatment engaged in more assimilation of the therapist (i.e., projected a dominant RO theme onto the therapist, no matter the therapist's traits). Later in treatment as the client experienced more of the real therapist, clients engaged in more accommodation of the therapist (i.e., projected an RO theme that was more fitting of the therapist's traits). Hence, this study highlighted how transference is a bipersonal phenomenon.

Does the Client's Experience of Transference Matter?

Researchers have examined how transference amount and valence (positive or negative) are related to session and treatment outcome and the psychotherapy process. Gelso et al. (1997) found that the amount of transference was not associated with treatment outcome, whereas Marmarosh et al. (2009)

found it was negatively related to symptom change. Specifically, higher negative transference predicted less symptom change from the beginning to the end of treatment. Although these two studies had contradictory findings, Gelso et al. (1991) and Gelso et al. (1997) revealed that the variable of client insight appears to play an important role in understanding the association between transference and outcome. They found that the best session and treatment outcomes occurred when both client insight and negative transference were high, whereas the worst outcomes occurred when client insight was weak and negative transference was strong. Hence, it appears that negative transference can be beneficial to the client if insight is attained but detrimental if the client is not insightful.

When examining the psychotherapy process, Gelso et al. (2005) and Markin et al. (2013) studied session smoothness in relation to the amount and valence of transference. Both studies found that higher negative transference was related to a rougher, rockier session. Interestingly, Markin et al. found that higher positive transference was related to a deeper session. In a classic study by Strupp et al. (1969) that focused on the client's view of treatment process and outcome, these researchers highlighted how cases in which the client had severe negative transference reactions were never able to work through them, preventing the therapy from progressing in any meaningful way. Hence, this cluster of studies highlights how intense negative transference has the potential to be particularly damaging to the treatment.

Because all but one of these studies used the therapist's assessment of transference, more research on the client's perspective is warranted. Although the client perspective is limited to that of which clients are consciously aware, future research questions that could illuminate more about the client's experience and contribution to transference include the following: Are there ways in which you have misperceived your therapist at the beginning, middle, and/or end of your treatment? If so, how has this affected your therapy? Did your therapist remind you of any other important relational figures in your life? If yes, how so? How do you think these similarities influenced your experience of therapy?

Countertransference: The Therapist's Vulnerabilities in Response to the Client and the Therapy Situation

As transference is conceptualized as primarily emerging from the client, countertransference (CT) is seen as primarily emerging from the therapist. However, as we have expressed in our discussion on transference, the client's and therapist's dynamics interact throughout the psychotherapy process. Hence, the transference and CT elements of the therapy relationship do not operate in a vacuum but are deeply synergistic. Although Freud's (1959) original 1910 conceptualization of CT defined it as an unconscious reaction to the client's transference neurosis, later psychoanalytic thinkers expanded the definition to include all of a therapist's attitudes and feelings toward the client—known as the totalistic view. A third and fourth wave of CT conceptions emerged: the complementary and relational viewpoints, both of which emphasized the two-person nature of CT. That is, the client elicits certain therapist reactions and vice versa (Gelso & Hayes, 2007). In addition to what CT encompasses and how it emerges in psychotherapy, another contention between early and later psychoanalytic thinkers is the extent to which CT is seen as helpful versus hindering to the treatment. Classical analysts believed CT was something to avoid or repel, whereas later analysts believed CT could be used to benefit the work.

In their book on CT, Gelso and Hayes (2007) developed a CT conceptualization integrating important historical concepts. They defined CT as "the therapist's internal and external reactions that are shaped by the therapist's past and present emotional conflicts and vulnerabilities" (p. 25). In their integrative framework, CT may be conscious or unconscious and is a reaction to the client's transference or other clinically relevant material and situations—what may be termed *acute CT reactions*. In addition, therapists may have chronic CT that consists of general reactions to the therapy frame and therefore occur across clients. For example, the therapist may respond with excessive supportiveness to all clients, where this ultra-supportiveness is tied to unresolved issues in the therapist. Most important, a therapist's unresolved conflicts and vulnerabilities are always implicated in CT. Nevertheless, CT is best understood in terms of what Gelso and Hayes termed the *countertransference interaction hypothesis* (i.e., the interaction of a client's dynamics or actions with a therapist's inner conflicts and vulnerabilities). In their integrative conception, CT can improve understanding of the client and help guide the therapy if managed properly.

Although CT originated in psychoanalysis, it is currently recognized as a pantheoretical construct (Gelso & Hayes, 2007). Therapists of all theoretical persuasions have their own conflicts and vulnerabilities that can influence their work with clients. These conflicts and vulnerabilities may manifest differently in various types of treatment (e.g., a humanistic therapist may struggle more to be a congruent presence with a particular client) or given a different name in different types of treatment (e.g., *therapeutic belief system* by some cognitive behavioral theorists). Nevertheless, whoever the therapist is and whatever therapy framework they employ, clinical and empirical evidence suggest that CT reactions can influence psychotherapy treatment for better or worse (Hayes et al., 2019). Researchers have examined CT from the therapist's perspective using qualitative methods (Hayes et al., 1998) and quantitative measures (e.g., State Anxiety Inventory [Hayes & Gelso, 1991]; Therapist Appraisal Questionnaire [Fauth & Hayes, 2006]). In addition, observer measures have been used, for instance, the Inventory of CT Behavior, which allows supervisors and research observers to assess a therapist's CT during therapy sessions (Fuertes et al., 2015). Unfortunately, little empirical research exists on the client's perspective of CT. Hence, our discussion on the client's experience of and contribution to CT is largely based on clinical experience.

The Client's Experience of and Contribution to Countertransference

Although CT is fundamentally a therapist variable, the client is the recipient of CT and is therefore affected by it, especially if CT goes unmanaged by the therapist. How might a client experience CT? From clinical experience, two important variables influencing the client's experience include the intensity and persistence of CT. If a therapist's CT reactions are of high intensity and/or long lasting, this could have an injurious impact on the client and ultimately the treatment. CT of high intensity might be experienced by the client as behavior that deviates from the therapist's norm. Sometimes a client will even highlight this distinguishable behavior. One of the second author's (subsequently referred to in the first person) favorite examples of this is drawn from my brief work with a university student in which my own unresolved issues surrounding relationship boundaries were triggered by an event in the client's life.

The client started the session by talking about how distressed she felt by her dad's incessant phone calls incited by his need to discuss his anguish about potentially divorcing the client's mom. This dynamic between my client and her dad happened often, and she was beginning to feel very depressed about her inability to help her parents and guilty for not wanting to answer her dad's calls. In response I became protective of my client, implying that she should not feel guilty about not wanting to answer the phone (rather than exploring the guilt) and jumping to action mode for what she could do to stop her dad from calling her about the potential divorce. As this CT reaction emerged, my client interrupted me, saying, "Wow, I've never seen you talk this much in our sessions. You must deal with a lack of boundaries in your family too." She was not wrong. My client's calling me out provided the signal I needed to begin engaging in some CT management. Fortunately, I was able to manage this CT trigger from that point on in the therapy. I always chuckled at how this client noticed my CT reaction given how much it stood in contrast to my typical therapist behavior.

As one of the first large empirical studies to investigate the client's perspective on their treatment, Strupp et al. (1969) asked clients posttreatment if their therapist ever said or did anything that decreased the client's self-respect. Although this question alone cannot confirm that CT was implicated, one client's response—shared in the following quote—sheds light on what it was like for her to be the recipient of what seemed to be a CT reaction. We see that her therapist's "slip" was painful yet also generated profound growth:

> I consider this one of the turning points of my treatment. Through an inadvertent slip one day, the therapist did say something that absolutely crushed me for a day or so. This happened as I was leaving and in the intervening two days between this visit and the next I grew up at least ten years. I learned that, though hurt, I still lived, that someone for whom I had great regard could make a mistake too and that I could get angry without the world coming to an end or lightning striking me dead! In my next visit, the therapist explained it was a slip and apologized (incidentally, the only time he ever made a reference to himself) and I further realized I could forgive someone for hurting me. (Strupp et al., 1969, p. 22)

Persistence is the second major variable that can influence a client's experience of CT. If a CT behavior lasts for a long period of time, then the client may experience this as being in a stalemate with the therapist. For example, a client experiencing a therapist's persistent CT reaction may feel unable to talk about a particular issue with the therapist. An example from a male second-year doctoral student therapist supervised by the second author sheds light on this phenomenon. The male trainee continued getting stuck with his male clients when the client became emotional in session. During supervision, the supervisee discussed how uncomfortable he felt experiencing more vulnerable emotions with another man, which he believed prevented him from exploring topics that invoked sadness in his male clients. On video recordings of his sessions, he became visibly uncomfortable and asked questions to direct these clients away from the emotionally laden topic. During his termination session for what was mostly a successful treatment with one of his male clients, the supervisee asked the client what was helpful and hindering in their working together. After discussing several helpful aspects, the client gently noted that there was a topic he avoided that was too emotionally raw because he began to see therapy as a place to discuss "deep but not too deep things." Hence, it appeared that the client himself gathered the supervisee's discomfort with emotion throughout the treatment, thereby preventing the client from discussing a particular issue.

An example from Strupp et al. (1969) highlights how a therapist appeared to have a strong CT with one client, Carole, whose treatment failed. Carole described her therapist as "passive, stiff and formal, cold, and unaccepting" (p. 30), adding that "he was cordial, but never gave me any encouragement." The same therapist treated another client, William, who rated his treatment as largely successful. William described the therapist as "understanding and warm" and "admired his sense of humor" (p. 33). Although there were likely client differences (e.g., transference) that contributed to their different feelings toward the therapist, the therapist himself indicated that he stuck to a standard psychoanalytic model with Carole, versus a "largely supportive" model with William that later became psychoanalytic. Hence, it is worth wondering why this therapist decided against providing Carole with the degree of support she needed to succeed in therapy. It is possible that CT played a role in these two clients' perspectives that ultimately contributed to one treatment's failure and the other's success.

One can see that a client's experience of CT may affect their contribution in terms of how they respond to the CT in therapy. Using earlier examples from the second author, a client may highlight the CT for the therapist, thereby helping the therapist to manage it. Alternatively, a client may respond by withdrawing when they notice the therapist's CT. Depending on the therapist's awareness of this withdrawal or of their own CT, the therapist may either continue engaging in the CT or begin to manage it. In addition to the client's contribution in terms of their response to CT, there are also client factors that underlie how CT manifests in the therapist.

Client Factors in Countertransference

What client factors underlie the nature and intensity of CT? Research and clinical literature suggest three primary variables: client personality pathology, personality structure, and attachment style. The degree of personality pathology has been empirically and clinically discovered to be associated with the intensity of CT reactions. In their systematic review of the literature on CT and client personality, Stefana et al. (2020) found that a client's personality pathology was negatively associated with therapist feelings of confidence and positively associated with therapist feelings of helplessness and being overwhelmed. Hence, as has been spoken of in clinical experience (e.g., McWilliams, 2011), clients with greater personality pathology elicit difficult CT reactions in therapists. This can contribute to the level of difficulty in treating clients with more profound or severe personality pathology. Interestingly, Stefana et al. (2020) also found that personality pathology was negatively associated with a therapist's feelings of boredom and tiredness. At face value, feeling less bored or tired with a client would be a positive CT experience. However, we speculate that this finding speaks to how clients with more severe personality pathology keep therapists on their toes. In a similar review, Colli and Ferri (2015) found that personality pathology was positively associated with therapists' difficult emotional reactions (i.e., feeling inadequate, guarded, rejected, criticized, and disorganized). Furthermore, their review findings indicated that symptom severity was not a strong mediator between personality pathology and CT, suggesting that personality pathology alone (i.e., dysfunctional schemas of self, other, and interpersonal interactions) is related to CT. Last, this review included studies across theoretical orientations and found that CT occurred across all kinds of therapy and is independent of a therapist's theoretical preferences.

Clinical literature has discussed associations between client personality type and type or quality of CT (McWilliams, 2011). For example, narcissistic, obsessive–compulsive, and depressive personalities have been linked with bored, ineffective, and sympathetic CT reactions, respectively. The empirical literature is somewhat mixed on these connections. Researchers speculate that the mixed findings could be explained by *DSM* personality clusters used in studies not being adequately refined (Colli & Ferri, 2015). Thus, although there may be some CT similarities within the clusters, there is also likely variation. For example, although borderline and narcissistic personalities are Cluster B (dramatic/overly emotional) disorders, narcissistic personalities are notorious for the boredom they can incite in therapists, whereas borderline personalities are not (McWilliams, 2011). There are some preliminary findings suggesting that odd/eccentric clients evoke distance and disconnection, emotionally dysregulated clients evoke anxiety and incompetence, and withdrawn and anxious clients evoke sympathy and concern (Stefana et al., 2020). Again, these findings pointed to the likelihood that therapist CT to the three clusters of a client's personality type were independent of theoretical orientation.

Researchers have also begun to examine how client attachment style is correlated with CT. Westerling et al. (2019) examined the association between client attachment style toward romantic partners and therapist CT. They found that initial (i.e., rated at the beginning of therapy) client attachment anxiety was positively associated with initial protective/parental, special/overinvolved, and overwhelmed/disorganized therapist-rated CT. In addition, initial client attachment anxiety was negatively associated with protective/parental and special/overinvolved CT across time but positively associated with overwhelmed/disorganized CT across time. The researchers speculate that this last result could be indicative of clients engaging in projective identification, leading the therapists to absorb the client's attachment insecurities. Mohr et al. (2005) investigated the interaction of the client and therapist attachment style in relation to CT. They found that CT was highest when the client had an anxious attachment pattern, and the therapist had a fearful or dismissing attachment pattern. Overall, there is growing empirical evidence that client attachment style is implicated in CT reactions.

Does the Client's Experience of Countertransference Matter?

Hayes et al.'s (2019) meta-analyses provide compelling evidence that CT reactions, and implicitly the client's experience of CT, matter for psychotherapy outcome. They found that CT reactions are negatively and modestly related to psychotherapy outcomes ($r = -.16$, $p = .002$, 95% CI [$-.26$, $-.06$], $k = 10$ studies, $N = 769$) and that managing CT successfully is highly related to better psychotherapy outcomes ($r = .56$, $p = .000$, 95% CI [.40, .73] $k = 7$ studies, $N = 478$). Hence, it seems that a therapist's inability to manage CT, and therefore clients being exposed to it, is negatively related to the success of treatment. For future research, important questions to garner more understanding of the client's perspective of CT include the following: Did you have a sense that your therapist's own issues affected your work with your therapist? What factors did you notice in your therapist that gave you this impression? Did you bring this up? How did your therapist react to that?

CONCLUSION

The therapy relationship is a deeply bipersonal construct, created and fostered by both the therapist and the client. Because of this fact, it is difficult to disentangle the role and contributions of the therapist and client. Still, the client indeed has a role, naturally a crucial one. Over the years, this role has often been ignored, and in this sense, our conceptualizing about the relationship has too often been therapist centric. In the present chapter, we have focused on the client's role, including their experience of and contributions to the therapy relationship (real relationship, working alliance, transference, and countertransference) and to treatment outcome.

We have relied on a combination of clinical experience, theory, and empirical research in framing this chapter. However, it needs to be underscored that there is a meager amount of empirical work from the client's perspective, and the work that does exist usually uses measures constructed by therapy researchers, naturally from their own perspective about what clients think and experience. Sorely needed is research from the client's perspective, especially qualitative work in which clients can present their views and experiences in their own words and where conclusions are drawn inductively based on clients' viewpoints rather than predetermined researcher-framed hypotheses and measures. Interestingly, this kind of work had appeared some time ago in studies of clients' views of their therapy, as noted earlier in this chapter (e.g., Ryan & Gizynski, 1971; Strupp et al., 1969). But this kind of work seemed to have stopped or perhaps continued at a very low rate. More recent studies have now been done (see review by Bedi & Hayes, 2020) and need to be continued. The goal would be to develop a science of clients' perspectives on the therapy relationship and other elements of psychotherapy. In this way, the input factor referred to at the beginning of the chapter would be given the scientific attention it warrants.

REFERENCES

Andersen, S. M., & Przybylinski, E. (2012). Experiments on transference in interpersonal relations: Implications for treatment. *Psychotherapy, 49*(3), 370–383. https://doi.org/10.1037/a0029116

Arachtingi, B., & Lichtenberg, J. W. (1999). Self-concept and self-esteem as moderators of client transference. *Psychotherapy, 36*(4), 369–379. https://doi.org/10.1037/h0087749

Bachelor, A. (1995). Clients' perception of the therapeutic alliance: A qualitative analysis. *Journal of Counseling Psychology, 42*(3), 323–337. https://doi.org/10.1037/0022-0167.42.3.323

Barber, J. P., Foltz, C., & Weinryb, R. M. (1998). The Central Relationship Questionnaire: Initial report. *Journal of Counseling Psychology, 45*(2), 131–142. https://doi.org/10.1037/0022-0167.45.2.131

Bedi, R., & Hayes, S. (2020). Clients' perspectives on, experiences of, and contributions to the working alliance: Implications for clinicians. In J. N. Fuertes (Ed.), *Working alliance skills for mental health professionals* (pp. 111–136). Oxford University Press.

Bedi, R. P. (2006). Concept mapping the client's perspective on counseling alliance formation. *Journal of Counseling Psychology, 53*(1), 26–35. https://doi.org/10.1037/0022-0167.53.1.26

Bedi, R. P., Davis, M. D., & Williams, M. (2005). Critical incidents in the formation of the therapeutic alliance from the client's perspective. *Psychotherapy, 42*(3), 311–323. https://doi.org/10.1037/0033-3204.42.3.311

Bhatia, A., & Gelso, C. J. (2018). Therapists' perspective on the therapeutic relationship: Examining a tripartite model. *Counselling Psychology Quarterly, 31*(3), 271–293. https://doi.org/10.1080/09515070.2017.1302409

Birkhäuer, J., Gaab, J., Kossowsky, J., Hasler, S., Krummenacher, P., Werner, C., & Gerger, H. (2017). Trust in the health care professional and health outcome: A meta-analysis. *PLOS ONE, 12*(2), e0170988. https://doi.org/10.1371/journal.pone.0170988

Bordin, E. S. (1979). The generalizability of the psychoanalytic concept of the working alliance. *Psychotherapy, 16*(3), 252–260. https://doi.org/10.1037/h0085885

Bordin, E. S. (1994). Theory and research on the therapeutic working alliance: New directions. In A. O. Horvath & L. S. Greenberg (Eds.), *The working alliance: Theory, research, and practice* (pp. 13–37). Wiley.

Bowlby, J. (1982). *Attachment and loss: Vol. 1. Attachment* (2nd ed.). Basic Books.

Bowlby, J. (1988). *A secure base: Parent–child attachment and healthy human development.* Basic Books.

Bradley, R., Heim, A. K., & Westen, D. (2005). Transference patterns in the psychotherapy of personality disorders: Empirical investigation. *The British Journal of Psychiatry, 186*(4), 342–349. https://doi.org/10.1192/bjp.186.4.342

Colli, A., & Ferri, M. (2015). Patient personality and therapist countertransference. *Current Opinion in Psychiatry, 28*(1), 46–56. https://doi.org/10.1097/YCO.0000000000000119

Connolly, M. B., Crits-Christoph, P., Barber, J. P., & Luborsky, L. (2000). Transference patterns in the therapeutic relationship in supportive–expressive psychotherapy for depression. *Psychotherapy Research, 10*(3), 356–372. https://doi.org/10.1093/ptr/10.3.356

Eubanks, C. F., Muran, J. C., & Safran, J. D. (2019). Repairing alliance ruptures. In J. C. Norcross & M. J. Lambert (Eds.), *Psychotherapy relationships that work: Vol. 1. Evidence-based therapist contributions* (3rd ed., pp. 549–579). Oxford University Press. https://doi.org/10.1093/med-psych/9780190843953.003.0016

Falkenström, F., Hatcher, R. L., Skjulsvik, T., Larsson, M. H., & Holmqvist, R. (2015). Development and validation of a 6-item working alliance questionnaire for repeated administrations during psychotherapy. *Psychological Assessment, 27*(1), 169–183. https://doi.org/10.1037/pas0000038

Fauth, J., & Hayes, J. A. (2006). Counselors' stress appraisals as predictors of countertransference behavior with male clients. *Journal of Counseling and Development, 84*(4), 430–439. https://doi.org/10.1002/j.1556-6678.2006.tb00427.x

Fitzpatrick, M. R., Janzen, J., Chamodraka, M., Gamberg, S., & Blake, E. (2009). Client relationship incidents in early therapy: Doorways to collaborative engagement. *Psychotherapy Research, 19*(6), 654–665. https://doi.org/10.1080/10503300902878235

Fitzpatrick, M. R., Janzen, J., Chamodraka, M., & Park, J. (2006). Client critical incidents in the process of early alliance development: A positive emotion–exploration spiral. *Psychotherapy Research, 16*(4), 486–498. https://doi.org/10.1080/10503300500485391

Flückiger, C., Del Re, A. C., Wampold, B. E., & Horvath, A. O. (2019). Alliance in adult psychotherapy. In J. C. Norcross & M. J. Lambert (Eds.), *Psychotherapy relationships that work: Vol. 1. Evidence-based therapist contributions* (3rd ed., pp. 24–78). Oxford University Press. https://doi.org/10.1093/med-psych/9780190843953.003.0002

Freud, S. (1888). Hysteria. In J. Strachey (Ed.), *The standard edition of the complete psychological works of Sigmund Freud* (pp. 41–57). Hogarth Press.

Freud, S. (1959). Future prospects of psychoanalytic psychotherapy. In *The standard edition of the complete psychological works of Sigmund Freud* (Vol. 11; J. Strachey, Ed. & Trans.; pp. 139–151). Hogarth Press.

Fuertes, J. N., Gelso, C. J., Owen, J. J., & Cheng, D. (2015). Using the Inventory of Countertransference Behavior as an observer-rated measure. *Psychoanalytic Psychotherapy, 29*(1), 38–56. https://doi.org/10.1080/02668734.2014.1002417

Fuertes, J. N., Mele, P., & Rapaport, J. (2020). Working alliance skills for healthcare professionals: Introduction. In J. Fuertes (Ed.), *Working alliance skills for mental health professionals* (pp. 1–10). Oxford University Press. https://doi.org/10.1093/med-psych/9780190868529.003.0005

Fuertes, J. N., Mislowack, A., Brown, S., Gur-Arie, S., Wilkinson, S., & Gelso, C. (2007). Correlates of the real relationship in psychotherapy: A study of dyads. *Psychotherapy Research, 17*(4), 423–430. https://doi.org/10.1080/10503300600789189

Gelso, C. (2014). A tripartite model of the therapeutic relationship: Theory, research, and practice. *Psychotherapy Research, 24*(2), 117–131. https://doi.org/10.1080/10503307.2013.845920

Gelso, C. J. (2011). *The real relationship in psychotherapy: The hidden foundation of change.* American Psychological Association. https://doi.org/10.1037/12349-000

Gelso, C. J. (2019). *The therapeutic relationships in psychotherapy practice: An integrative perspective.* Routledge.

Gelso, C. J., & Bhatia, A. (2012). Crossing theoretical lines: The role and effect of transference in nonanalytic psychotherapies. *Psychotherapy, 49*(3), 384–390. https://doi.org/10.1037/a0028802

Gelso, C. J., & Carter, J. A. (1985). The real relationship in counseling and psychotherapy: Components, consequences, and theoretical antecedents. *The Counseling Psychologist, 13*(2), 155–243. https://doi.org/10.1177/0011000085132001

Gelso, C. J., & Carter, J. A. (1994). Components of the psychotherapy relationship: Their interaction and unfolding during treatment. *Journal of Counseling Psychology, 41*(3), 296–306. https://doi.org/10.1037/0022-0167.41.3.296

Gelso, C. J., & Hayes, J. (2007). *Countertransference and the therapist's inner experience: Perils and possibilities.* Routledge. https://doi.org/10.4324/9780203936979

Gelso, C. J., & Hayes, J. A. (1998). *The psychotherapy relationship: Theory, research, and practice.* Wiley.

Gelso, C. J., Hill, C. E., & Kivlighan, D. M., Jr. (1991). Transference, insight, and the counselor's intentions during a counseling hour. *Journal of Counseling and Development, 69*(5), 428–433. https://doi.org/10.1002/j.1556-6676.1991.tb01539.x

Gelso, C. J., Kelley, F. A., Fuertes, J. N., Marmarosh, C., Holmes, S. E., Costa, C., & Hancock, G. R. (2005). Measuring the real relationship in psychotherapy: Initial validation of the therapist form. *Journal of Counseling Psychology, 52*(4), 640–649. https://doi.org/10.1037/0022-0167.52.4.640

Gelso, C. J., Kivlighan, D. M., Jr., Busa-Knepp, J., Spiegel, E. B., Ain, S., Hummel, A. M., Ma, Y. E., & Markin, R. D. (2012). The unfolding of the real relationship and the outcome of brief psychotherapy. *Journal of Counseling Psychology, 59*(4), 495–506. https://dx.doi.org/10.1037/a0029838

Gelso, C. J., Kivlighan, D. M., Jr., & Markin, R. D. (2018). The real relationship and its role in psychotherapy outcome: A meta-analysis. *Psychotherapy, 55*(4), 434–444. https://doi.org/10.1037/pst0000183

Gelso, C. J., Kivlighan, D. M., Wine, B., Jones, A., & Friedman, S. C. (1997). Transference, insight, and the course of time-limited therapy. *Journal of Counseling Psychology, 44*(2), 209–217. https://doi.org/10.1037/0022-0167.44.2.209

Gelso, C. J., & Kline, K. V. (2019). The sister concepts of the working alliance and the real relationship: On their development, rupture, and repair. *Research in Psychotherapy: Psychopathology, Process and Outcome, 22*(2), 142–149. https://doi.org/10.4081/ripppo.2019.373

Gelso, C. J., & Samstag, L. W. (2008). A tripartite model of the therapeutic relationship. In S. Brown & R. Lent (Eds.), *Handbook of counseling psychology* (4th ed., pp. 267–283). Wiley.

Gelso, C. J., & Silberberg, A. (2016). Strengthening the real relationship: What is a psychotherapist to do? *Practice Innovations, 1*(3), 154–163. https://doi.org/10.1037/pri0000024

Graff, H., & Luborsky, L. (1977). Long-term trends in transference and resistance: A report on a quantitative-analytic method applied to four psychoanalyses. *Journal of the American Psychoanalytic Association, 25*(2), 471–490. https://doi.org/10.1177/000306517702500210

Greenson, R. R. (1967). *The technique and practice of psychoanalysis* (Vol. 1). Universities Press.

Hayes, J. A., & Gelso, C. J. (1991). Effects of therapist-trainees' anxiety and empathy on countertransference behavior. *Journal of Clinical Psychology, 47*(2), 284–290. https://doi.org/10.1002/1097-4679(199103)47:2<284::AID-JCLP2270470216>3.0.CO;2-N

Hayes, J. A., Gelso, C. J., Kivlighan, D. M., & Goldberg, S. B. (2019). Managing countertransference. In J. Norcross & M. Lambert (Eds.), *Psychotherapy relationships that work* (3rd ed., Vol. 1, pp. 522–548). Oxford University Press. https://doi.org/10.1093/med-psych/9780190843953.003.0015

Hayes, J. A., McCracken, J. E., McClanahan, M. K., Hill, C. E., Harp, J. S., & Carozzoni, P. (1998). Therapist perspectives on countertransference: Qualitative data in search of a theory. *Journal of Counseling Psychology, 45*(4), 468–482. https://doi.org/10.1037/0022-0167.45.4.468

Horvath, A. O., Del Re, A. C., Flückiger, C., & Symonds, D. (2011). Alliance in adult psychotherapy. In J. C. Norcross (Ed.), *Psychotherapy relationships that work* (2nd ed., pp. 26–69). Oxford University Press. https://doi.org/10.1093/acprof:oso/9780199737208.003.0002

Horvath, A. O., & Greenberg, L. S. (1989). Development and validation of the Working Alliance Inventory. *Journal of Counseling Psychology, 36*(2), 223–233. https://doi.org/10.1037/0022-0167.36.2.223

Kelley, F. A., Gelso, C. J., Fuertes, J. N., Marmarosh, C., & Lanier, S. H. (2010). The real relationship inventory: Development and psychometric investigation of the client form. *Psychotherapy, 47*(4), 540–553. https://doi.org/10.1037/a0022082

Kernberg, O. (2004). Borderline personality disorder and borderline personality organization: Psychopathology and psychotherapy. In J. J. Magnavita (Ed.), *Handbook of personality disorders: Theory and practice* (pp. 92–119). Wiley.

Kivlighan, D. M., Jr. (1990). Relation between counselors' use of intentions and clients' perception of working alliance. *Journal of Counseling Psychology, 37*(1), 27–32. https://doi.org/10.1037/0022-0167.37.1.27

Levy, K. N., Kivity, Y., Johnson, B. N., & Gooch, C. V. (2018). Adult attachment as a predictor and moderator of psychotherapy outcome: A meta-analysis. *Journal of Clinical Psychology, 74*(11), 1996–2013. https://doi.org/10.1002/jclp.22685

Levy, K. N., & Scala, J. W. (2012). Transference, transference interpretations, and transference-focused psychotherapies. *Psychotherapy, 49*(3), 391–403. https://doi.org/10.1037/a0029371

Luborsky, L., & Crits-Christoph, P. (1990). *Understanding transference: The core conflictual relationship theme method.* Basic Books.

Luborsky, L. L. (1976). Helping alliances in psychotherapy. In J. L. Cleghorn (Ed.), *Successful psychotherapy* (pp. 92–116). Brunner/Mazel.

Markin, R. D., McCarthy, K. S., & Barber, J. P. (2013). Transference, countertransference, emotional expression, and session quality over the course of supportive expressive therapy: The raters' perspective. *Psychotherapy Research, 23*(2), 152–168. https://doi.org/10.1080/10503307.2012.747013

Marmarosh, C. L., Gelso, C. J., Markin, R. D., Majors, R., Mallery, C., & Choi, J. (2009). The real relationship in psychotherapy: Relationships to adult attachments, working alliance, transference, and therapy outcome. *Journal of Counseling Psychology, 56*(3), 337–350. https://doi.org/10.1037/a0015169

McCarthy, K. S., Connolly Gibbons, M. B., & Barber, J. P. (2008). The relation of rigidity across relationships with symptoms and functioning: An investigation with the revised Central Relationship Questionnaire. *Journal of Counseling Psychology, 55*(3), 346–358. https://doi.org/10.1037/a0012578

McWilliams, N. (1999). *Psychoanalytic case formulation.* Guilford Press.

McWilliams, N. (2011). *Psychoanalytic diagnosis: Understanding personality structure in the clinical process.* Guilford Press.

Mohr, J. J., Gelso, C. J., & Hill, C. E. (2005). Client and counselor trainee attachment as predictors of session evaluation and countertransference behavior in first counseling sessions. *Journal of Counseling Psychology, 52*(3), 298–309. https://doi.org/10.1037/0022-0167.52.3.298

Moore, S. R., & Gelso, C. J. (2011). Recollections of a secure base in psychotherapy: Considerations of the real relationship. *Psychotherapy, 48*(4), 368–373. https://doi.org/10.1037/a0022421

Norcross, J. C., & Lambert, M. J. (Eds.). (2019). *Psychotherapy relationships that work: Vol. 1. Evidence-based therapist contributions.* Oxford University Press.

Rhodes, R. H., Hill, C. E., Thompson, B. J., & Elliott, R. (1994). Client retrospective recall of resolved and unresolved misunderstanding events. *Journal of Counseling Psychology, 41*(4), 473–483. https://doi.org/10.1037/0022-0167.41.4.473

Ryan, V. L., & Gizynski, M. N. (1971). Behavior therapy in retrospect: Patients' feelings about their behavior therapies. *Journal of Consulting and Clinical Psychology, 37*(1), 1–9. https://doi.org/10.1037/h0031293

Safran, J. D., & Muran, J. C. (2000). *Negotiating the therapeutic alliance: A relational treatment guide*. Guilford Press.

Stefana, A., Bulgari, V., Youngstrom, E. A., Dakanalis, A., Bordin, C., & Hopwood, C. J. (2020). Patient personality and psychotherapist reactions in individual psychotherapy setting: A systematic review. *Clinical Psychology & Psychotherapy, 27*(5), 697–713. https://doi.org/10.1002/cpp.2455

Stiles, W. B., Glick, M. J., Osatuke, K., Hardy, G. E., Shapiro, D. A., Agnew-Davies, R., Rees, A., & Barkham, M. (2004). Patterns of alliance development and the rupture-repair hypothesis: Are productive relationships U-shaped or V-shaped? *Journal of Counseling Psychology, 51*(1), 81–92. https://doi.org/10.1037/0022-0167.51.1.81

Strupp, H. H., Fox, R. E., & Lessler, K. (1969). *Patients view their psychotherapy*. The Johns Hopkins University Press.

Tellides, C., Fitzpatrick, M., Drapeau, M., Bracewell, R., Janzen, J., & Jaouich, A. (2008). The manifestation of transference during early psychotherapy sessions. *Counselling & Psychotherapy Research, 8*(2), 85–92. https://doi.org/10.1080/14733140802014331

Tryon, G. S., Blackwell, S. C., & Hammel, E. F. (2008). The magnitude of client and therapist working alliance ratings. *Psychotherapy, 45*(4), 546–551. https://doi.org/10.1037/a0014338

Westerling, T. W., III, Drinkwater, R., Laws, H., Stevens, H., Ortega, S., Goodman, D., Beinashowitz, J., & Drill, R. L. (2019). Patient attachment and therapist countertransference in psychodynamic psychotherapy. *Psychoanalytic Psychology, 36*(1), 73–81. https://doi.org/10.1037/pap0000215

Wiseman, H., Barber, J. P., Raz, A., Yam, I., Foltz, C., & Livne-Snir, S. (2002). Parental communication of Holocaust experiences and interpersonal patterns in offspring of Holocaust survivors. *International Journal of Behavioral Development, 26*(4), 371–381. https://doi.org/10.1080/01650250143000346

Woodhouse, S. S., Schlosser, L. Z., Crook, R. E., Ligiero, D. P., & Gelso, C. J. (2003). Client attachment to therapist: Relations to transference and client recollections of parental caregiving. *Journal of Counseling Psychology, 50*(4), 395–408. https://doi.org/10.1037/0022-0167.50.4.395

Zilcha-Mano, S., McCarthy, K. S., Dinger, U., & Barber, J. P. (2014). To what extent is alliance affected by transference? An empirical exploration. *Psychotherapy, 51*(3), 424–433. https://doi.org/10.1037/a0036566

8

Client-Focused Assessment and Intervention

Tailoring the Work to the Client

James F. Boswell and Adela Scharff

Each psychotherapy client is unique. Although psychotherapy is effective on average, a psychotherapist does not usually treat an average client. Therefore, despite this general effectiveness, most, but not all, clients benefit from psychotherapy (Lambert, 2010), including in research-supported bona fide psychotherapies (Lambert, 2013). One method for improving the effectiveness of psychotherapy involves the development of new (and presumably better) treatments. The past several decades have witnessed a proliferation of new treatments, a pursuit that has certainly generated knowledge and clinical innovation. For example, the field of psychotherapy has made strides in addressing certain presenting problems that were once considered by many to be intractable, such as dialectical behavior therapy for borderline personality disorder (Linehan, 1993). However, new treatments have not necessarily raised the overall effectiveness of psychotherapy at a population level (Wampold & Imel, 2015).

A complementary approach to the development of more effective treatments is to increase the *precision* of psychotherapy. Typically, the development of a new treatment is tied to a discrete presenting problem, or diagnosis. On the "front lines" of clinical practice, the presenting diagnosis is often expected to be the primary factor that guides treatment (or treatment package) selection. While clarifying the nature of the diagnosis is important, treatment tailoring by way of categorical diagnosis alone is rather blunt and likely to be insufficient (Pincus et al., 2010). As such, the National Institutes of Health's division entitled Precision Medicine Initiative (PMI) aims to study and promote a more

https://doi.org/10.1037/0000303-009
The Other Side of Psychotherapy: Understanding Clients' Experiences and Contributions in Treatment, J. N. Fuertes (Editor)

precise measurement of health-related factors (spanning genetics to environ-mental and behavioral factors), in order to redefine notions of etiology, main-tenance, and health care outcomes. The PMI Working Group (2015) asserted that "this understanding will lead to more accurate diagnoses, more rela-tional disease prevention strategies, better treatment selection, and the devel-opment of novel therapies" (p. 1). Although primarily motivated to focus on cancer, mental health care is certainly in the orbit of this initiative (Delgadillo & Lutz, 2020).

It is probably not controversial to acknowledge the importance of tailoring psychotherapy to the individual client. Trained psychotherapists are naturally responsive to clients and the unfolding context (Stiles et al., 1998). Moreover, psychotherapy research has long been interested in determining the individual differences that are associated with better or poorer treatment outcomes. Practically speaking for psychotherapists, this means personalization by tailor-ing assessment and treatment to the individual client. When psychotherapists rely on a primary diagnosis to inform initial treatment selection (which is not necessarily a bad idea), this is far from the only factor that guides treatment decision making. The American Psychological Association (APA) defined *evidence-based practice* as the "integration of the best available research with clinical expertise in the context of client characteristics, culture, and prefer-ences" (APA Presidential Task Force on Evidence-Based Practice, 2006, p. 273). Historically, such client-focused tailoring has concentrated on treatment selection based on the client's baseline characteristics, such as preferences and readi-ness to change (Beutler & Harwood, 2000). Recent decades have witnessed the development of client-centered prediction models that can help to inform clinical decision making over the course of a given client's psychotherapy (e.g., things are on track, so stay the course, or things are off track, so consider making a change to the treatment; Howard et al., 1996; Lambert, 2010). Even more recently, attempts have been made to integrate clinical assessment feed-back to inform both at initial treatment selection and during treatment decision making (e.g., Lutz et al., 2019).

While the importance of tailoring and acknowledging a trained psycho-therapist's natural tendency to do so may be uncontroversial, it is much more problematic to operationalize this responsiveness. Appeals to "good clinical judgment" are a start but ultimately insufficient. In practice, psychotherapists use a variety of tools—both explicit and implicit—to inform treatment deci-sions. Applied research demonstrates that the accuracy of a clinical judgment is generally improved when augmented by actuarial data (Garb, 2005; Hannan et al., 2005). Whether based on careful clinical observation or validated by self-report measures, assessment is a critically important component of the clinical decision-making process. The what, when, and how of a client-focused assessment and treatment decision making are often more complicated.

The goal of this chapter is to provide an overview of important factors when navigating client-focused assessment and assessment-informed intervention. Client-focused assessment includes a mix of nomothetic (generalizing to all clients) and idiographic (focusing on the individual) methods to inform both early treatment decision making (e.g., should therapy begin with a more action- or insight-oriented approach?) and adaptive intervention decision making throughout a course of treatment (e.g., staying the course or trying something different). The use of the phrase *client-focused assessment* is intended to emphasize the importance of tailoring the assessment approach to the individual client where possible. This could be as simple as adjusting the frequency of assessment among different clients or could involve more sophisticated tailoring, such as computer adaptive testing methods (Gibbons et al., 2016).

We begin by briefly addressing what we view as a false dichotomy between assessment and treatment. We then address the importance and function of both baseline and ongoing, within-treatment assessment. Specifically, we review the use of routine outcome monitoring (ROM), a client-centered approach to obtaining routine feedback about how therapy is progressing from the client's perspective. Throughout the chapter, we attempt to highlight the role of culture and identity in the assessment and intervention process. We also present sample client–therapist dialogues to illustrate key concepts.[1] In terms of what to measure, we focus our attention on select client characteristics that (a) have received more attention in the psychotherapy process-outcome literature, (b) have relevance that is not tied to a particular diagnosis or treatment model, and (c) are feasible to assess in routine practice through interview and/or self-report measure methods. This chapter is not intended to be an exhaustive review of the underlying process-outcome literature itself (see Constantino et al., 2021). In the spirit of evidence-based tailoring, arguably any individual difference that has an association with a valued process or outcome is worthy of assessment. While a large number of potentially valuable assessment targets are available, it is important to prioritize those with the greatest relevance to a given patient's needs and goals. In addition to practical constraints for both psychotherapists and clients, a "kitchen sink" approach to assessment will have limited utility for decision making.

In addition to the *what* or *focus* of the assessment, assessment processes as an activity (the how) are often taken for granted. Consequently, there is limited targeted research on the assessment-outcome relationship (Garb, 2005). There are, however, some exceptions to this. When applicable, we will highlight assessment processes that have demonstrated associations with treatment outcome.

ASSESSMENT AS TREATMENT

The boundary between assessment and intervention can be fuzzy (Schön, 1983), as effective clinical assessment is likely to serve some therapeutic function (Eisen et al., 2000). In fact, this assumption has led to models developed for

---

[1]Clinical examples in this chapter are fictitious clinical amalgams or disguised versions of interactions with one or more clients.

this explicit purpose. Arguably the most well-known model is therapeutic assessment (TA), which is a method of semistructured collaborative psychological assessment that explicitly aims for therapeutic impact in addition to gathering information (De Saeger et al., 2016; Finn & Tonsager, 1997). The TA assessor's primary goal is to work collaboratively with the client to help them gain new information that could help improve the client's quality of life. The process includes formulating individualized assessment questions (e.g., "Why do I feel so wimpy right now?" or "Why don't I feel like I have control over my life and my future?"; Smith & George, 2012), in order to orient the *testing phase* and develop an individualized assessment intervention session, followed by an interactive summary and discussion session (Aschieri et al., 2016). Accordingly, assessment is client focused rather than test focused (Finn, 2020; Finn & Tonsager, 1997). TA feedback is often formatted as a personal letter, which many clients find meaningful. As one woman who received TA while waiting for personality disorder treatment reflected, "The therapist gave me a narrative that fit me completely. . . . Afterwards she even wrote it in a letter. I had no more questions about myself. I just had to look at the letter" (De Saeger et al., 2016, p. 476).

Preliminary evidence supports TA as an effective tool to foster treatment engagement and even symptom reduction (Smith et al., 2010; Tharinger et al., 2009). A series of single-case experiments have also demonstrated significant symptom improvement following the initiation of TA in adults (Aschieri & Smith, 2012; Hinrichs, 2016; Smith & George, 2012; Tarocchi et al., 2013). Case studies have been published documenting TA with diverse populations and presenting problems, for example, with a young African American foster child in a community clinic and in an inpatient setting with a man diagnosed with narcissistic personality disorder (e.g., Fantini, 2016; Guerrero et al., 2011; Hinrichs, 2016). In these case studies, improvement was measured with respect to symptom and functioning domains tied to the initial assessment questions identified collaboratively by the client and assessor (e.g., "I am hard on myself" or "I recognize others' love and affection for me" as rated on a Likert scale; Aschieri & Smith, 2012).

Controlled research on the use of TA with adults supports the efficacy of TA in increasing client treatment engagement. In randomized, controlled studies, TA reduced symptomatic distress and increased self-esteem in college students on the wait list for services at university-based counseling centers (Finn & Tonsager, 1992; Newman & Greenway, 1997). Among individuals seeking treatment for personality disorders, pretreatment TA was associated with better outcome expectancies and superior client perceptions of progress toward treatment, as well as marginally superior client alliance to the clinician, relative to a goal-focused pretreatment intervention (De Saeger et al., 2014). Qualitatively, clients report a range of positive experiences with TA, including a positive relationship with the assessor and gaining insight, empowerment, and validation (De Saeger et al., 2016). In an example of empowerment, one client stated, "I noticed later in [subsequent] therapy that I had more self-confidence compared to my group members, as if I was less busy searching for . . . [approval]" (p. 476).

Given the mounting evidence base for TA, the direct therapeutic benefits of assessment are an area that warrants further exploration. For example, little is known about which specific elements of the TA process are most effective for clients or about the potential benefits associated with assessment beyond the TA framework. In addition to the aforementioned benefits of TA, the assessment also shows the therapist's interest in accurately understanding their client's experience. This may be particularly relevant with respect to issues of cultural identity. By incorporating questions about cultural identity into routine assessment, a therapist can demonstrate cultural comfort or the willingness to explore and understand important aspects of a client's background, identity, and values (Owen et al., 2016; Tao et al., 2015).

CLIENT-FOCUSED ASSESSMENT

Clinical assessment is nearly always intended, or assumed, to be client focused. As such, it might be useful to consider strategies or elements that make an assessment more or less client focused, beginning with what a client-focused assessment likely is not. A client-focused assessment is not a one-sided process where a therapist asks a series of questions to "check off the box." This, admittedly, can be difficult to avoid when conducting a more structured interview. This one-sided approach can also show up when a client is given a stack of initial paperwork and self-report measures, with little explanation or discussion. In contrast, a client-focused assessment is collaborative and intends to engage the client as a partner in the activity. For example, a therapist might say to a new client,

> I ask new clients to complete some standard paperwork and questionnaires, but I understand that the purpose of this can be confusing and some parts might not seem like a good fit. I do need to gather some basic information at the start but perhaps we should briefly review what is in here. I can try to answer any questions you might have, and we might find that one or two things in here don't seem like a great fit, so we can put them aside. How does that sound?

The importance of collaboration is also emphasized when asking a client, subsequent to the completion of an assessment, "What was that like for you?" We've observed that failure to engage the client in these basic ways can lead to strains in the working alliance (Bugatti & Boswell, 2016). For example, after being asked to complete a series of self-report measures on multiple occasions, more than one client has stated some version of "I've never really understood these questions. They don't seem relevant, so I'm not sure how useful they are to you. Though I assume you are finding it useful for some reason." Within a working alliance framework, such statements indicate a disagreement on the tasks of therapy (Eubanks et al., 2018).

In addition, a client-focused, collaborative assessment does not over-generalize from observed broad characteristics. A classic example is tailoring treatment selection on the basis of initial diagnosis alone. It is, of course, useful to know if a client meets criteria for panic disorder. However, research has demonstrated that panic disorder patients with severe adult separation anxiety are less likely to respond to manualized cognitive behavior therapy (CBT; Aaronson et al., 2008). Thus, a therapist would do well to inquire about separation anxiety with clients who endorse panic symptoms. A client's separation anxiety does not mean a CBT therapist will need to go back to the drawing board, but it does indicate that some adjustment to the standard protocol (e.g., attending to interpersonal issues) may be necessary (e.g., Busch & Milrod, 2013).

Another example of overgeneralization can occur when gathering baseline information on demographic and identity characteristics. Initial paperwork might ask a new client to check off their race/ethnicity, and in the United States, the form might provide an option for only "African American" rather than "Black." However, many individuals who identify with the umbrella term of "Black" are from a different descent in the African diaspora (e.g., Afro Latinx) and may not identify as African American. A client might experience alienation in such instances when a therapist fails to inquire about their identity and subjective experiences on the topic. To rectify this, a therapist might explain, "We have labels and categories in the field that can miss the mark for many people. I am interested to hear about your identification and experience in your own words." Awareness of individual differences both within and between cultures is important on its own. Creating a space to discuss identity and culture can also combat biases or stereotypes a therapist may hold relative to client demographic characteristics—for example, over-diagnosis of schizophrenia with African American clients (Gara et al., 2019).

In short, a truly client-focused assessment is collaborative and attempts to understand the client as a unique individual, even when you've "seen it a thousand times" or the research literature tells you something about the average (e.g., on average, a client who is less ready to change is unlikely to benefit from action-oriented strategies). In our view, this helps support a more responsive (and, in turn, more effective) psychotherapy, in terms of both initial intervention selection and the tailoring of the treatment over the course of the psychotherapy.

CLIENT-FOCUSED BASELINE ASSESSMENT

We view the terms *baseline* and *initial* assessment as largely interchangeable and will use the term *baseline* throughout this chapter to maintain consistency. A baseline assessment conducted in the first one or more appointments with a new client is important for understanding the client, the nature of their concerns, and their preferences and expectations for the therapy. The information gathered at the baseline assessment informs diagnosis, prognosis, and initial intervention selection.

In previous reviews that focus on associations between client factors and psychotherapy process and outcome (see Boswell et al., 2016; Constantino et al., 2021), we have found it useful to divide client characteristics into broader categories, such as demographic variables (e.g., race/ethnicity, gender, age), beliefs and preferences (e.g., expectancies, credibility, preferences), and intrapsychic traits (e.g., stage of change, reactance). Although many factors within each of these client categories are certainly relevant to decision making over the course of treatment, several of these factors strike us as particularly important to assess, in some form, in the baseline or early phase of the psychotherapy. Next, we address the baseline assessment of selected client characteristics within these broad categories, as well as the implications for matching interventions to those selected client characteristics.

Demographics

We have already touched on some of the pitfalls of noncollaborative assessment of demographic characteristics, including the increased likelihood of overgeneralizing from broad identity categories. In our community-based university training clinic, we do ask new clients to self-report characteristics, such as race and ethnicity, gender, and age, as part of routine administrative paperwork. In addition to a "forced choice" format, there is open space to provide some additional information. However, in our experience, this opportunity is rarely taken. Therefore, we also walk through the responses with the client in the room, in order to (a) confirm that the information is accurate and (b) provide an opportunity for them to describe themselves in their own words. If a question or set of response options misses the mark, then this opens the door to potentially fruitful discussion. For example, a client is given the opportunity to share, "The form doesn't provide an option for my gender identity, so I left it blank." It is conceivable that a novice trainee could interpret the missing information as an indication that this is a complicated issue for the client, which could lead to avoiding the topic ("I better tread lightly"). Such avoidance might leave the client feeling invalidated. We have also conceived of these initial "strains" as a type "double alliance rupture" because the unspoken client concern involves the treatment setting (i.e., the clinic "owns" the assessment procedures) as well as the therapist.

THERAPIST: I see that the section on the form that asks about ethnicity is blank. I wonder if it was difficult to know how to respond, or if in the seemingly infinite number of questions, you might have . . .

CLIENT: I saw it. It's just complicated, and I didn't want to mark anything down.

THERAPIST: I see.

CLIENT: The options provided also didn't seem relevant, so . . .

THERAPIST: I'm glad you're telling me this because it's important. If it is OK with you, I would like to try to understand the complication that you mentioned.

Hopefully, it is clear that such discussions represent an integration of assessment and treatment. Clarity regarding demographic characteristics and identity can guide a personalized understanding of the case and treatment plan. However, research on the association between demographic characteristics and outcome is mixed, at best (Boswell et al., 2016; Constantino et al., 2021). Nonetheless, the implicit and explicit valuing of the client's subjective experience itself can help foster a positive initial working alliance (Tao et al., 2015).

In a summary of multiple studies involving large naturalistic samples, Lambert (2010) concluded that client age, sex, and ethnicity provided no predictive utility over and above initial symptom severity in the prediction of treatment change trajectories. However, in their meta-analysis, Swift and Greenberg (2012) found a small effect of age on premature termination ($d = 0.16$), such that younger clients had a greater probability of dropout. Importantly, results from these reviews provide potentially useful *prognostic information*—the likelihood that any treatment will produce a benefit. This is relevant information yet does not directly inform intervention selection. Demographic characteristics have failed to emerge as consistent moderators of specific treatment effects (e.g., clients with X characteristics tend to experience more benefit from Treatment A vs. Treatment B). The absence of clear relationships to inform tailoring could be an artifact of the pitfalls of how psychotherapy research typically assesses demographic characteristics. Nevertheless, some findings point to the utility of adapting treatment to the client's identified culture.

Smith et al. (2011) conducted a meta-analysis of culturally adapted treatments relative to treatment-as-usual (TAU). Adaptations included providing psychotherapy in the client's native language and using culturally appropriate examples and metaphors. The treatment effect of adaptive therapies was moderated by ethnicity. Asian Americans demonstrated the largest benefit ($d = 1.18$), followed by Hispanic and African American clients (both $d = 0.47$) and Native Americans ($d = 0.22$). Client age was a moderator of treatment outcome, such that younger adults benefited less than older adults. Overall, results support the use of culturally adapted therapy approaches, particularly for older adults who may be less assimilated into the dominant culture. The small effects with Native American clients may indicate that alternative or additional adaptations are necessary.

Beliefs and Preferences

Although relevant throughout the course of psychotherapy, clients enter psychotherapy with a set of beliefs about the nature of psychotherapy and their likelihood of benefit. In addition, clients often enter psychotherapy with a set of preferences for the nature of the psychotherapy and the style and behavior of the psychotherapist. Belief and preference factors are important individual difference variables that should be attended to early in the process of assessment and treatment planning.

Expectancies

Psychotherapy-related expectancies are a common factor that can shape client experiences, motivations, and outcomes (Constantino et al., 2011; Constantino, Coyne, et al., 2018). Two general expectancy types are outcome expectancy—a prognostic belief about the degree to which one will benefit from a current or pending treatment—and treatment expectancy—beliefs about a current or pending treatment's nature and processes. Treatment expectancies can be about the respective roles that the client and therapist will adopt, the contents of treatment, and/or the format or duration of treatment.

We generally assess expectancies in two ways at the beginning of therapy. First, we ask the client to complete a brief self-report measure, the Credibility/Expectancy Questionnaire (CEQ; Devilly & Borkovec, 2000). This is the most commonly used measure of expectancies in psychotherapy research and practice. This brief, face-valid instrument is in the public domain, and it can be adapted for different disorders and treatments. The outcome expectancy subscale includes three items, including one that is commonly used on its own to assess outcome expectancies (Constantino, Vîslă, et al., 2018): "By the end of the therapy period, how much improvement in your [anxiety] symptoms do you think will occur?" Second, informed by their responses on the CEQ, we discuss both outcome and treatment-related expectancies with the client within the first couple of sessions. This is particularly important because the CEQ does not directly assess treatment-related expectancies.

Collaborative discussions regarding outcome expectancies typically begin with the therapist asking the less direct question "What do you hope to achieve in therapy?" And then inquiring, "Are you feeling hopeful that you'll be able to achieve [goal] by the end of our work together?" For clients who express an uncertain or pessimistic view about therapy being helpful, it is important empathize with the client's concerns or ambivalence. We also believe the client's perspective deserves exploration. For example, are negative outcome expectancies driven by previous unhelpful therapy experiences? Or is this expressed pessimism consistent with a working conceptualization that the client's presenting problem is a persistent major depressive disorder, and they are carrying a general feeling of hopelessness about the future?

Clients can possess "generic" outcome and treatment-related expectancies (e.g., enter therapy with generally positive expectancies for therapy, regardless of the nature of the therapy or therapist), as well as outcome and treatment-related expectancies that are more specific to the treatment in question. As noted, treatment-related expectancies can include the respective roles that the client and therapist will adopt, the contents of treatment, and/or the format or duration of treatment. Although such expectations likely intersect with client treatment preferences, these factors are distinguishable, and we address client preferences later. In our experience, a collaborative assessment and discussion of treatment-related expectancies is most fruitful when the treatment plan begins to take shape. After gathering information about the client's history and presenting concerns, an exchange such as the following may take place:

THERAPIST: Based on the concerns you've described and what brought you to therapy now, I think I'm starting to get a better understanding of how best to help you. Although every person is unique, there are well-researched approaches that have been found to be quite helpful for people with similar concerns. I have some experience with these approaches that could be a good fit, but I want to make sure this fits with what you've been expecting.

CLIENT: Okay. I appreciate that. I suppose I haven't been sure what to expect from this.

THERAPIST: I understand, which is why this discussion is important. As a start, what I'm envisioning would be an active, problem-focused approach, with a structure that we will collaboratively develop for each session. It would also involve asking you to monitor and practice things outside of session. This approach is also designed to be time limited, in the ballpark of 15 to 20 weekly appointments. Any reactions or concerns about any of that?

CLIENT: I guess I don't have concerns. I just wasn't sure. I suppose it is a relief to know I won't need to be in therapy forever.

Results from a recent meta-analysis demonstrated a small-to-moderate association between clients' more positive presenting or early treatment outcome expectancies and their posttreatment improvement ($r = 0.18$; Constantino, Vîslă, et al., 2018). However, associations between treatment expectancies and outcome have been less clear and consistent, relative to the evidence for outcome expectancies (Constantino et al., 2011). In the case that a therapist's treatment recommendation is inconsistent with a client's expectancy, it is better to be aware of the disconnect and discuss it than to simply assume parties are on the same page. In terms of matching, however, there is limited evidence on which psychotherapies work best for clients with particular expectancies. We are aware of no studies for which clients' presenting expectations moderate a treatment effect; that is, they serve as a specific condition under which one treatment outperforms one or more others. This is an area in need of research: It may be the case that having a particular role, process, or duration expectation when arriving for therapy provides a context that allows one treatment to perform better, on average, than another.

Treatment Credibility

Client-perceived treatment credibility is how logical, suitable, and effective a given intervention seems (Devilly & Borkovec, 2000). Similar to expectancies, we assess treatment credibility with the CEQ and in session with new clients, typically after an initial treatment rationale has been discussed. Using anxiety as an example, the three credibility items are "At this point, how logical does the therapy offered seem to you?" "At this point, how successful do you think this treatment will be in reducing your anxiety symptoms?" and "How confident would you be in recommending this treatment to a friend who experiences anxiety?"

More broadly, treatment credibility centers on a client's current "answer" to some variation of the question "To what extent does this therapy make sense to me as a way to get better?" We will pose the question directly to the client. For example,

> In the context of your anxiety, you have noted an increasing degree of avoidance. Consistent with this, I use a CBT approach to treatment that emphasizes the reduction of avoidance behaviors and getting back to doing the things that are important to you. Does this seem like a good fit to you?

Constantino, Coyne, et al. (2018) conducted the first meta-analysis of studies that tested the relation between clients' early therapy perception of treatment credibility and outcome. The analysis yielded a small but significant positive effect ($r = 0.12$). Similar to expectancies, however, no clear tailoring variables emerged; that is, there is little evidence to guide the decision to adopt a particular intervention (or avoid another) in the context of lower or higher perceived treatment credibility. The basic principle remains that higher perceived credibility is generally associated with better outcomes, so when a client does not perceive the suggested approach as credible, then the therapist should work with the client to find an approach that is perceived to be a better fit. In response to a perceived lack of credibility, therapists may want to respond initially with foundational clinical skills like empathy, validation, and evocation to gain a clearer understanding of a client's credibility belief.

Preferences

Preference assessment is a critical piece of evidence-based treatment selection and planning (APA Presidential Task Force on Evidence-Based Practice, 2006). Swift et al. (2011, 2018) grouped client preferences into three categories: (a) *activity preferences* are the client's desire for psychotherapy to include specific elements and therapist behaviors/interventions; (b) *treatment preferences* are the client's desire for a specific type of intervention to be used, such as a preference for CBT versus person-centered therapy; and (c) *therapist preferences* are the client's desire to work with a therapist who possesses specific characteristics (e.g., a certain gender or interpersonal style or a racial match; Ward, 2005).

In our experience, even clients with a prior history of psychotherapy struggle to articulate treatment preferences in the form of specific models (e.g., CBT vs. person-centered therapy). We tend to learn more about treatment preferences by attending to activity preferences and then assessing the client's perception of treatment credibility after hearing an initial description of a treatment approach that is likely to be a good fit. We have adopted the

Cooper-Norcross Inventory of Preferences (C-NIP; Cooper & Norcross, 2016) to assess activity-related preferences at the start of treatment.

The C-NIP can be used to facilitate an initial dialogue with clients about their therapy preferences. It consists of two parts. The first part invites clients to indicate their preferences for how they would like a psychotherapist to work with them. The 18 items are grouped into four bipolar scales: Therapist Directiveness versus Client Directiveness, Emotional Intensity versus Emotional Reserve, Past Orientation versus Present Orientation, and Warm Support versus Focused Challenge. The second part asks multiple open-ended questions about client preferences. For instance, clients are asked if they have strong preferences for the length of therapy, therapy format/modality, or anything they would particularly *dislike*. Completion and scoring of the C-NIP typically take approximately 5 minutes.

In practice, we have either asked clients to complete the measure before the first or second session and then reviewed their responses in the session or collaboratively completed the C-NIP as an activity in an early session. This might be introduced by the therapist: "Therapy is not a one-size-fits-all activity, so I would like to understand any preferences you might have for our work together."

THERAPIST: It sounds like you want me to be less directive in here and be sure to let you take the lead. Is that right?

CLIENT: Yes, I think that would be a better fit for me.

THERAPIST: Do you have a sense of why that would be a better fit?

CLIENT: I've had more structured therapy in the past, with a therapist who took charge. That was helpful, to an extent, but it felt like there was no room for me. Does that make sense?

THERAPIST: Yes, that makes sense. That's important to hear. My natural tendency is to be more directive, but I take your preference seriously and can adjust my style. This might be a difficult question, but do you think you would feel comfortable to let me know if I'm not giving you enough room in here?

CLIENT: Yes, I think I can do that.

Because some clients are rather uncertain about their preferences, we have had positive experiences with using the C-NIP as an early in-session activity with clients. Similar to perceived treatment credibility, taking client preferences seriously can lead to some difficult decisions for the client and therapist. For example, if a therapist has a strong allegiance to a particular model that is not perceived as credible by the client, how should the therapist respond? Similarly, how should a therapist respond if a client expresses a strong preference for a directive and structured approach, yet the therapist strongly believes that a nondirective approach is best and they are not comfortable adopting a directive and structured approach? In some instances, these present opportunities for a trainee (or even experienced therapist) to learn how to adapt. In other instances, referral to a different therapist is likely indicated. This may also be indicated when a client has *therapist* preferences that cannot be accommodated. Of course, such decisions will be less disruptive if they are openly discussed and negotiated at the time of taking an initial referral (e.g., whether or not the potential new client has a strong preference for a therapist of a particular gender or ethnicity that you are unable to accommodate; see Ward, 2005).

In a meta-analysis of the preference accommodation–outcome literature, the overall preference effect (clients who were given their preferred psychotherapy or choice of treatment condition) was significant ($d = 0.28$; Swift et al., 2018). Furthermore, clients who were not matched to their preferred treatment condition or were not given a choice of treatment condition were 1.79 times more likely to drop out than clients who were matched to their preferred treatment. These results highlight the importance of assessment and trying one's best to accommodate client preferences.

Intrapsychic Traits

For a comprehensive review of intrapsychic traits and their process–outcome associations, please see Constantino et al. (2021). Within the scope of this chapter, we focus on two traits that are particularly relevant for client-focused baseline assessment and that have received significant conceptual and empirical attention: *stage of change* and *reactance*.

Stage of Change

Clients vary in their preparation and/or readiness for change, and such variability can influence psychotherapy outcome (Krebs et al., 2018). A common operationalization of change stages is as follows: *precontemplation* (no problem awareness or intention to change in the near future), *contemplation* (problem awareness and consideration of change but no current commitment to action), *action* (overt behavioral change steps with commitment), and *maintenance* (efforts to consolidate gains and prevent relapse). See Chapter 3 in this volume for more details about the stages of change.

The transtheoretical model (Prochaska & DiClemente, 1982) predicts that certain intervention strategies are differentially effective for clients in certain stages of change. For example, strategies aimed at raising awareness and problem clarification are most likely to be helpful for those in the precontemplation and contemplation stages. For a client who presents with anger problems, the therapist might ask, "You've mentioned that you've noticed a lot of angry feelings. I wonder how your anger affects you and those around you?" In contrast, clients in the action stage are more likely to benefit from learning and practicing new behaviors, through strategies such as exposure and behavioral activation.

Similar to belief and preference factors, we assess client stage of change with a mix of questionnaire and in-session discussion. When using a self-report measure, we commonly employ the University of Rhode Island Change Assessment (McConnaughy et al., 1989). This measure includes 32 items that yield scores on four subscales of precontemplation, contemplation, action, and maintenance. If the client's highest score is in the contemplation stage, for example, we view it as a likely marker of ambivalence about change and/or their perceived capacity for change. Before attempting more directive and action-oriented strategies, we will initially pull from motivational interviewing principles to better understand and explore this potential ambivalence (Boswell, Bentley, et al., 2015).

In a meta-analysis of theoretically diverse psychotherapies, researchers found a moderate association between stage of change and outcome; patients farther along the stage continuum at the start of treatment evidenced more improvement ($d = 0.41$; Krebs et al., 2018). Although this association is worthy of note, Krebs et al. (2018) could not identify any controlled research studies of matching the treatment strategy to the specific client stage of change. In addition, there remains little information on the mechanisms through which stages of change operate on improvement. Nonetheless, understanding a patient's stage of change provides some initial guidance to therapists on how to adapt and individualize their approach; for example, insight-oriented and motivation-enhancement strategies are likely a good place to begin for clients in the precontemplation and contemplation stages (see Westra et al., 2016).

Reactance

Reactance represents the emotional arousal that people experience when another is hindering their freedom and their motivation to reclaim that freedom (Brehm & Brehm, 1981). Scholars have framed reactance as a more trait-like variable, with some people exhibiting higher reactance across varied situations than others—termed *reactance potential* (Beutler & Consoli, 1993). Theory and research have focused on the interaction between a client's presenting reactance level and the therapist's intervention style, with the idea that higher therapist directiveness is a better match for low reactance clients, whereas therapist nondirectiveness is a better fit for high reactance clients.

In practice, we assess client reactance less directly in at least two ways. First, useful information on reactance can be gathered during discussions of treatment expectations and preferences. As noted, the C-NIP inquires about the degree to which a client prefers to direct the sessions versus prefers for the therapist to direct the sessions. A client who expresses a strong preference for the therapist to be more directive, for the therapy to be more problem and action oriented, and for the therapy to involve homework is judged to be relatively lower in reactance, and a more directive approach would be indicated. Conversely, a client who expresses a preference for the therapist to be less directive, for the therapy to be more insight oriented, and for the therapy to involve minimal expectations for between-session assignments is judged to be relatively higher in reactance, and a less directive approach would be indicated.

In a meta-analysis, Beutler et al. (2018) found that patients with higher reactance had better outcomes when their therapist took a less directive approach ($d = 0.79$). Conversely, as theory and correlational logic would also suggest, patients with lower reactance had better outcomes when their therapist adopted a more directive approach. Thus, a client's reactance level is worthy of attention, and this can inform intervention selection and/or the adjustment of the general therapeutic stance.

Summary

Thus far, we have attended to client-focused baseline assessment. Admittedly, far from providing an exhaustive list of client characteristics, we have highlighted the relevance of select demographic, belief and preference, and intrapsychic characteristics. Underscoring the importance of collaboration for client-focused assessment, we have discussed the usefulness of addressing these factors in session with the client when possible, rather than relying solely on pre-treatment or presession questionnaires. Interestingly, even the most well-researched client factors are presently limited to prognostic utility. That is, they provide the therapist with more information about the likelihood that any treatment approach will produce a benefit. For example, negative outcome expectancies are associated with poorer treatment outcome, yet there is little evidence to guide the selection of a specific treatment strategy (vs. some alternative), beyond recognition that some attempt at expectancy enhancement is needed ("I can see that change seems nearly impossible, and I can only imagine what that feels like. I'd like to understand this better.") Clearly, more research is needed to understand the comparative effectiveness of specific strategies in addressing low outcome expectancies, low perceived treatment credibility, and stage of change.

Preferences, in some ways by definition, carry more *prescriptive utility*—they provide some indication of expected differential benefit from specific treatment approaches. Clients will benefit more from receiving a treatment (or working with a therapist) that matches their preferences, relative to a treatment that does not match their preferences. Understanding client preferences (by using a measure such as the C-NIP, for example) can also provide useful information about treatment expectancies and client reactance potential. The prescriptive utility of reactance is on relatively firm ground, suggesting that the therapist should adjust their level of directiveness as a function of client reactance (Beutler & Harwood, 2000).

Underscoring the importance of client collaboration, and as a segue to the next section on within-treatment assessment (i.e., ongoing assessment subsequent to the baseline period), it is important to remind ourselves as therapists that the conclusions we draw from baseline assessment should not be "written in stone" (another form of overgeneralization). On more than one occasion, we have had a client who initially expresses a preference for the therapist to be more directive and pleads to learn skills and be given tasks between sessions (i.e., perceived to possess low reactance potential), who then proceeds not to complete between-session homework. This does not, on its own, indicate that the initial impression of a low reactance client was incorrect. However, it does indicate a need for discussion.

THERAPIST: When we started working together, it seemed like there was a preference for me to take more of the lead and to suggest things to do outside of the session. Now that we've started to do some of that, I'm wondering what it's been like for you.

CLIENT: I know. I'm not being a very good client.

THERAPIST: Hmm. I'm not sure that I see it that way, but that feeling you're expressing seems important. Sometimes we don't know what we don't know. It was all theoretical when we first discussed it, right?

CLIENT: Right. I think I was being honest, but now it seems like I'm less clear. Homework and things like that still make sense to do, but I'm finding it hard to get to it for some reason.

THERAPIST: I appreciate that. First, adjustments are expected in here. Second, I think being less clear is an important observation that we should explore today. Would that be OK?

CLIENT: I think that would be useful, yes.

THERAPIST: OK. I also want to do a better job of checking in that we are on the same page.

CLIENT-FOCUSED WITHIN-TREATMENT ASSESSMENT

We use the phrase *within-treatment assessment* to indicate client-focused assessments within the course of the treatment itself, subsequent to the baseline assessment/initial evaluation. Such assessments can occur during or immediately before or after a session or at one or more time points between two consecutive sessions. The nature and frequency of a within-treatment assessment should be collaboratively determined between the client and psychotherapist. For example, here is a discussion regarding within-treatment assessment of depression symptoms with a standardized self-report measure:

THERAPIST: In order to track how you are feeling, as well as how things are progressing in our work together, I think it would be important to assess your symptoms and how they're affecting you. That can be useful feedback in my experience. We would use a questionnaire like this [*shows a copy of a questionnaire*].

CLIENT: Sure, OK, that seems like a good idea.

THERAPIST: The research also shows that monitoring how you are doing increases the likelihood of benefiting from therapy. We have some options though. This measure here is relatively short, five questions [*hands a copy to the client*]. This measure here is a bit longer but more specific [*hands a copy to the client*]. I've used both of these before with clients. The main benefit of the shorter one is that it usually takes only about a minute to answer the questions.

CLIENT: I can see that. But it seems like the longer one maybe provides more information?

THERAPIST: Yes, you read my mind. Although it's longer, I might recommend going with the longer one because we can add up your ratings to get an overall score for tracking, while also getting more detailed information on things like your sleep. The other measure doesn't ask about your sleep or concentration, specifically, and I know those are concerns for you.

CLIENT: Exactly. I think the longer one is a better fit.

THERAPIST: OK. That will also probably take no longer than 5 minutes. I typically ask clients to complete this before each session if possible, coming in a few minutes early for that in the waiting area. Would that work for you?

CLIENT: Um. I'm not sure. Given my schedule, I don't think I can get here early each week. Maybe every other week?

THERAPIST: That seems like a good start. Shall we plan for that and see how it goes?

This example also illustrates how the information obtained through the baseline assessment (i.e., that this client is concerned about sleep quality and concentration) can inform the subsequent within-treatment assessment. Within-treatment assessment is important because it gives the psychotherapist (and the client) critical information about the status of the treatment and progress, or lack thereof, in previously identified valued domains. The process of determining what to assess during treatment can be initiated by asking the client, "What would it look like if you are making the progress that you are looking for in here?" or "How would we know if we're on the right track in here?"

Although we describe more sophisticated progress tracking approaches later, this is a good opportunity to state that a more basic approach can be used effectively:

THERAPIST: How would we know if you are making progress in therapy?

CLIENT: I think a lot of it comes down to self-esteem. If I can increase my self-esteem, that would be good progress to me. That is my main issue, I think.

THERAPIST: OK. Let's come up with a measure of that. What about take a scale of 0 to 10? A zero would be having no self-esteem, and a 10 would be having the maximum self-esteem.

CLIENT: Well, I don't know. I don't want to be all full of myself, so a 10 wouldn't necessarily be good.

THERAPIST: Great point. What if we consider a 10 relative to you, specifically? A 10 would represent the optimal amount of self-esteem for you—a marker of reaching your goal.

CLIENT: Oh, I get that. That makes sense.

THERAPIST: So, if 0 is no self-esteem, and 10 is optimal self-esteem, what would you rate yourself at this point?

CLIENT: I don't think I have *no* self-esteem, so probably a 3.

THERAPIST: OK, so I will check in for your rating on that 0-to-10 scale each week, and we'll track your progress. Sound good?

A side effect of tracking self-esteem in this case is that shared, ongoing awareness of progress on the valued outcome can also inform decisions regarding termination. For example,

> We've had a couple of sessions in a row now with a "9" rating. You've been working very hard and the progress is clear, from my perspective. Perhaps we are approaching a natural end to your work in here. What do you think about putting a discussion of that on the agenda?

Conversely, if the hypothetical client remains stuck at a 4 for several weeks, this might prompt a discussion of the lack of progress. For example,

> We've been at a "4" for several weeks now. I'd like to press the 'pause button' and talk about that if it's OK with you? I want to make sure we are taking the best path in here. What is your experience of where things are at?

By far, the most common approach to within-treatment assessment of this kind in psychotherapy is routine progress and outcome monitoring (Wampold, 2015). Early developments in this area led to the apt label of *patient-focused research* (Howard et al., 1996) because the collection of data for a given client can then inform therapy decisions for that given client. This emphasis is somewhat different from choosing a particular standardized treatment approach for the client and assuming it will be effective based on the existing treatment literature (i.e., Treatment A is an evidence-based treatment for clients with similar presenting problems, so if I apply Treatment A, then my client will experience improvement).

Routine Outcome Monitoring Feedback

ROM systems allow therapists to assess and respond to an individual client's evolving progress, nonresponse, or deterioration in real time (Lambert et al.,

2018). ROM systems involve the regular completion of standardized client self-report symptom/functioning measures, which produce clinically relevant data that are provided to therapists (and in some cases to clients as well) in the form of feedback messages of both a descriptive type (e.g., a simple line graph depicting problem levels over time) and a predictive type (e.g., a warning signal that a client is statistically likely to drop out or deteriorate based on comparisons with other clients with similar levels of presenting distress being treated in similar contexts; Boswell, Kraus, et al., 2015). Although the call for using such systems is not new (e.g., Howard et al., 1996), it has been only in recent years that comprehensive ROM systems have been refined and rigorously tested (Wampold, 2015).

As we have inquired rhetorically elsewhere (Boswell, Kraus, et al., 2015; Muir et al., 2019), what would happen if therapists did not monitor client progress/outcome? Evidence suggests that therapists tend to overestimate their client improvement rates and to notably underestimate the deterioration rates for their caseload (Walfish et al., 2012). Moreover, at the case level, clinicians using solely their clinical judgment appear to be poor at noticing warning signs that clients are at risk for a negative outcome. In one study, therapists accurately forecasted harm in just one of 40 cases that ultimately went on to deteriorate (Hannan et al., 2005). Therapists appear to miss cues that could help them adjust the treatment when replaying on clinical judgment alone.

An illustration of this comes from a client in a community mental health center who was asked to complete one such ROM tool, the Treatment Outcome Package (TOP; Kraus et al., 2005). The TOP collects information on multiple symptom and functioning domains (e.g., depression, substance use, sleep, quality of life) and can be completed via paper-and-pencil or online. Completed forms are scored by the developer's software and a feedback report is generated, which includes a figure that graphically depicts a client's score in each domain in the form of standard deviations relative to a nonclinical population mean of 0 (higher positive scores indicating greater severity). The client was asked to complete the TOP prior to the first appointment in the waiting area, and the therapist brought the ensuing feedback report into the appointment. The therapist and client examined the report together in session, and both noted that the client's most clinically elevated domains were depression and anxiety. Although less severe, the client's profile was also slightly above the nonclinical population norm on the substance use and social conflict subscales. The client reported that the information in the feedback report seemed on target from his perspective. Among other questions, the therapist inquired about the client's substance use. The client reported that he drinks alcohol, typically consuming one or two beers in a sitting, two or three nights a week. The client also noted that he had previous periods of heavy drinking, but he has "gotten it under control."

The client and therapist proceeded to work from a broadly CBT orientation, with a focus on emotion awareness and regulation skills, decreasing experiential avoidance, and increasing cognitive flexibility. The client attended sessions regularly and seemed engaged; he made good faith attempts at trying new things between sessions. However, subsequent TOP administrations (completed every other week, prior to the session) did not indicate much change in the initially clinically elevated domains. At the eighth session, the therapist observed on the TOP report that the client was approximately five standard deviations above the nonclinical population on the substance use scale. As usual, the therapist brought the report into session for review.

THERAPIST: I appreciate your willingness to continue to track how things are going on this measure. For today, the main thing that sticks out to me is the elevation in the substance area, as you can see here.

CLIENT: Yeah [*looks away*].

THERAPIST: Can we talk about what might be going on?

CLIENT: I've been drinking. A lot. Every night after work, and I was called out one day earlier this week because of it. I'm not sure what's going on, but I know it's not good.

THERAPIST: I'm hearing that you've been struggling, but you're not sure what's contributing to that. I appreciate that you're communicating that to me now. I understand that's not easy. Let's try to understand this together and explore some of our options.

CLIENT: I would appreciate that.

Routinely completing the TOP allowed the therapist and client to immediately identify an important deviation from the client's typical behavior. The therapist conceptualized the client's drastic increase in alcohol consumption as a form of self-medication and avoidance. In-session exploration revealed that the client was feeling overwhelmed with work and a romantic relationship. On the one hand, psychotherapy was motivating the client to overcome avoidance and take on more challenges; on the other hand, because of this increased engagement, the client reported feeling more "flooded." The therapist and client discussed slowing the pace of the work somewhat and introducing some new coping strategies to help manage stress.

Meta-analyses and systematic reviews have generally supported the benefits of ROM (Fortney et al., 2017; Lambert et al., 2018). Lambert et al. (2018) examined the comparative effect on the outcome of therapists (and in some cases clients) receiving ROM-generated progress feedback versus TAU without feedback. Overall, results showed that ROM feedback promoted significantly better outcomes than TAU, to a small-to-moderate degree. In addition, among the studies that examined treatment outcomes specifically for those clients identified as statistically at risk for a negative outcome, the feedback condition (a) outperformed TAU to a moderate degree on posttreatment outcome, (b) reduced the likelihood of deterioration, and (c) increased the likelihood that clients would achieve reliable and clinically significant improvement by posttreatment (Muir et al., 2019).

The feedback that a given course of treatment is not on track for a positive outcome is important information on its own. However, psychotherapists have expressed concerns about the ultimate utility of this information in the absence of guidance on how to be responsive to this feedback ("It looks like we are off track, but I have no idea why or what to do to get back on track"). An important innovation in ROM-feedback work has been the development of targeted clinical supportive tools (CSTs; brief guidelines helping therapists to identify and solve problems that may have plausibly precipitated clients' risk for deterioration). CSTs are integrated when a client is determined to be "not on track." When this risk of a negative outcome is detected, the therapist is asked to conduct a follow-up assessment to help determine the potential cause of the nonresponse or deterioration, such as asking the client to complete a working alliance assessment. If the quality of the alliance seems poor, then the therapist can access alliance-enhancement resources, such as strategies for repairing alliance ruptures (Eubanks et al., 2018).

Lambert et al. (2018) also meta-analyzed ROM studies that involved CSTs. Among the studies that compared the effects of feedback + CSTs to TAU for clients identified as at risk, the feedback + CST condition (a) outperformed TAU to a moderate degree on posttreatment outcome, (b) reduced the likelihood of deterioration, and (c) increased the likelihood that clients would achieve reliable and clinically significant improvement. These meta-analyses provide relatively strong evidence that providing therapists with ROM-based feedback (especially in combination with CSTs) results in better outcomes, particularly for those clients who are statistically determined to be at risk for harm.

Enhancing the Client Centeredness of ROM

Work in the area of ROM feedback has largely focused on symptoms, functioning, and general distress domains, using a standardized, nomothetic approach. That is, for standardized ROM tools, all clients are expected to complete the same measures. When trying to optimize assessments to fit individual clients, even multidimensional ROM tools can miss the mark in some cases. There is increasing interest in augmenting standardized, nomothetic outcome assessments with idiographic approaches (Boswell, 2020; Bugatti & Boswell, in press).

Nomothetic assessment procedures such as self-report questionnaires yielding norm-referenced, standardized scores feature several advantages, including consistency within each course of treatment, the population, and norm-referenced comparisons (Scott & Lewis, 2015). Nonetheless, nomothetic measures are less easily tailored to individual clients. Psychotherapists typically address hypothesized underlying psychological processes that might differ in importance and relevance among different clients. As a complement to the use of nomothetic assessments, *idiographic measures* enable clinicians to monitor client-specific treatment factors, such as client goals, needs, values, and skills, based on assessment targets that are most relevant to the specific context of each client (Scott & Lewis, 2015). Research on the use of idiographic measures for ROM is still sparse, yet this area appears promising (Edbrooke-Childs et al., 2015; Lindhiem et al., 2016). Interestingly, some research findings show that clinicians report more positive attitudes toward idiographic than nomothetic measures (Jensen-Doss, Smith, et al., 2018).

The example client from earlier who would like to prioritize improving self-esteem is a good candidate for using an idiographic outcome measure. The therapist might explain the augmented assessment by saying,

> I understand that you are ultimately interested in reducing your anxiety and depression symptoms. We can use this assessment measure to track progress in this area. It can also be useful to also incorporate a progress tracking item or two that more closely fits your specific concerns and interests. You mentioned that avoiding social plans is both a cause and consequence of your anxiety. Perhaps we can track how often you are avoiding and canceling plans and see if we notice a pattern with your anxiety along the way. How does that sound?

Summary

Based on the research evidence and our own clinical experience with outcome monitoring and feedback, we strongly recommend incorporating monitoring practices in psychotherapy. Although most research has focused on standardized ROM-feedback systems, evidence is mounting for the use of more idiographic outcome monitoring. We see value in this simpler approach, including greater ease of integration into routine practice for a psychotherapist less familiar with standardized assessment tools. The idea that a collaborative approach involves negotiating the nature and frequency of the assessment bears repeating. In our view, it is better to track within-treatment progress occasionally than not at all. In addition, ideally, trainee therapists will be exposed to the implementation of both standardized outcome monitoring approaches and more idiographic assessment approaches, based on the expressed priorities of the client.

Interestingly, survey research generally demonstrates that therapists endorse positive attitudes toward routine client assessment with standardized measures; however, actual utilization rates (e.g., use of a ROM-feedback system) remain low (Jensen-Doss, Haimes, et al., 2018; Wright et al., 2020). For therapists, the disconnection between attitudes and behavior is likely explained, at least in part, by resource and logistical constraints. The development of web-based assessment tools that involve automated scoring and feedback are a significant innovation in this regard (see Lyon et al., 2016, for a more comprehensive list of existing tools). Admittedly, such assessment platforms can be rather expensive, an implementation challenge that needs to be addressed in some form (Lyon et al., 2016). Insurance reimbursement for such client-focused assessment is one policy that would mitigate overall costs to the clinician or an agency.

CONCLUSION AND FUTURE DIRECTIONS

Baseline assessment can confer therapeutic benefits and help to guide the selection of treatment approaches and therapeutic styles (e.g., level of directiveness), and within-treatment assessment can ensure therapists are aware of client progress and improve responsiveness when a client is not receiving the expected benefits of therapy. By tracking outcomes over time, moreover, a clinician can identify their particular clinical strengths and areas for growth. Much is unknown, however, about how feedback is used by therapists (Wampold, 2015). This area is receiving more attention (e.g., de Jong et al., 2012), as is the expansion of variables that should be considered for baseline and within-treatment assessment (Constantino et al., 2013).

Regarding baseline assessment, client factors such as outcome expectancies and perceived treatment credibility can inform prognostic judgments, yet the research base remains mixed in the area of intervention tailoring. Regardless, the evidence to date suggests that clients generally endorse positive attitudes toward completing assessments and report feeling more involved in their treatment, as well as more respected by providers, when they are asked to participate in assessments (Eisen et al., 2000; Moltu et al., 2018). Clients report that assessment communicates that clinicians are taking them seriously and the belief that assessment information leads to better treatment decisions (Dowrick et al., 2009). The important observation that client-focused assessment is indeed experienced as client centered should not be trivialized. Our hope is that you can see how the distinction between assessment and intervention is not as clear as it may seem a first glance, and potential therapeutic benefits of assessment can be harnessed by engaging in a more client-focused assessment.

Our view is that the "siloing" of assessment and intervention may be reinforced early on in graduate training (e.g., there are assessment courses and practica, and there are psychotherapy courses and practica). We are not arguing that narrowly focused coursework and training should not exist; however, for psychotherapy courses/practica, in particular, the integration of client-focused assessment methods is consistent with the evidence base and would likely enhance the training experience. For example, practicum supervisors can establish that some degree of progress and outcome monitoring is expected with training cases (whether standardized or idiographic). While initially focused on ROM, the skills of (a) introducing the rationale for assessment, (b) implementing the assessment, and (c) integrating the assessment results are generalizable to the implementation of other assessment methods. Familiarity would, in turn, likely promote more positive attitudes toward routine assessment and the use of such methods after training.

Although we clearly see the value in client-focused assessment and intervention and the integration of client-focused assessment methods in training, significant research and knowledge gaps should be acknowledged. For example, evidence generally supports the use of ROM feedback in psychotherapy, particularly for cases that are at risk for nonresponse. However, what therapists do with the feedback is largely taken for granted. In other words, more research is needed to understand how therapists interpret, respond to, and make use of (or do not use) outcome monitoring feedback. A similar statement could be made about most forms of assessment-derived feedback in psychotherapy. For example, it is important to know that a client's stage of change and early treatment outcome expectancies are, generally, associated with outcome. However, it remains largely unknown at this time whether the assessment process itself (i.e., conducting a more formal assessment of readiness to change and expectancies through interview and self-report methods vs. not conducting such assessments) accounts for any incremental outcome benefits. Results from a comparative trial with an additive design (e.g., treatment as usual alone vs. treatment as usual plus formal client-focused assessment methods) might begin to address this knowledge gap.

In addition, relative to the prognostic utility of client characteristics, there is less evidence to guide treatment selection. For some client factors, the absence of more direct evidence is perplexing. For example, therapists can look to theory and research from social and personality psychology to inform strategies for enhancing outcome expectations or the perceived credibility of a treatment model. However, little to no research has "packaged" derived principles (e.g., a credibility enhancement module) and tested them rigorously in actual clinical contexts (e.g., involving real vs. analogue clients). This area is ripe for development and testing.

REFERENCES

Aaronson, C. J., Shear, M. K., Goetz, R. R., Allen, L. B., Barlow, D. H., White, K. S., Ray, S., Money, R., Saksa, J. R., Woods, S. W., & Gorman, J. M. (2008). Predictors and time course of response among panic disorder patients treated with cognitive-behavioral therapy. *The Journal of Clinical Psychiatry, 69*(3), 418–424. https://doi.org/10.4088/JCP.v69n0312

APA Presidential Task Force on Evidence-Based Practice. (2006). Evidence-based practice in psychology. *American Psychologist, 61*(4), 271–285. https://doi.org/10.1037/0003-066X.61.4.271

Aschieri, F., Fantini, F., & Smith, J. D. (2016). Collaborative/Therapeutic Assessment: Procedures to enhance client outcomes. In S. Maltzman (Ed.), *The Oxford handbook of treatment processes and outcomes in psychology* (pp. 241–269). Oxford University Press.

Aschieri, F., & Smith, J. D. (2012). The effectiveness of therapeutic assessment with an adult client: A single-case study using a time-series design. *Journal of Personality Assessment, 94*(1), 1–11. https://doi.org/10.1080/00223891.2011.627964

Beutler, L. E., & Consoli, A. J. (1993). Matching the therapist's interpersonal stance to clients' characteristics: Contributions from systematic eclectic psychotherapy. *Psychotherapy, 30*(3), 417–422. https://doi.org/10.1037/0033-3204.30.3.417

Beutler, L. E., Edwards, C., & Someah, K. (2018). Adapting psychotherapy to patient reactance level: A meta-analytic review. *Journal of Clinical Psychology, 74*(11), 1952–1963. https://doi.org/10.1002/jclp.22682

Beutler, L. E., & Harwood, T. M. (2000). *Prescriptive psychotherapy: A practical guide to systematic treatment selection.* Oxford University Press. https://doi.org/10.1093/med:psych/9780195136692.001.0001

Boswell, J. F. (2020). Monitoring processes and outcomes in routine clinical practice: A promising approach to plugging the holes of the practice-based evidence colander. *Psychotherapy Research, 30*(7), 829–842. https://doi.org/10.1080/10503307.2019. 1686192

Boswell, J. F., Bentley, K. H., & Barlow, D. H. (2015). Motivation facilitation in the Unified Protocol for Transdiagnostic Treatment of Emotional Disorders. In H. Arkowitz, W. Miller, & S. Rollnick (Eds.), *Motivational interviewing in the treatment of psychological problems* (2nd ed., pp. 33–57). Guilford Press.

Boswell, J. F., Constantino, M. J., & Anderson, L. M. (2016). Potential obstacles to treatment success in adults: Client characteristics. In S. Maltzman (Ed.), *The Oxford handbook of treatment processes and outcomes in psychology* (pp. 183–205). Oxford University Press.

Boswell, J. F., Kraus, D. R., Miller, S. D., & Lambert, M. J. (2015). Implementing routine outcome monitoring in clinical practice: Benefits, challenges, and solutions. *Psychotherapy Research, 25*(1), 6–19. https://doi.org/10.1080/10503307.2013.817696

Brehm, J. W., & Brehm, S. S. (1981). *Psychological reactance: A theory of freedom and control.* Academic Press.

Bugatti, M., & Boswell, J. F. (2016). Clinical errors as a lack of context responsiveness. *Psychotherapy, 53*(3), 262–267. https://doi.org/10.1037/pst0000080

Bugatti, M., & Boswell, J. F. (in press). Clinician perceptions of nomothetic and individualized patient-reported outcome measures in measurement-based care. *Psychotherapy Research.*

Busch, F. N., & Milrod, B. L. (2013). Panic-focused psychodynamic psychotherapy-extended range. *Psychoanalytic Inquiry, 33*(6), 584–594. https://doi.org/10.1080/ 07351690.2013.835166

Constantino, M. J., Boswell, J. F., Bernecker, S. L., & Castonguay, L. G. (2013). Context-responsive psychotherapy integration as a framework for a unified psychotherapy and clinical science: Conceptual and empirical considerations. *Journal of Unified Psychotherapy and Clinical Science, 2*(1), 1–20.

Constantino, M. J., Boswell, J. F., & Coyne, A. E. (2021). Patient, therapist, and relational factors. In M. Barkham, W. Lutz, & L. G. Castonguay (Eds.), *Bergin and Garfield handbook of psychotherapy and behavior change* (7th ed., pp. 225–262). Wiley & Sons.

Constantino, M. J., Coyne, A. E., Boswell, J. F., Iles, B. R., & Vîslă, A. (2018). A meta-analysis of the association between patients' early perception of treatment credibility and their posttreatment outcomes. *Psychotherapy, 55*(4), 486–495. https://doi.org/ 10.1037/pst0000168

Constantino, M. J., Glass, C. R., Arnkoff, D. B., Ametrano, R. M., & Smith, J. Z. (2011). Expectations. In J. C. Norcross (Ed.), *Psychotherapy relationships that work: Evidence-based responsiveness* (2nd ed., pp. 354–376). Oxford University Press. https://doi.org/ 10.1093/acprof:oso/9780199737208.003.0018

Constantino, M. J., Vîslă, A., Coyne, A. E., & Boswell, J. F. (2018). A meta-analysis of the association between patients' early treatment outcome expectation and their posttreatment outcomes. *Psychotherapy, 55*(4), 473–485. https://doi.org/10.1037/pst0000169

Cooper, M., & Norcross, J. C. (2016). A brief, multidimensional measure of clients' therapy preferences: The Cooper–Norcross Inventory of Preferences (C-NIP). *International Journal of Clinical and Health Psychology, 16*(1), 87–98. https://doi.org/10.1016/ j.ijchp.2015.08.003

de Jong, K., van Sluis, P., Nugter, M. A., Heiser, W. J., & Spinhoven, P. (2012). Understanding the differential impact of outcome monitoring: Therapist variables that moderate feedback effects in a randomized clinical trial. *Psychotherapy Research, 22*(4), 464–474. https://doi.org/10.1080/10503307.2012.673023

Delgadillo, J., & Lutz, W. (2020). A development pathway towards precision mental health care. *JAMA Psychiatry, 77*(9), 889–890. https://doi.org/10.1001/jamapsychiatry. 2020.1048

De Saeger, H., Bartak, A., Eder, E. E., & Kamphuis, J. H. (2016). Memorable experiences in Therapeutic Assessment: Inviting the patient's perspective following a pretreatment randomized controlled trial. *Journal of Personality Assessment, 98*(5), 472–479. https://doi.org/10.1080/00223891.2015.1136314

De Saeger, H., Kamphuis, J. H., Finn, S. E., Smith, J. D., Verheul, R., van Busschbach, J. J., Feenstra, D. J., & Horn, E. K. (2014). Therapeutic assessment promotes treatment readiness but does not affect symptom change in patients with personality disorders: Findings from a randomized clinical trial. *Psychological Assessment, 26*(2), 474–483. https://doi.org/10.1037/a0035667

Devilly, G. J., & Borkovec, T. D. (2000). Psychometric properties of the credibility/expectancy questionnaire. *Journal of Behavior Therapy and Experimental Psychiatry, 31*(2), 73–86. https://doi.org/10.1016/S0005-7916(00)00012-4

Dowrick, C., Leydon, G. M., McBride, A., Howe, A., Burgess, H., Clarke, P., Maisey, S., & Kendrick, T. (2009). Patients' and doctors' views on depression severity questionnaires incentivised in UK quality and outcomes framework: Qualitative study. *BMJ, 338*(7697), b663. https://doi.org/10.1136/bmj.b663

Edbrooke-Childs, J., Jacob, J., Law, D., Deighton, J., & Wolpert, M. (2015). Interpreting standardized and idiographic outcome measures in CAMHS: What does change mean and how does it relate to functioning and experience? *Child and Adolescent Mental Health, 20*(3), 142–148. https://doi.org/10.1111/camh.12107

Eisen, S. V., Dickey, B., & Sederer, L. I. (2000). A self-report symptom and problem rating scale to increase inpatients' involvement in treatment. *Psychiatric Services, 51*(3), 349–353. https://doi.org/10.1176/appi.ps.51.3.349

Eubanks, C. F., Muran, J. C., & Safran, J. D. (2018). Repairing alliance ruptures. In J. C. Norcross & B. E. Wampold (Eds.), *Psychotherapy relationships that work: Evidence-based responsiveness* (3rd ed., pp. 549–579). Oxford University Press.

Fantini, F. (2016). Family traditions, cultural values, and the clinician's countertransference: Therapeutic assessment of a young Sicilian woman. *Journal of Personality Assessment, 98*(6), 576–584. https://doi.org/10.1080/00223891.2016.1178128

Finn, S. E. (2020). *Our clients' shoes: Theory and techniques of Therapeutic Assessment.* Routledge. https://doi.org/10.4324/9781003064459

Finn, S. E., & Tonsager, M. E. (1992). Therapeutic effects of providing MMPI-2 test feedback to college students awaiting therapy. *Psychological Assessment, 4*(3), 278–287. https://doi.org/10.1037/1040-3590.4.3.278

Finn, S. E., & Tonsager, M. E. (1997). Information-gathering and therapeutic models of assessment: Complementary paradigms. *Psychological Assessment, 9*(4), 374–385. https://doi.org/10.1037/1040-3590.9.4.374

Fortney, J. C., Unützer, J., Wrenn, G., Pyne, J. M., Smith, G. R., Schoenbaum, M., & Harbin, H. T. (2017). A tipping point for measurement-based care. *Psychiatric Services, 68*(2), 179–188. https://doi.org/10.1176/appi.ps.201500439

Gara, M. A., Minsky, S., Silverstein, S. M., Miskimen, T., & Strakowski, S. M. (2019). A naturalistic study of racial disparities in diagnoses at an outpatient behavioral health clinic. *Psychiatric Services, 70*(2), 130–134. https://doi.org/10.1176/appi.ps.201800223

Garb, H. N. (2005). Clinical judgment and decision making. *Annual Review of Clinical Psychology, 1*(1), 67–89. https://doi.org/10.1146/annurev.clinpsy.1.102803.143810

Gibbons, R. D., Weiss, D. J., Frank, E., & Kupfer, D. (2016). Computerized adaptive diagnosis and testing of mental health disorders. *Annual Review of Clinical Psychology, 12*(1), 83–104. https://doi.org/10.1146/annurev-clinpsy-021815-093634

Guerrero, B., Lipkind, J., & Rosenberg, A. (2011). Why did she put nail polish in my drink? Applying the Therapeutic Assessment model with an African American foster child in a community mental health setting. *Journal of Personality Assessment, 93*(1), 7–15. https://doi.org/10.1080/00223891.2011.529002

Hannan, C., Lambert, M. J., Harmon, C., Nielsen, S. L., Smart, D. W., Shimokawa, K., & Sutton, S. W. (2005). A lab test and algorithms for identifying clients at risk for treatment failure. *Journal of Clinical Psychology, 61*(2), 155–163. https://doi.org/10.1002/jclp.20108

Hinrichs, J. (2016). Inpatient therapeutic assessment with narcissistic personality disorder. *Journal of Personality Assessment, 98*(2), 111–123. https://doi.org/10.1080/00223891.2015.1075997

Howard, K. I., Moras, K., Brill, P. L., Martinovich, Z., & Lutz, W. (1996). Evaluation of psychotherapy: Efficacy, effectiveness, and patient progress. *American Psychologist, 51*(10), 1059–1064. https://doi.org/10.1037/0003-066X.51.10.1059

Jensen-Doss, A., Haimes, E. M. B., Smith, A. M., Lyon, A. R., Lewis, C. C., Stanick, C. F., & Hawley, K. M. (2018). Monitoring treatment progress and providing feedback is viewed favorably but rarely used in practice. *Administration and Policy in Mental Health, 45*(1), 48–61. https://doi.org/10.1007/s10488-016-0763-0

Jensen-Doss, A., Smith, A. M., Becker-Haimes, E. M., Mora Ringle, V., Walsh, L. M., Nanda, M., Walsh, S. L., Maxwell, C. A., & Lyon, A. R. (2018). Individualized progress measures are more acceptable to clinicians than standardized measures: Results of a national survey. *Administration and Policy in Mental Health, 45*(3), 392–403. https://doi.org/10.1007/s10488-017-0833-y

Kraus, D. R., Seligman, D. A., & Jordan, J. R. (2005). Validation of a behavioral health treatment outcome and assessment tool designed for naturalistic settings: The Treatment Outcome Package. *Journal of Clinical Psychology, 61*(3), 285–314. https://doi.org/10.1002/jclp.20084

Krebs, P., Norcross, J. C., Nicholson, J. M., & Prochaska, J. O. (2018). Stages of change and psychotherapy outcomes: A review and meta-analysis. *Journal of Clinical Psychology, 74*(11), 1964–1979. https://doi.org/10.1002/jclp.22683

Lambert, M. J. (2010). *Prevention of treatment failure: The use of measuring, monitoring, and feedback in clinical practice.* American Psychological Association. https://doi.org/10.1037/12141-000

Lambert, M. J. (2013). The efficacy and effectiveness of psychotherapy. In M. J. Lambert (Ed.), *Bergin and Garfield's handbook of psychotherapy and behavior change* (6th ed., pp. 169–218). Wiley & Sons.

Lambert, M. J., Whipple, J. L., & Kleinstäuber, M. (2018). Collecting and delivering progress feedback: A meta-analysis of routine outcome monitoring. *Psychotherapy, 55*(4), 520–537. https://doi.org/10.1037/pst0000167

Lindhiem, O., Bennett, C. B., Orimoto, T. E., & Kolko, D. J. (2016). A meta-analysis of personalized treatment goals in psychotherapy: A preliminary report and call for more studies. *Clinical Psychology: Science and Practice, 23*(2), 165–176. https://doi.org/10.1111/cpsp.12153

Linehan, M. M. (1993). *Cognitive-behavioral treatment of borderline personality disorder.* Guilford Press.

Lutz, W., Rubel, J. A., Schwartz, B., Schilling, V., & Deisenhofer, A.-K. (2019). Towards integrating personalized feedback research into clinical practice: Development of the Trier Treatment Navigator (TTN). *Behaviour Research and Therapy, 120*, 103438. https://doi.org/10.1016/j.brat.2019.103438

Lyon, A. R., Lewis, C. C., Boyd, M. R., Hendrix, E., & Liu, F. (2016). Capabilities and characteristics of digital measurement feedback systems: Results from a comprehensive review. *Administration and Policy in Mental Health, 43*(3), 441–466. https://doi.org/10.1007/s10488-016-0719-4

McConnaughy, E. A., DiClemente, C. C., Prochaska, J. O., & Velicer, W. F. (1989). Stages of change in psychotherapy: A follow-up report. *Psychotherapy, 26*(4), 494–503. https://doi.org/10.1037/h0085468

Moltu, C., Veseth, M., Stefansen, J., Nøtnes, J. C., Skjølberg, Å., Binder, P. E., Castonguay, L. G., & Nordberg, S. S. (2018). This is what I need a clinical feedback system to do for me: A qualitative inquiry into therapists' and patients' perspectives. *Psychotherapy Research, 28*(2), 250–263. https://doi.org/10.1080/10503307.2016.1189619

Muir, H. J., Coyne, A. E., Morrison, N. R., Boswell, J. F., & Constantino, M. J. (2019). Ethical implications of routine outcomes monitoring for patients, psychotherapists, and mental health care systems. *Psychotherapy, 56*(4), 459–469. https://doi.org/ 10.1037/pst0000246

Newman, M. L., & Greenway, P. (1997). Therapeutic effects of providing MMPI-2 test feedback to clients at a university counseling service: A collaborative approach. *Psychological Assessment, 9*(2), 122–131. https://doi.org/10.1037/1040-3590.9.2.122

Owen, J., Tao, K. W., Drinane, J. M., Hook, J., Davis, D. E., & Kune, N. F. (2016). Client perceptions of therapists' multicultural orientation: Cultural (missed) opportunities and cultural humility. *Professional Psychology, Research and Practice, 47*(1), 30–37. https:// doi.org/10.1037/pro0000046

Pincus, A. L., Lukowitsky, M. R., & Wright, A. G. C. (2010). The interpersonal nexus of personality and psychopathology. In T. Millon, R. F. Krueger, & E. Simonsen (Eds.), *Current directions in psychopathology: Scientific foundations for the* DSM-V *and* ICD-11 (pp. 523–552). Guilford Press.

Precision Medicine Initiative (PMI) Working Group. (2015). *The Precision Medicine Initiative Cohort Program: Building a research foundation for 21st century medicine.* National Institutes of Health. https://acd.od.nih.gov/documents/reports/PMI_WG_report_2015-09-17-Final.pdf

Prochaska, J. O., & DiClemente, C. C. (1982). Transtheoretical therapy: Toward a more integrative model of change. *Psychotherapy, 19*(3), 276–288. https://doi.org/10.1037/ h0088437

Schön, D. (1983). *The reflective practitioner: How professionals think inaction.* Temple Smith.

Scott, K., & Lewis, C. C. (2015). Using measurement-based care to enhance any treatment. *Cognitive and Behavioral Practice, 22*(1), 49–59. https://doi.org/10.1016/j.cbpra. 2014.01.010

Smith, J. D., & George, C. (2012). Therapeutic assessment case study: Treatment of a woman diagnosed with metastatic cancer and attachment trauma. *Journal of Personality Assessment, 94*(4), 331–344. https://doi.org/10.1080/00223891.2012.656860

Smith, J. D., Handler, L., & Nash, M. R. (2010). Therapeutic assessment for preadolescent boys with oppositional defiant disorder: A replicated single-case time-series design. *Psychological Assessment, 22*(3), 593–602. https://doi.org/10.1037/a0019697

Smith, T. B., Domenech Rodríguez, M. M., & Bernal, G. (2011). Culture. In J. C. Norcross (Ed.), *Psychotherapy relationships that work: Evidence-based responsiveness* (pp. 316–335). Oxford University Press. https://doi.org/10.1093/acprof:oso/9780199737208.003.0016

Stiles, W. B., Honos-Webb, L., & Surko, M. (1998). Responsiveness in psychotherapy. *Clinical Psychology: Science and Practice, 5*(4), 439–458. https://doi.org/10.1111/ j.1468-2850.1998.tb00166.x

Swift, J. K., Callahan, J. L., Cooper, M., & Parkin, S. R. (2018). The impact of accommodating client preference in psychotherapy: A meta-analysis. *Journal of Clinical Psychology, 74*(11), 1924–1937. https://doi.org/10.1002/jclp.22680

Swift, J. K., Callahan, J. L., & Vollmer, B. M. (2011). Preferences. *Journal of Clinical Psychology, 67*(2), 155–165. https://doi.org/10.1002/jclp.20759

Swift, J. K., & Greenberg, R. P. (2012). Premature discontinuation in adult psychotherapy: A meta-analysis. *Journal of Consulting and Clinical Psychology, 80*(4), 547–559. https://doi.org/10.1037/a0028226

Tao, K. W., Owen, J., Pace, B. T., & Imel, Z. E. (2015). A meta-analysis of multicultural competencies and psychotherapy process and outcome. *Journal of Counseling Psychology, 62*(3), 337–350. https://doi.org/10.1037/cou0000086

Tarocchi, A., Aschieri, F., Fantini, F., & Smith, J. D. (2013). Therapeutic assessment of complex trauma: A single-case time-series study. *Clinical Case Studies, 12*(3), 228–245. https://doi.org/10.1177/1534650113479442

Tharinger, D. J., Finn, S. E., Gentry, L., Hamilton, A., Fowler, J., Matson, M., Krumholz, L., & Walkowiak, J. (2009). Therapeutic Assessment with children: A pilot study of treatment acceptability and outcome. *Journal of Personality Assessment, 91*(3), 238–244. https://doi.org/10.1080/00223890902794275

Walfish, S., McAlister, B., O'Donnell, P., & Lambert, M. J. (2012). An investigation of self-assessment bias in mental health providers. *Psychological Reports, 110*(2), 639–644. https://doi.org/10.2466/02.07.17.PR0.110.2.639–644

Wampold, B. E. (2015). Routine outcome monitoring: Coming of age—with the usual developmental challenges. *Psychotherapy, 52*(4), 458–462. https://doi.org/10.1037/pst0000037

Wampold, B. E., & Imel, Z. E. (2015). *Counseling and psychotherapy. The great psychotherapy debate: The evidence for what makes psychotherapy work* (2nd ed.). Routledge/Taylor & Francis Group.

Ward, E. C. (2005). Keeping it real: A grounded theory study of African American clients engaging in counseling at a community mental health agency. *Journal of Counseling Psychology, 52*(4), 471–481. https://doi.org/10.1037/0022-0167.52.4.471

Westra, H. A., Constantino, M. J., & Antony, M. M. (2016). Integrating motivational interviewing with cognitive-behavioral therapy for severe generalized anxiety disorder: An allegiance-controlled randomized clinical trial. *Journal of Consulting and Clinical Psychology, 84*(9), 768–782. https://doi.org/10.1037/ccp0000098

Wright, C. V., Goodheart, C., Bard, D., Bobbitt, B. L., Butt, Z., Lysell, K., McKay, D., & Stephens, K. (2020). Promoting measurement-based care and quality measure development: The APA mental and behavioral health registry initiative. *Psychological Services, 17*(3), 262–270. https://doi.org/10.1037/ser0000347

Rethinking Therapists' Responsiveness to Center Clients' Experiences of Psychotherapy

Heidi M. Levitt, Kathleen M. Collins, Javier L. Rizo, and Ally B. Hand

For many years, the psychotherapy literature has focused on therapists' theories of psychopathology and of their clients' change processes. It is therapists' interpretations, conceptualizations, and interventions that are foundational in most theories of psychotherapy and psychotherapy research endeavors. Although their perspectives have advanced the development of the field of psychotherapy, this focus historically has excluded the other contributor to change in therapy—namely, the client. It is only within the last 50 years that research on clients' experiences of psychotherapy has begun to blossom (Levitt, 2015). Foregoing the perspective of clients in our representations of the coconstructed process of change has meant that the self-healing activities of clients and their efforts to manage the therapeutic encounter are rarely integrated into our professional understanding of what psychotherapy entails (Gordon, 2012). Although clients have been found to contribute most to the variance in client change scores (e.g., Wampold & Imel, 2015), they remain the neglected factor in psychotherapy research (Bohart & Tallman, 2010). In this chapter, we argue that an understanding of clients' experiences provides necessary guidance for the training and practice of responsive therapists. We first consider what the literature on clients' experiences teaches us about the skills that therapists need, both to implement interventions responsively and to support clients' self-healing efforts, and then make recommendations for practice, training, and research. We draw primarily on the findings from an omnibus qualitative meta-analysis (Levitt, Pomerville, & Surace, 2016)

https://doi.org/10.1037/0000303-010
The Other Side of Psychotherapy: Understanding Clients' Experiences and Contributions in Treatment, J. N. Fuertes (Editor)

to describe what qualitative researchers have learned from clients' descriptions of their experiences in psychotherapy. If therapists are able to identify and understand these experiences, they will be better able to apply skills and shape interventions that can support clients' self-healing process.

CENTERING THE CLIENT IN CONSIDERATIONS OF THERAPIST RESPONSIVENESS

The neglect of the research on clients' therapy experiences may seem surprising in light of the rapidly growing interest in therapists' responsiveness (e.g., see reviews of this literature by Kramer & Stiles, 2015; Wu & Levitt, 2020), which has described therapists' ability to tailor modes of relating and interventions to the needs of their clients. Responsiveness processes have gained attention in part because of the finding that differences between therapists appear to account for clients' change (meaning that some therapists tend to perform reliably better than others) more than differences between therapy orientations, which have been found to have little effect (e.g., Saxon et al., 2017). These findings have led researchers to wonder why some therapists might be more responsive than others. An understanding of a client's internal experiences would seem requisite to the process of responsiveness.

Stiles et al. (1998) described responsiveness as a problem for research that conceptualizes therapy as the study of fixed therapist behaviors and their effects (e.g., clinical trials and intervention research). The process of therapists continually adapting interventions to clients would confound findings, making it impossible to know if effects were due to a targeted intervention or due to processes inherent in its adjustment. Indeed, the adaptation of therapy interventions by therapists appears to be pervasive; even in highly manualized treatments in clinical trials, clinicians have been found to import techniques from other approaches (Berg, 2020). In response, *therapist responsiveness* was offered as a term that describes the reality of how therapists shape their interventions. It was defined by Stiles et al. (1998) as

> behavior that is affected by emerging context, including emerging perceptions of others' characteristics and behavior . . . involving bidirectional causation and feedback loops. . . . It may include treatment selection and planning based on clients' problems and characteristics as well as the timing and phrasing of interventions based on clients' level of understanding and emotional state. (p. 439)

Given this problem, some psychotherapy researchers have developed alternative strategies for studying therapy responsiveness (see Kramer & Stiles, 2015, and Watson & Wiseman, 2021, for descriptions of some approaches and findings, which include process measure research and qualitative analyses). In this chapter, we use a variety of terms to reflect the actions that therapists are taking while being responsive, such as *tailoring, adjusting, importing,* and *adapting* interventions and interactional styles.

What distinguishes therapists from other interlocutors is that they use theory to guide their listening. They attend not only to clients' speech but also to nonverbal information and processes that reveal the clients' implicit beliefs and internal experiences. Responsiveness is impossible without recognizing how often clients' experiences are masked in sessions because they wish to please their therapists and work actively to maintain a strong alliance (Bohart & Tallman, 2010; Rennie, 1994) or because they do not feel confident about expressing their internal experiences (Rennie, 2007). It is when therapists are attuned to these dynamics in-session that they are able to shape their interventions in an especially responsive manner.

In this chapter, we suggest that a productive way to move forward in understanding the role of responsiveness in treatment is to illuminate client processes that can guide therapists in their application of skills and the shaping of their intentions. After all, if the clients' in-session experiences and efforts are not understood and accounted for, there is no way of directing responsiveness efforts to meet their needs. For this reason, we encourage an augmentation to the concept of responsiveness so that it is reenvisioned as therapists' adjustment of their responses to better meet clients' needs via (a) adjusting and tailoring their interventions to the needs of the client and (b) supporting their clients' self-healing processes in therapy (see also Chapter 6, this volume, for more details about clients' self-healing processes and activities). In both regards, clients' needs are key for therapists' responsiveness. The latter function of responsiveness requires more attention, however, as the research on clients' agency in sessions, spearheaded by Arthur Bohart and David Rennie (Bohart & Tallman, 2010; Gordon, 2012; Levitt, Pomerville, & Surace, 2016; Rennie, 1994; Williams & Levitt, 2007), has not yet been well integrated into mainstream psychotherapy research.

Intervention training can provide therapists with routes to reach their goals that can be helpful, especially in early training. However, when considering responsiveness in training, teaching therapist intentions may be even more valuable (Levitt et al., 2006). In contrast to teaching behaviors and rules, helping novice therapists understand the intentions that guide expert therapists' actions can provide them with guidance while permitting many varied routes to the same end (Braithwaite, 2002). Because therapy interactions occur within highly nuanced and contextualized exchanges, having trainees focus on their intentions (e.g., intentions to stimulate client curiosity, to identify patterns in functioning, to explore the therapist-client relationship, to support clients' agency) can support them to shape interventions responsively in session. Thus, the focus on training may be to teach the clinical intentions that guide their implementation (see Levitt & Piazza-Bonin, 2017, on the intentions of therapists known for their clinical wisdom).

One reason why clients' experiences have not been centered in the understandings of responsiveness is the way that they have been conceptualized as a factor in our analyses—typically as a property of therapist effects (e.g., Castonguay & Hill, 2017). Although this approach makes perfect sense in enabling statistical analyses to study therapist behaviors, it divorces responsiveness from its holistic lived experience. When we examine the qualitative and mixed methods literature on responsiveness, it becomes evident that responsiveness, as a process, is a property of therapy that is rooted in the process of clients and therapists understanding one another (Wu & Levitt, 2020). Therapists are responsive when they sense what is happening inside the client in a given moment, which is often influenced by how the client is understanding the therapist in turn. In this way, therapists are not just responsive to a fixed property of the client but to the shifting cycle of the relational dynamics, which may be influenced by experiences both within and outside the dyad.

AN ORIENTATION TO THE META-ANALYSIS OF CLIENTS' THERAPY EXPERIENCES

Because a detailed description of the method used in the publication of the meta-analysis is beyond our scope, this chapter will provide a brief summary of the key points for readers' orientation (refer to Levitt, Pomerville, & Surace, 2016, for more details). The meta-analytic method examined 109 studies that used a broad range of qualitative methods, including grounded theory, phenomenological, consensual qualitative, and thematic analyses, among others. It summarized the qualitative psychotherapy research on clients' experiences published before 2013 and was based on the study of 1,414 clients in total. Studies included in the meta-analysis were focused on individual adult psychotherapy and were published in English. The average number of clients included in these studies was 13, and the studies originated from researchers located across 13 countries. Even though many studies (38) did not report therapists' psychotherapy orientations, it was evident from the clients' reports that they received treatment within a wide variety of approaches, including humanistic–existential (38 studies), psychodynamic approaches (37 studies), cognitive behavioral approaches (37 studies), and eclectic/integrated approaches (15).

The method of analysis was based on a critical-constructivist version of grounded theory (Levitt, 2021), in which findings from the primary studies were summarized and labeled. Then, the authors compared each of these findings with the others, identifying common themes and creating initial categories with labels that reflected them. The initial categories then were compared with each other, and higher-order categories were formed to reflect overarching common patterns. This process continued until a hierarchy developed that had, at its apex, one central core category. The hierarchy appeared to be comprehensive because the final 20 studies within the grounded theory analysis did not result in the creation of new categories, indicating theoretical saturation.

Although there were six levels of the hierarchy, the lower levels are subsumed by the conceptualizations of the higher levels, and so there is no need to describe them all. In our discussion of the hierarchy, we will describe each cluster in turn, identifying some skills and intentions that therapists might draw from the insights therein, and then describe the core category that was developed from considering the clusters. To avoid having to repeatedly reference this study through the chapter, we simply refer to it as "the meta-analysis" going forward. See Table 9.1 for a summary of the clusters, the clients' needs, and the foundational skills that therapists require to support those client needs.

TABLE 9.1. Clusters, Clients' Needs, and Foundational Therapist Skills

Cluster title	Clients' experiences and needs	Foundational skills supporting responsiveness
Cluster 1: Therapy Is a Process of Change Through Structuring Curiosity and Deep Engagement in Pattern Identification and Narrative Reconstruction	To benefit from therapy, clients need to learn to become curious about their own functioning and to engage in introspection so that they can identify problematic patterns of functioning that can be adjusted.	• Developing Radical Reflexivity and Metacommunication • Fostering Curiosity About Patterns of Functioning • Assisting Clients to Integrate Insight Holistically
Cluster 2: Caring, Understanding, and Accepting Therapists Allow Clients to Internalize Positive Messages and Enter the Change Process of Developing Self-Awareness	Clients need to feel accepted, understood, and cared for so that they are comfortable entering the threatening process of self-exploration and maintaining this connection. This process allows them to internalize a more accepting sense of their own experiences and themselves.	• Supporting Secure Attachment and Rupture Resolution in Therapeutic Relationships • Developing Empathy and Mentalization Skills
Cluster 3: Professional Structure Creates Credibility and Clarity but Casts Suspicion on Care in the Therapeutic Relationship	Clients value therapists' expertise and professionalism but at the same time they worry that the therapists' care may be inauthentic and, so, to find trust in the relationship, they monitor the relationship carefully for evidence.	• Demonstrating a Deliberated Flexibility in Boundaries • Practicing Genuineness and Appropriate Self-Disclosure
Cluster 4: Therapy Progresses as a Collaborative Effort With Discussion of Differences	Clients need healthy ways of addressing differences in power within the therapy relationships so they can maintain a sense of being understood, accepted, and cared for in the therapy relationship, despite the differences and gaps that exist between clients' and therapists' knowledge and experiences.	• Acknowledging and Processing Professional Power Differences • Acknowledging and Processing Cultural Power Differences
Cluster 5: Recognition of the Client's Agency Allows for Responsive Interventions That Fit the Client's Needs	Clients need to be supported to set their own goals, reach insights, and become self-determining and can independently develop solutions that work for them in their own cultural and interpersonal contexts.	• Developing Confidence in Self-Referencing • Engaging Therapist Responsiveness

CLUSTER 1: THERAPY IS A PROCESS OF CHANGE THROUGH STRUCTURING CURIOSITY AND DEEP ENGAGEMENT IN PATTERN IDENTIFICATION AND NARRATIVE RECONSTRUCTION

The first cluster that we present describes therapist skills and intentions that correspond with the repeated finding that therapy helps clients to identify and shift a variety of psychological patterns. This client perspective was recognized in 71 of the psychotherapy research studies included in the meta-analysis and was found in studies across therapeutic orientations, including relational dynamics (Lilliengren & Werbart, 2005), thought patterns (Göstas et al., 2013), styles of emotional engagement (Henretty et al., 2008), and behavioral habits (Clarke et al., 2004).

In stark contrast to therapists' conceptualization of change as tied to the faculty most associated with their theoretical orientation (e.g., psychodynamic therapists targeting relational change, cognitive therapists producing cognitive change, humanistic therapists as focused on emotional change), clients experienced therapeutic change as holistic and as contributing to greater self-understanding, regardless of the therapeutic approach used by their therapist (Levitt, Pomerville, & Surace, 2016). For instance, gaining insight into thought patterns in the course of cognitive therapy may help clients have new emotional reactions, behavioral responses, and relate differently with significant others, generating new self-narratives. Across 48 studies, findings indicated that clients reported an experience of change that became integrated into their broader sense of themselves and their self-narrative. Understanding clients' experience of the change process enhances the therapists' ability to stretch beyond the limits of a therapy orientation to better help their clients to integrate insights holistically, by pointing out how patterns influence their thoughts, emotions, and interpersonal dynamics. In this way, therapist responsiveness was characterized by the stimulation of clients' radical reflexivity, curiosity, and insight.

Developing Radical Reflexivity and Metacommunication

The majority of studies in the meta-analysis found that therapy helped clients to develop the ability to self-reflect both inside and outside of the therapy room (Levitt, Pomerville, & Surace, 2016). Clients' ability to become aware of, to monitor, and to deliberately alter their self-awareness (supporting its discussion in therapy) has been called *radical reflexivity* (Rennie, 2007). Clients expressed that as a result of therapy, they deepened their capacity for reflexive thinking, leading them to observe when, why, and how different internal experiences arise and to realize that they have the capacity to change their experiences. When asked about her experiences of psychotherapy, a client described this recognition: "I want to emphasize the most, that I have learned to see patterns in how I behave and why I behave in that way, which makes it possible to avoid doing it in that way the next time" (Lilliengren & Werbart, 2005, p. 332).

A key skill that therapists can use to foster radical reflexivity in their clients is *metacommunication*, that is, talking about the process of communicating (Rennie, 2007). For instance, therapists might share their thoughts or motivations behind a question that they ask a client, they might explain their reactions to what a client has said, or they may invite the client to share their own reactions to something they have said. Metacommunication can both model reflexive thinking to the client and structure the conversation so that clients are encouraged to not only express their internal experience but also to notice their thoughts and feelings about that experience. Clients often find it particularly helpful when therapists move beyond an abstract discussion to bring attention to what is happening at the moment between them:

> I am one of those who overly compensate. And, I didn't realize I was doing it, and one day I brought her candy. . . . She said, "See, you are doing it to me." That was kind of like a true example. It was just like a turning point I think, because I really believed her because it was right there in front of me. (Levitt et al., 2006, p. 321)

Responsiveness here was characterized by metacommunication, which could be encouraged directly in session or outside of a session through the use of feedback forms, questionnaires, or interviews about their therapy experience (Flückiger et al., 2012).

Therapists also can ask clients to reflect on what it feels like to talk about the therapeutic relationship or to make progress in therapy. Inviting clients' metacommunication, by asking them to describe how recognizing patterns in one area (e.g., thoughts, relationships, emotions) might lead to shifts across any of these domains, may allow both therapists and clients to better recognize clients' internal experiences. Also, supporting clients to develop reflexive skills can deepen the integration of new insights that occur.

Fostering Curiosity About Patterns of Functioning

Across studies, clients reported that they not only strengthened their ability to self-reflect through the course of psychotherapy, but they also strengthened their sense of curiosity about themselves (Levitt, Pomerville, & Surace, 2016). Curiosity as both a trait and a transient state has been found to motivate exploratory and growth-oriented behaviors, which promote a sense of well-being and authenticity (Kashdan & Steger, 2007; Spielberger & Reheiser, 2009). Just as reflexive thinking becomes more natural as clients engage in psychotherapy, so can the practice of being curious about oneself. Adopting a "not-knowing" stance of curiosity about clients' experiences can allow therapists to be more receptive to hearing their clients' perspectives (Bateman & Fonagy, 2013) and also to model this inquiry into clients' experiences.

Regardless of therapists' theoretical orientation or clients' therapy goals, therapists tend to ignite curiosity in their clients. There are many ways in which therapists do this naturally, such as by using nonverbal cues (e.g., tone, posture) to indicate their interest in their clients and to reinforce clients' direct expressions of curiosity about themselves (Waehler, 2013). The use of exploration skills, such as empathic listening, reflecting client feelings, and asking open-ended questions, has been found to encourage clients' self-reflection and convey that a therapist is genuinely interested in and attuned to their exploration (Hill, 2009). A client described the process of learning to ask questions about herself and her patterns:

> Whenever [my therapist] asks me questions like that, when she kind of recaps it, it makes me feel a lot better. . . . What I think she's trying to do is trying to challenge me to . . . put things in a different perspective. It just makes me feel a lot better because then I can kind of tie stuff in, as far as like what she and I are talking about, and see how it's relating to me as far as why I'm [in therapy]. (Henretty et al., 2008, p. 251)

Therapists' responsiveness to clients' self-healing capacity can increase clients' curiosity about themselves and heighten their awareness of their internal feelings and experiences. This practice gradually increases clients' skills at introspection and their self-confidence about the knowledge that they gain about themselves. As clients come to rely on their own self-knowledge, they are better able to direct their process of growth.

Assisting Clients to Integrate Insight Holistically

The ability to facilitate insight is widely regarded as an essential helping skill within the mental health professions (Hill, 2009). In addition to gaining insight into a specific issue or aspect of psychological experiences, however, clients within 58 studies described an increased self-awareness across multiple psychological domains that helped them construct a more comprehensive understanding of themselves and others.

Although change occurs when therapists have a strong allegiance to one bona fide therapeutic approach (Wampold & Imel, 2015), this appears to be bolstered by the work clients do to integrate insights into a cohesive self-narrative. Thus, therapists may want to consider the specific techniques within a given approach (e.g., cognitive restructuring in cognitive therapy, transference interpretations in psychodynamic therapy) as one pathway to assisting clients in identifying change patterns. Once a pattern is recognized, its exploration may be augmented by deliberate work to support clients in processing the insight holistically so that its influence becomes broadly understood. Many paths may lead to a similar understanding of a problematic pattern in this manner. Therapists might begin treatment by responsively selecting interventions that are consistent with the change processes associated with their therapeutic orientation but then intentionally supporting their clients to translate this change across various domains (Boswell et al., 2010). For instance, cognitive therapists might ask their clients how their work to correct a cognitive bias has influenced their emotional experience or their relational dynamics.

For instance, in one therapy case, a client began counseling with a cognitive-focused goal of increasing "positive thinking," although his therapist did not work from a primarily cognitive model and did not introduce this concept. Over the course of therapy, the client also reported several noncognitive changes, including improvements with self-esteem and healthy boundary setting. When asked about changes from therapy, the client-participant noted, "The more positive mental attitude from earlier sessions has sneaked into my self-understanding" (Mackrill, 2008, p. 446). This case demonstrates how, regardless of the specific aspect of change or the therapeutic orientation, therapeutic change tends to happen more holistically. Therapists can guide the clients' journey of developing curiosity and insights across their emotional, cognitive, relational, and behavioral patterns toward change in their broader self-concept. This approach views responsiveness as prioritizing the clients' experience of growth, rather than remaining focused on the type of interventions that are prioritized by therapists.

CLUSTER 2: CARING, UNDERSTANDING, AND ACCEPTING THERAPISTS ALLOW CLIENTS TO INTERNALIZE POSITIVE MESSAGES AND ENTER THE CHANGE PROCESS OF DEVELOPING SELF-AWARENESS

Consistent with many models of therapeutic change (e.g., Gendlin, 2003; Hill, 2009; Rogers, 1957), intersubjective exploration can facilitate clients' insight, although entering into this process can be threatening for many clients. The second cluster, based on 82 studies in the meta-analysis, described the repeated finding that clients' experiences of being understood and validated by a caring and genuine therapist allowed them the safety to engage in exploration. A client described the powerful effects of this connection:

> It felt as though my counsellor, without breaching boundaries, went beyond a professional level/interest and gave me such a human, compassionate response, something I couldn't put a price on. . . . I think I had only ever expected to receive from her professional self. . . . [I] felt like she was giving from her core. (Knox, 2008, p. 185)

Conversely, the experience of feeling misunderstood or feeling that the therapist was remote caused strain in the therapeutic alliance and led clients to withdraw or close off emotionally.

Understanding clients' concerns about intersubjective exploration can help therapists develop therapeutic trust and be in a better position to be responsive to clients who are withdrawing or closing off. When these concerns were recognized, clients became less fearful of negative judgments from their therapists, less defensive, and better able to engage in introspection and reflection. As the security and trust in the therapeutic relationship deepened, clients began to internalize positive self-appraisals from their therapist. Beyond the dyad, clients' positive sense of self could strengthen other interpersonal relationships as well. In the following two subsections, we explore two sets of skills that therapists can use to enhance this relationship-exploration cycle of change (see Levitt & Williams, 2010, for a description of this cycle from the perspective of expert therapists).

Supporting Secure Attachment and Rupture Resolution in Therapeutic Relationships

In 61 studies included in the meta-analysis, clients who felt that their therapists authentically cared for them reported being better able to engage in vulnerable discussions without fear of abandonment. Clients highlighted honesty and safety as qualities of their therapist that fostered a "true" connection in their relationship.

> From the moment I ever had a first session with him, he was completely open with me about everything. . . . And I told him a lot of things about me . . . things that I had done that . . . I regretted and he never blinked an eye, I never heard him say anything under his breath. . . . He always listened to me, you know, he always encouraged me to express my feelings, he always encouraged me. (Levitt et al., 2006, p. 318)

Therapy was a context for clients to meaningfully grow and come to accept themselves.

In psychotherapy, the bond between clients and therapists could be healing in its own right, but it can also contribute to clients engaging in self-exploration, awareness, and acceptance. Keeping in mind how threatening this work can be for clients may guide therapists to conceptualize their relationships in light of attachment theory. For instance, stronger therapeutic relationships may be more easily built with clients who have had secure attachments (Mallinckrodt & Jeong, 2015). Therapists can better facilitate a sense of connection between themselves and their clients by being responsive to clients' attachment style (Wiseman & Tishby, 2014).

Therapists can develop skills to interpret how clients' attachment styles (e.g., secure, dismissing, preoccupied) might influence their present internal experience in psychotherapy (Talia et al., 2019). By noticing when clients are seeking proximity, maintaining contact, avoiding contact, or resisting therapists' interventions, therapists may develop a more nuanced understanding of clients' experience in sessions. Noticing clients' attachment behaviors can help therapists provide responsive support and guide their development of self-awareness.

Considering clients' internal experience of attachment also may be helpful when repairing ruptures in the relationship. In 25 of the studies in the meta-analysis, clients said that feeling unheard, misunderstood, or unappreciated challenged the therapeutic alliance. Recommended strategies for therapists are to respond by communicating concern and caring as well as to invite and accept the clients' emotional reactions (e.g., for descriptions of such responses to ruptures, see Muran & Eubanks, 2020). Ruptures, however, are not inherently problematic. In fact, repairing them can even deepen the therapeutic relationship (Miller-Bottome et al., 2018), reduce feelings of threat among clients, encourage client self-exploration, and help clients to internalize a more positive sense of self.

Developing Empathy and Mentalization Skills

A finding from 56 studies of the meta-analysis indicated that when clients feel deeply understood and accepted by their therapists, they are able to engage in self-reflection nondefensively and increase their self-awareness. One client described how she felt when her therapist reflected back her experience to her:

> It made you feel as though somebody had taken on board what you had been saying . . . to hear that back, what you'd told somebody, was, you know, quite emotional really . . . in a good way, because it made you feel heard, and that was nice. (Shine & Westacott, 2010, p. 169)

Both empathy and mentalization can be used by therapists responsively to support clients to engage in self-exploration and circumvent their defensiveness and self-criticism.

The importance of empathy to clients cannot be overstated. Clients have expressed that the act of a therapist attempting to understand their internal experience is therapeutic in and of itself. Empathic responses from therapists let clients feel validated and communicate to clients that it is safe to explore sensitive topics in sessions. A recent quantitative meta-analysis by Elliott et al. (2018) found that empathy accounted for about 9% of the variance in therapy outcome. It is no surprise that the leading factor in understanding therapy outcome, with a contribution that has surpassed that of the working alliance, is one in which therapists are working to understand the internal experience of clients in session. Empathy enables therapists to refine their attunement to their clients' experiences and to provide responsive interventions.

Humanist and psychodynamic theorists have developed theories and practices that enhance empathic capacity and communication (e.g., Bohart & Greenberg, 1997; Elliott et al., 2018). These skills include developing a rich conceptualization of emotional experiences and processes of change in therapy (such as in emotion-focused therapy; Elliott & Greenberg, 2007), attending to unspoken dynamics, naming experiential states, learning to tolerate painful emotions, formulating conceptualizations of clients' issues, empathic responding, symbolizing inchoate emotions, and demonstrating nonverbal cues that convey therapists' authentic care (e.g., Muntigl et al., 2014; Watson & Greenberg, 2009; Watson et al., 2019).

When engaged empathically, therapists are primed to respond to clients with genuine caring and nonjudgmental attitudes (Hill, 2009). Such an attitude supports clients' capacity to contact painful thoughts, emotions, and memories and then to accept them (Elliott & Greenberg, 2007). Often clients struggled with whether to admit or accept a part of their experience, and an empathic response can model self-acceptance and may be transformative. In 18 of the studies, findings revealed that internalizing the messages from an affirming therapist allowed clients to increase their self-acceptance and strengthen their external relationships. One client described the power of a validating response: "I had the feeling that the counsellor accepts these feelings, and then these feelings disappeared" (Timulák & Lietaer, 2001, p. 68). In this way, therapists' empathy decreases clients' self-critical attitudes, enabling more secure relationships with others as well.

In addition to empathy, clients benefit from learning mentalization skills from their therapists. Mentalization is the process by which people interpret and symbolize their own (or others') intentions, mental states, and actions (Bateman et al., 2009). Once clients learn these skills, they are better able to communicate their experiences in therapy and in other relationships. For instance, a client described the impact of therapy on his relationships:

> It felt very meaningful to be in therapy, and it became an important channel of sorts. I started almost purposefully to influence my family to start talking about deeper feelings. And that I could talk about things with my sister and my parents that we have never touched on before has been very important to me personally. (Lilliengren & Werbart, 2005, p. 331)

When clients feel understood in therapy, they develop trust (or *epistemic trust*; Fonagy & Allison, 2014) with their therapists, which stimulates cognitive flexibility and a greater openness to new social experiences. Just as therapists' empathy and acceptance can foster clients' self-compassion, clients' mentalization can lead to a greater capacity for relational attunement. Repeatedly in the meta-analysis, clients described how caring and accepting therapists allowed them to better engage in self-exploration and to develop self-acceptance. Therapists' empathic attunement and mentalization skills can help them better understand their clients' internal experiences, which can allow them to responsively support their clients to develop both self-awareness and self-compassion.

CLUSTER 3: PROFESSIONAL STRUCTURE CREATES CREDIBILITY AND CLARITY BUT CASTS SUSPICION ON CARE IN THE THERAPEUTIC RELATIONSHIP

Clients across 54 studies examined in the meta-analysis expressed that the professional structure of therapy influenced their experience in therapy and their outcomes. On one hand, therapists' professional status and training gave clients confidence. On the other hand, because the therapy relationship is in a professional context, it led clients to wonder whether their therapists truly cared about them as people. As a result, therapists' professional status increased their credibility yet also could undermine clients' trust in therapists and their belief in their therapists' authenticity.

Clients described a variety of ways in which therapists could structure therapeutic boundaries to strengthen trust. Having a clear structure of psychotherapy, including preset session lengths, scheduling, and payment arrangements, increased clients' perception of therapist competency as well as their trust in the therapeutic process. However, when the therapy structure is rigid and inflexible, it can become a barrier to fostering client trust and helping the client feel cared for in the therapeutic alliance. A client conveyed how bending boundaries helped:

> He ran overtime, big time, that session, which impressed the hell out of me. . . . He didn't look at the clock. . . . He genuinely cared what was happening in the room at the moment . . . [and] treated me like a real person. (Levitt et al., 2006, p. 319)

In the forthcoming sections, we discuss the use of flexible boundaries and include demonstrations of genuineness in relation to these concepts.

Demonstrating a Deliberated Flexibility in Boundaries

Psychotherapy studies across orientations have shown that having some flexibility in professional boundaries in therapy can foster an environment that supports clients' capacity to discuss sensitive topics and to disclose deeply personal thoughts and feelings (Levitt, Minami, et al., 2016). Binder et al. (2009) presented a client's positive experience of accommodating professional boundaries:

> When I was in crisis, he was flexible . . . I was allowed to come every day for a week or so. At the same time, he was very professional. He was able to use examples from his own life, and still stay professional—it is a very thin line out there. . . . Some doctors are just so distanced . . . but he was very professional, and at the same time he was a real person. (p. 253)

Knowing how to set boundaries and being able to recognize instances in which they can be appropriately transgressed is a specific skill that therapists can hone to increase their clients' trust in the therapy process. Extending the time or increasing the scheduling of sessions was frequently described as evidence of care that was meaningful to clients.

Clients also described appreciating when therapists were flexible by adjusting payments. This practice is complicated because, although therapy costs can undermine a therapeutic relationship or make it difficult for clients to continue therapy, therapists also require an income to provide services. Acknowledging and openly discussing the financial burden of therapy to low-income clients, and developing an accommodating payment structure, can contribute to positive client experiences (Thompson et al., 2015) by reflecting a therapist's desire to be accessible and sensitive to clients' financial situations. A client in Thompson et al.'s (2015) study described deeply appreciating their therapist's payment flexibility:

> When I lost insurance, I was really freaked out about how I was going to pay for [therapy], and I clearly needed it. My therapist was very understanding, and was willing to work with me on it, and went to a sliding scale fee. We spent a lot of time in session talking about how stressful it was for me not to have the answers about where I could go and how I was going to deal with this on a long-term basis. (p. 216)

When possible, flexible payment structures communicate to clients that they mean more to the therapist than a weekly fee and allow clients to pay in accordance with their means. Attention to the impact of boundaries can expand therapist responsiveness, perhaps at times when it is needed most.

Practicing Genuineness and Appropriate Self-Disclosure

Because clients want to feel connected to and cared for by their therapist yet are concerned that the therapy relationship is professional, they are sensitive to demonstrations of authentic care (Pope-Davis et al., 2002). Genuineness is integral to cultivating the trust and comfort that clients desire and is an important relational quality across psychotherapy orientations (Kolden et al., 2018). While definitions of genuineness may vary, Carl Rogers (1957) described it as therapists being authentic in their self-expression and communications to clients and often used the term *congruence* to signify this alignment. A meta-analysis has suggested that congruence accounts for 5.3% of the variance of client outcome (Kolden et al., 2018), and the literature has indicated that when therapists exhibit congruence, they increase clients' perceptions of their trustworthiness (Schnellbacher & Leijssen, 2009).

Clients interpret therapist congruence as a sign of genuineness in the therapeutic relationship (Thompson et al., 2015; Knox, 2008). To increase congruence, therapists can benefit from developing and practicing skills such as providing honest feedback, using "I" statements, and displaying their emotions in front of clients. Knox (2008) presented a client's experience of their therapist's genuineness: "It was that feeling of her bringing herself into the counselling session, not remaining apart, separate—as though she was giving me of her actual self, her human, caring self" (p. 105). Findings from a meta-analysis demonstrated a strong relationship between therapist genuineness and the strength of the therapeutic alliance (Nienhuis et al., 2018).

Therapist self-disclosure also can cultivate feelings of genuineness among clients. Clients have expressed that their therapists' self-disclosure, especially disclosure that conveys similarity between the client and the therapist and/or humanizes the therapist, is key to fostering a genuine relationship (Audet, 2011; Levitt, Minami, et al., 2016). Meta-analyses of studies exploring therapist self-disclosure have found repeatedly that self-disclosure has an overall positive effect on clients (Henretty et al., 2014; Henretty & Levitt, 2010; Hill et al., 2018). Self-disclosure can increase clients' perceptions of their therapist's warmth and also encourages clients to self-disclose (Henretty & Levitt, 2010; Hill et al., 2018). It can create a safe, nonjudgmental environment for clients with marginalized identities, such as when LGBTQ+ therapists self-disclose their sexual orientation with LGBTQ+ clients (Henretty & Levitt, 2010).

Clients have reported negative views of therapists who did not seem professional, so therapists should be aware of the risks of overdisclosing or sharing information that might compromise the therapy relationship and use their clinical judgment accordingly (Levitt, Minami, et al., 2016). Audet (2011) described a client's experience of their therapist's self-disclosure: "The professional boundary is there, but you're still connecting as human beings and a little personal sharing enhances the experience" (p. 94). When used appropriately, self-disclosure can be a sign of genuineness and flexibility that powerfully conveys therapists' care for their clients. In any case, understanding that clients often harbor suspicions about the authenticity of their therapists' feelings toward them can better enable therapists to respond with skills that foster feelings of genuineness among clients and allay these concerns.

CLUSTER 4: THERAPY PROGRESSES AS A COLLABORATIVE EFFORT WITH DISCUSSION OF DIFFERENCES

Psychotherapy is a mutual process between the client and the therapist, in which they are both focused on the clients' healing. Yet, it is a process that unfolds in a context characterized by power dynamics that exist at the individual, interpersonal, and structural levels. Within 59 research studies reviewed in the meta-analysis, clients described that differences and similarities between therapist and client in professional power (e.g., the therapist having expertise and professional credentials that the client typically lacks) and in cultural power (e.g., power instilled by virtue of demographic qualities such as gender, race, ethnicity, socioeconomic status, and sexual orientation) impacted their perceptions of their therapists, their engagement in the therapeutic process, and the strength of the therapeutic relationship (Levitt, Pomerville, & Surace, 2016). In the following sections, we explore key skills that enable therapists to respond and facilitate meaningful discussions of differences with their clients, increase collaboration in the therapeutic process, and attend to the multifaceted and layered impact of power in psychotherapy.

Acknowledging and Processing Professional Power Differences

Although research shows that clients want to be actively engaged in therapy (Levitt, Pomerville, & Surace, 2016), clients often do not know what to expect from a therapeutic relationship and may be unsure of their role (Geller & Farber, 2020). This uncertainty can create a power imbalance in which clients may believe that their role in therapy is similar to their role with a medical doctor—to view the professional as the authority and to submit to the plan and strategies indicated (Rennie, 1994). In therapy, however, where interventions typically are coconstructed, this expectation can reduce clients' feelings of safety and agency, limit therapists' tailoring of interventions, and lead clients to terminate therapy prematurely (Swift et al., 2012).

Therapists can reduce clients' deference (a strategy that clients often use to preserve the therapeutic alliance; Levitt & Morrill, 2021; Rennie, 1994) and address professional power differences in the dyad by directly discussing the therapy process with their clients from the first session, exploring their clients' expectations about therapy, and providing psychoeducation about the therapeutic process (e.g., see the creative script by Geller & Farber, 2020, used to orient clients to their role in therapy). Overtly emphasizing the client's role as an agentic collaborator in intake sessions can encourage an egalitarian power distribution in the therapeutic relationship from the start. One client described the value of this equalization:

> I think it's very important for me to have a therapist I feel equal to. Power dynamics are a very important thing that I have. I have control issues and I'm dealing with power struggles between men and women and I don't want to have that between my therapist and I too. It's just like another battle. So I think that's very important for me to feel comfortable. (Pope-Davis et al., 2002, p. 377)

Clients who experienced an egalitarian power distribution in the therapeutic relationship have been found to be less likely to prematurely terminate therapy and more likely to provide constructive feedback to their therapist (Pope-Davis et al., 2002). Therapists can reply strategically to issues of power and control in the session by checking with clients on their perception of their role and their engagement in therapy. This responsiveness may strengthen the relationship and lead to deeper and fruitful discussions.

Acknowledging and Processing Cultural Power Differences

Clients want to feel seen, understood, and accepted by their therapists. However, cultural differences between clients and therapists can pose a barrier to clients feeling comfortable in therapy. When therapists display a lack of awareness and knowledge about their clients' cultural context, it can leave clients feeling misunderstood, disconnected, and as though their experiences are being trivialized (Chang & Berk, 2009). Feelings of cultural distance also can prevent clients from openly discussing racial, ethnic, and cultural issues (i.e., experiences of discrimination/oppression and family dynamics) with their therapist (Chang & Yoon, 2011).

Therapists can minimize these power differentials and their clients' perceptions of cultural distance by responding with an open discussion about culture in the dyad and encouraging the client to discuss their cultural worldview and experiences (Chang & Berk, 2009; Pope-Davis et al., 2002). Clients view therapists who acknowledge and invite discussion of the complexities of their identities (e.g., intersections between race, ethnicity, class, sexual orientation) and the cultural differences that exist in the dyad as more sensitive, warm, accepting, trustworthy, and competent (Chang & Berk, 2009; Levitt, Pomerville, & Surace, 2016; Owen et al., 2011; Pope-Davis et al., 2002). Rogers-Sirin et al. (2015) reported the experience of a first-generation Trinidadian immigrant working with a White therapist:

> The fact that I noticed it [her race] didn't make her uncomfortable. Um, the fact that she acknowledged one, that my experience was real, and two, acknowledged that her experience was different from mine and that it was ok for me to say how I felt from my perspective. (p. 263)

Additionally, clients who perceived their therapists as possessing multicultural competence have reported fewer racial microaggressions in general and fewer negative impacts when racial microaggressions occurred (Hook et al., 2016), stronger working alliances with their therapists (Hook et al., 2013), more positive therapy outcomes (Owen et al., 2016), and a greater likelihood of treatment completion (Anderson et al., 2019).

Historically, psychotherapy research has focused on forms of professional and cultural power in isolation. However, we recommend considering their intersectional and coconstitutive effects both in practice and in research. Clients from varied cultural backgrounds may interpret professional power and their role differently, and professional power may exacerbate feelings of difference that are due to cultural power. Therapist responsiveness here would benefit from the conceptual and intervention skills to comfortably talk about both the therapists' power and the influence of the clients' culture and identities on the therapy relationship in-session. The therapist could demonstrate to clients that it is safe to discuss these issues, support and allow clients to bring their entire selves into therapy, and make it easier to resolve misunderstandings when they occur (Levitt, Pomerville, & Surace, 2016).

CLUSTER 5: RECOGNITION OF THE CLIENT'S AGENCY ALLOWS FOR RESPONSIVE INTERVENTIONS THAT FIT THE CLIENT'S NEEDS

The fifth cluster in the meta-analysis reflected a concept that is fundamental to this volume and was described within 72 studies in this cluster, namely, that clients are agents of change in psychotherapy and not passive recipients of interventions by their therapist (Levitt, Pomerville, & Surace, 2016). Indeed, clients described a desire to bring their extensive self-knowledge into the therapeutic exploration and to take the lead in the development of insights. These client reports align with the humanistic insight that clients have a natural capacity and drive for self-directed healing and thus are "active self-healers" (whether this is recognized by therapists or not; see the groundbreaking work in this area by Bohart & Tallman, 2010). As one client in a recent qualitative study noted, "It's 50% me and 50% her. . . . She could help me and I don't mean take problems off me and deal with them for me. She can direct me in how I can help myself" (Brooks et al., 2021, p. 6). Therapists can encourage clients to take an active role in therapy directly or to invite this more subtly through the way they respond to their clients, using the skills described in the following subsections.

It is worth noting that supporting clients' agency includes empowering them to decide when and how to engage in therapy, as well as to decide when they are unable to fully engage. For instance, some clients may feel uncomfortable or "put on the spot" if their therapist pushes them to talk about warded-off topics when they are not yet ready (Grafanaki & McLeod, 2002). Indeed, clients have been found to deliberately (e.g., changing the subject) or inadvertently (e.g., memory lapses) disengage with therapy as a way of titrating pain and preparing themselves for threatening work in the future (Frankel & Levitt, 2009). Discussing this form of agency may promote clients' self-awareness of their capacity for therapeutic work in a given moment and demonstrate therapists' attunement to their clients' experiences.

Developing Confidence in Self-Referencing

Clients who feel agentic in the therapy relationship tend to engage actively in self-exploration and to take responsibility for their role as a coconstructor of the therapy process. A key skill that therapists can use to increase a client's agency is to foster their ability to self-reference (Klein et al., 1986). *Self-referencing* is the ability to develop a comprehensive sense of one's internal experiences and to be able to draw meaning from that experience. Clients who are able to self-reference can check internally to decide if a concept is fully aligned with their experiences and, if not, consider how it would need to be changed to fit better. This ability to attune to oneself and to pose problems about one's experience is fundamental to gaining a sense of agency (Bandura, 2006):

> Once I figured [out why I was angry] I felt much better about letting myself be angry about it. But it was really good just to, to have her lead me on that path rather than telling me, well, clearly the reason you're so angry is that it's just, you know, the story of your life happening over and over again. It was good having her lead me in that direction but letting me figure it out on my own. And make it my own, I guess . . . It makes it my own realization. There's like a sense of agency. (Hoener et al., 2012, p. 76)

Clients become more agentic when they are able to focus on what they are experiencing in a given moment and subsequently make meaning from it.

One way in which therapists can respond to and foster their clients' ability to self-reference is through the use of *focusing* (Gendlin, 2003). This experiential approach encourages clients to contact and develop a "felt sense" for unclear emotions that are hard for them to understand (Elliott & Greenberg, 2007). Therapists use a gentle, exploratory tone to guide the client to sustain an internal focus on the troublesome issue and look to see what metaphors or images it inspires. As clients become better able to articulate their internal experiences, therapists may make empathic conjectures as to what the client is feeling, taking care to defer to clients' knowledge of what they are truly experiencing. Whether through the use of exercises, such as focusing, or by modeling, clients can be guided to develop the ability to look inward, pose questions about their internal experience, and develop solutions that are appropriate for their contexts. Indeed, clients may define therapy success as learning to process their experiences with greater complexity and attunement, both in therapy and across contexts, rather than as no longer experiencing any distress (Brooks et al., 2021). Confidence in this ability can support clients to be self-determining and to guide their own growth so they need not rely on their therapist.

Engaging Therapist Responsiveness

In addition to fostering self-referencing directly, therapists can subtly encourage clients' agency through their interactions with and responses to clients. Therapists naturally seek to be responsive by tailoring their treatment to clients' needs at the moment, current circumstances, and their own clinical intuitions (Kramer & Stiles, 2015). Thus, therapist responsiveness is a stance or guiding intention rather than a single behavior or intervention. The ongoing practice of responding to clients to facilitate their moment-to-moment processing has been thought to lead to the success of therapy more so than tailoring treatment based on factors such as diagnosis (Norcross & Wampold, 2018).

Clients sometimes make their needs readily apparent, such as through asking direct questions, as was the case with the following client-participant who invited her therapist to self-disclose:

> I asked her [the therapist] some questions, I wanted her to share something about herself with me, rather than me giving all the stuff. I wanted something back. And I felt she accepted me, because she was sharing something with me. And I felt good about that. I felt closer to her. (Grafanaki & McLeod, 2002, p. 27)

At other times clients may not convey their needs so directly, in which case the therapist must rely on their overall conceptualization of each client to respond to a client's unexpressed needs: "We were looking at diagrams . . . and I thought, 'Well, I can do this at home . . . I want you to come over my shoulder'. . . and there was the chair, she came over" (Fitzpatrick et al., 2009, p. 659). The client was pleased that the therapist could sense what was wanted. Because clients often are not explicit about their needs, therapists use a variety of skills to evaluate their responsiveness to clients, such as reflective listening, regular check-ins about the pace and progress of therapy, assessments of clients' readiness for receiving certain interpretations, and the use of self-disclosure to invite and model vulnerability in clients (Wu & Levitt, 2020).

Although clients in the studies examined within the meta-analysis repeatedly described desiring to have agency in sessions and to lead their process of self-exploration, the exception was when they felt stuck or were halting processing (e.g., Levitt et al., 2006). At these times, many clients welcomed encouragement to process difficult material or direction when they were engaging in previously identified nonproductive patterns (e.g., avoiding difficult material), as shown in the following quote: "I really liked that the therapist dared to be rather intrusive and put me on the spot and push things that used to be pretty hard for me. It helped me go deeper into things" (Palmstierna & Werbart, 2013, p. 28).

The findings from this cluster then suggest that it can be helpful for therapists to recognize that clients are central agents of change in therapy and to see their own role as providing unconditional guidance and support for their efforts. However, this must be done responsively, with the clients' current state, overall treatment goals, and strength of the therapeutic relationship in mind. Throughout the course of therapy, therapists can seek to develop clients' ability to self-reference, which may promote their self-healing capacities as well.

CORE CATEGORY: BEING KNOWN AND CARED FOR SUPPORTS CLIENTS' ABILITY TO AGENTICALLY RECOGNIZE OBSTRUCTIVE EXPERIENTIAL PATTERNS AND ADDRESS UNMET VULNERABLE NEEDS

The present core category summarizes the central experiences that clients reported as leading to change across therapy approaches and the sorts of skills that therapists can use to enhance their responsiveness to these experiences:

1. Authentic and caring therapists led clients to feel seen and accepted by them, having learned that they can repair ruptures and address cultural and professional differences that might exist between them.

2. To the extent that therapists encouraged clients' agency in the treatment, clients felt more confident in their ability to intentionally navigate their lives and more comfortable with self-discovery.

3. Having cultivated a secure frame, clients developed a curiosity about themselves and began to explore aspects of themselves and their relationships that might otherwise have been too threatening to consider.

4. Regardless of the form of pattern identification that was centralized in a given therapy approach (i.e., patterns in thinking, feeling, behavior, interpersonal responses, or self-narratives), the new awareness of maladaptive or nonoptimal ways of functioning allowed them to develop new holistic responses that might have previously felt vulnerable or unnatural.

5. Through the therapeutic relationship, clients began to internalize a more positive sense of themselves, which enabled them to grow more confident in their own self-exploration. As they developed a greater self-attunement that guided self-exploration, clients became more effective in solving their problems and meeting their needs independently, outside of the therapy context.

To foster these forms of client change, therapists will benefit from having the foundational skills described herein (see Table 9.1 for a summary of these). These include conceptual skills, such as helping clients to develop radical reflexivity, curiosity about their patterns of functioning, and a capacity for mentalization. They include relational skills, such as developing a secure attachment, repairing ruptures, forging an empathic and genuine connection, and the ability to process cultural and professional power differences. Also, they include intervention skills, such as guiding clients to integrate new insights in a holistic manner, forming appropriately flexible boundaries, and developing clients' confidence in their self-referencing. Because the meta-analysis was based on clients' experiences in a wide range of therapeutic approaches, the skills identified in this chapter will support clients across any psychotherapy orientation. They are compatible with a broad range of therapists' values and beliefs about mental health and healing.

All of these skills require, however, that therapists are attuned to their clients and are able to engage in a responsive manner. In keeping with our reenvisioning of responsiveness in relation to (a) adapting interventions to suit clients' needs and (b) the desire to increase their self-healing capacities, we encourage therapists to adopt a mindset that recognizes clients as collaborators in the therapy process. Developing an awareness of clients' agentic work in therapy can direct therapists to reconstrue what it means to be responsive. For instance, clients may have varying forms or levels of curiosity about themselves, their attachment capacities, their confidence in self-referencing, or their ability to form insight. Therapists will need to meet clients where they are and engage in a continual process of evaluation throughout sessions so as to deliberately facilitate their introspection, self-healing, and self-directive capacities. In the next section, we explore the implication of both forms of responsiveness.

IMPLICATIONS FOR PRACTICE, TRAINING, AND RESEARCH

In the spirit of encouraging therapists to conduct evidence-based practice, and to deliberately use a broad evidence base that includes both qualitative research and clients' perspectives, we focused our chapter on what can be learned from research on clients' experiences. In this section, we consider recommendations for practice, training, and research.

Recommendations for Practice

Despite working with therapists who represented varied theoretical directions, clients in the meta-analysis focused on shared change processes described in these stages of treatment. The strategies to further responsiveness that we have described are not exhaustive in supporting clients to feel connected and engaged in therapy, to explore their patterns and come to insights, or to recognize and address clients' unmet needs. Many of the skills (e.g., to develop clients' reflexive capacity, to process client–therapist differences, to support clients' self-referencing) may be carried out using an assortment of interventions, for example, working with alliance ruptures (Eubanks et al., 2018), unconditional positive regard (Bozarth, 2013), clients' expectations about psychological healing (Østlie et al., 2018), and transference, countertransference, and cultural identity (Baumann et al., 2020). These activities could be effective in practice and can be tailored for use within therapists' theoretical orientations or tailored for client characteristics.

This chapter can sensitize therapists to the internal experiences of their clients and the foundational skills needed to support responsive therapy. Given the dominant medicalized view in the field, in which therapy is defined by what therapists do in sessions (their interventions, their orientations), adopting the perspective of clients and recognizing their agentic work to preserve the alliance and to promote self-change is a radical departure. It may take deliberate practice to retain this understanding in session (Rousmaniere, 2017). While we recognize that learning specific behavioral interventions is useful, especially in initial training, we believe that interventions are best taught as guided by intentions that are focused on supporting clients' needs and their capacity to be both self-reflective and empowered to direct their own process of change. If therapists keep in mind that a central aspect of their mission is to use interventions responsively and to support their clients' self-healing, their clinical practice will be transformed and this perspective will eventually become a habit of character. Indeed, it will become an ethical position tied to the recognition of the client's personhood (Berg, 2020).

Recommendations for Training

Just as there are courses in virtually every graduate training program in psychotherapy that focus on theoretical orientations and interventions, dedicated training that teaches responsiveness to clients' experiences and to deliberately developing strategies toward building clients' self-healing should be a requisite for developing therapists. Centering client agency and viewing the goal of therapy as the empowerment of clients to trust their own experience and solve problems is key to responsive therapy and also requires humility (for more on cultural humility, see Davis et al., 2020). For example, culturally competent therapists often adopt a perspective that recognizes that clients are inevitably more attuned to the constraints and possibilities of their personal, cultural, and interpersonal contexts and therefore are more likely to develop successful solutions that will work in their lives. Rethinking our training to place therapists' skills in developing an intention-guided responsiveness to clients' experiences alongside use of interventions can be challenging but appears in keeping with the research on client change. This chapter and the others in this book can be a useful guide in that effort as can a curriculum developed for responsiveness training based on a meta-analysis of the responsiveness literature (Wu & Levitt, 2020).

Within training, we suggest that trainers teach novice therapists to understand the experience of being a client and the processes of change that clients find beneficial rather than focusing on teaching behaviorally defined interventions. We recommend the frequent use of roleplays so that trainees experience both what it is like to guide a client through the processes that we have described as well as what it is like to be in a client role and to encounter obstacles that need to be overcome. Within this context, interventions can be flexibly and responsively used to guide therapists-clients through a process of change, rather than applied rigidly across clients (see Elliott et al., 2004, for an example of how to teach change processes as guided by intentions). In this way, therapists can develop an understanding of responsiveness and psychotherapy that is rooted in the lived experience of the client.

Being able to discuss these experiences with trainers and fellow trainees within a supportive learning context can help therapists to develop skills related to empathy, self-referencing, and self-reflection and learn to apply them. Noticing when there are gaps between a mock-therapist's and a mock-client's experiences can provide immediate feedback that directs refinement in clinical style and delivery. The more practice with adapting a skill to clients' needs, the better integrated these intentions become within a therapist's repertoire. The better integrated these intentions are, the more interventions, relational strategies, and ways to support clients' self-healing will come to mind as a way to facilitate a given change process. For therapists who are no longer in training, these conversations can be beneficial when held with peer-supervisors.

Recommendations for Research

As a complement to quantitative meta-analysis, qualitative meta-analyses are also crucial to identifying central findings across the literature. The two methods complement each other and should be employed in synchrony when developing policy and recommendations for our diverse field of practitioners and clients. Whereas the former type of meta-analysis can affirm that a process is impactful in psychotherapy (e.g., empathy), it is the latter that describes how that process is experienced in session, what its function is, and when it is advised or ill advised.

For instance, the qualitative meta-analytic finding that clients integrate insights holistically may help to explain the repeated quantitative meta-analytic findings that common factors are the strongest predictor of psychotherapy outcome and that all psychotherapy orientations are equivalently effective despite their focus on different types of functional patterns (Wampold & Imel, 2015). After all, from a client's perspective, successful therapies across orientations are using many of the same mechanisms of change. The theoretical approaches all lead to clients' integrating new holistic patterns of functioning, rather than engaging specific mechanisms as typically theorized. Clients in all good therapies may internalize a more positive self-image, feel care, and become more agentic. Indeed, clients themselves may be seen as the common factor that undergirds the findings of psychotherapeutic equivalence (Levitt, 2016).

Given these insights, qualitative meta-analyses can build psychotherapy's evidence base and can provide invaluable guidance for clinical training and practice. They give researchers and therapists insight into the subjective experience of the client, which may be otherwise covert or deliberately hidden and, thus, not amenable to measurement or experimentation. Also, they have the potential to capture context-driven patterns that may shift across culture, time, and place and that are central to the way that therapy is performed.

These meta-analytic approaches can enable the development of principles of change and clinical practice guidelines that are based on a comprehensive review of a wide range of psychotherapy research methodologies and psychotherapy research cultures (which may value experimental, qualitative, and process measures differently from one another). A comprehensive understanding is vastly preferable as a basis for clinical practice rather than creating guidelines and lists of empirically based treatments derived from reviews of literature that ignore decades of rich and clinically meaningful research (or that demonstrate epistemological bias by focusing narrowly on one study design or emphasizing products of one psychotherapy research culture at the exclusion of others). As a field, psychologists gradually have become more aware of the diverse methods and epistemological approaches that can allow us to investigate questions with new thoroughness and rigor (e.g., American Psychological Association, 2020). Prominent methodologists across epistemological approaches have argued that methodological pluralism will advantage psychological science (Levitt et al., 2020; Shadish, 1986). We encourage the field to synthesize information collected by both qualitative and quantitative meta-analysis within integrative meta-analyses, especially when forming clinical practice guidelines for practitioners from a range of traditions (see Wu & Levitt, 2020, for an example of this approach).

In addition, these forms of reviews can assist researchers by identifying promising areas for future research. They can investigate types of change that are important not only to therapists (or insurance companies) but to clients as well. This chapter identifies five therapy change processes that could lead to fruitful research using a variety of methods, such as experimentation, process measure research, and qualitative approaches. The core category suggests an overarching understanding of the psychotherapy change process—as clients experience it—which may be relevant to most hypotheses and questions regarding therapy.

To support inquiry about clients' experiences of change, an outcome measure has been developed based on this line of research, the Client's Experience in Therapy Scale (CETS; Levitt et al., 2021). This measure can complement symptom-based understandings of progress in psychotherapy—allowing researchers to assess not only shifts in symptoms but also the extent to which clients were engaged in a high-quality process of psychotherapeutic change of varied forms that are central to them (e.g., insights, relational capacity, agency). The CETS items were formed from the categories in this meta-analysis and had strong psychometrics across exploratory and confirmatory factor analyses, revealing that the measure is equally appropriate across a broad range of psychotherapy orientations and client demographics. Since clients are a common factor across all theoretical orientations (and since the meta-analysis was based on studies of a diverse range of orientations and clients), it appears to hold relevance for assessing change as driven and experienced by clients in a wide range of clinical settings and contexts.

As clients have expressed repeatedly across a wide range of studies, using our therapeutic skills to responsively adapt interventions and to support their agency may be the best way to serve them. This perspective demands the consideration of clients' internal experiences in shaping our discipline's policies, in understanding what a comprehensive review of evidence entails, and in building practice guidelines based on comprehensive (quantitative, qualitative, and integrative) systematic reviews. The meaningful inclusion of client experiences in psychotherapy research will support an inclusive psychological science in which clients' efforts are better represented and therapists are better prepared to be responsive to their needs.

REFERENCES

American Psychological Association. (2020). *Publication manual of the American Psychological Association* (7th ed.). https://doi.org/10.1037/0000165-000

Anderson, K. N., Bautista, C. L., & Hope, D. A. (2019). Therapeutic alliance, cultural competence and minority status in premature termination of psychotherapy. *American Journal of Orthopsychiatry, 89*(1), 104–114. https://doi.org/10.1037/ort0000342

Audet, C. (2011). Client perspectives of therapist self-disclosure: Violating boundaries or removing barriers? *Counselling Psychology Quarterly, 24*(2), 85–100. https://doi.org/10.1080/09515070.2011.589602

Bandura, A. (2006). Toward a psychology of human agency. *Perspectives on Human Science, 1*(2), 164–180. https://doi.org/10.1111/j.1745-6916.2006.00011.x

Bateman, A., & Fonagy, P. (2013). Mentalization-based treatment. *Psychoanalytic Inquiry, 33*(6), 595–613. https://doi.org/10.1080/07351690.2013.835170

Bateman, A., Fonagy, P., & Allen, J. G. (2009). Theory and practice of mentalization-based therapy. In G. O. Gabbard (Ed.), *Textbook of psychotherapeutic treatments* (pp. 757–780). American Psychiatric Publishing.

Baumann, E. F., Ryu, D., & Harney, P. (2020). Listening to identity: Transference, countertransference, and therapist disclosure in psychotherapy with sexual and gender minority clients. *Practice Innovations (Washington, D.C.), 5*(3), 246–256. https://doi.org/10.1037/pri0000132

Berg, H. (2020). Virtue ethics and integration in evidence-based practice in psychology. *Frontiers in Psychology, 11*, 258. https://doi.org/10.3389/fpsyg.2020.00258

Binder, P. E., Holgersen, H., & Nielsen, G. H. (2009). Why did I change when I went to therapy? A qualitative analysis of former patients' conceptions of successful psychotherapy. *Counselling & Psychotherapy Research, 9*(4), 250–256. https://doi.org/10.1080/14733140902898088

Bohart, A. C., & Greenberg, L. S. (1997). *Empathy reconsidered: New directions in psychotherapy.* American Psychological Association. https://doi.org/10.1037/10226-000

Bohart, A. C., & Tallman, K. (2010). Clients: The neglected common factor in psychotherapy. In B. L. Duncan, S. D. Miller, B. E. Wampold, & M. A. Hubble (Eds.), *The heart and soul of change: Delivering what works in therapy* (pp. 83–111). American Psychological Association. https://doi.org/10.1037/12075-003

Boswell, J. F., Nelson, D. L., Nordberg, S. S., McAleavey, A. A., & Castonguay, L. G. (2010). Competency in integrative psychotherapy: Perspectives on training and supervision. *Psychotherapy: Theory, Research, & Practice, 47*(1), 3–11. https://doi.org/10.1037/a0018848

Bozarth, J. D. (2013). Unconditional positive regard. In M. Cooper, M. O'Hara, P. F. Schmid, & A. C. Bohart (Eds.), *The handbook of person-centred psychotherapy and counselling* (2nd ed., pp. 180–192). Palgrave Macmillan/Springer Nature. https://doi.org/10.1007/978-1-137-32900-4_12

Braithwaite, J. B. (2002). Rules and principles: A theory of legal certainty. *Australian Journal of Legal Philosophy, 27*. Advance online publication. https://doi.org/10.2139/ssrn.329400

Brooks, J., Bratley, R., Jones, L., King, N., & Lucock, M. (2021). Expectations and experiences of psychological therapy from the client perspective: A qualitative study. *British Journal of Guidance & Counselling*. Advance online publication. https://doi.org/10.1080/03069885.2019.1707167

Castonguay, L. G., & Hill, C. E. (Eds.). (2017). *How and why are some therapists better than others?: Understanding therapist effects.* American Psychological Association. https://doi.org/10.1037/0000034-000

Chang, D. F., & Berk, A. (2009). Making cross-racial therapy work: A phenomenological study of clients' experiences of cross-racial therapy. *Journal of Counseling Psychology, 56*(4), 521–536. https://doi.org/10.1037/a0016905

Chang, D. F., & Yoon, P. (2011). Ethnic minority clients' perceptions of the significance of race in cross-racial therapy relationships. *Psychotherapy Research, 21*(5), 567–582. https://doi.org/10.1080/10503307.2011.592549

Clarke, H., Rees, A., & Hardy, G. E. (2004). The big idea: Clients' perspectives of change processes in cognitive therapy. *Psychology and Psychotherapy: Theory, Research and Practice, 77*(1), 67–89. https://doi.org/10.1348/147608304322874263

Davis, D., DeBlaere, C., Hook, J. N., & Owen, J. (2020). *Mindfulness-based practices in therapy: A cultural humility approach.* American Psychological Association. https://doi.org/10.1037/0000156-000

Elliott, R., Bohart, A. C., Watson, J. C., & Murphy, D. (2018). Therapist empathy and client outcome: An updated meta-analysis. *Psychotherapy: Theory, Research, & Practice, 55*(4), 399–410. https://doi.org/10.1037/pst0000175

Elliott, R., & Greenberg, L. S. (2007). The essence of process-experiential/emotion-focused therapy. *American Journal of Psychotherapy, 61*(3), 241–254. https://doi.org/10.1176/appi.psychotherapy.2007.61.3.241

Elliott, R., Watson, J. C., Goldman, R. N., & Greenberg, L. S. (2004). *Learning emotion-focused therapy: The process-experiential approach to change.* American Psychological Association. https://doi.org/10.1037/10725-000

Eubanks, C. F., Muran, J. C., & Safran, J. D. (2018). Alliance rupture repair: A meta-analysis. *Psychotherapy: Theory, Research, & Practice, 55*(4), 508–519. https://doi.org/10.1037/pst0000185

Fitzpatrick, M. R., Janzen, J., Chamodraka, M., Gamberg, S., & Blake, E. (2009). Client relationship incidents in early therapy: Doorways to collaborative engagement. *Psychotherapy Research, 19*(6), 654–665. https://doi.org/10.1080/10503300902878235

Flückiger, C., Del Re, A. C., Wampold, B. E., Znoj, H., Caspar, F., & Jörg, U. (2012). Valuing clients' perspective and the effects on the therapeutic alliance: A randomized controlled study of an adjunctive instruction. *Journal of Counseling Psychology, 59*(1), 18–26. https://doi.org/10.1037/a0023648

Fonagy, P., & Allison, E. (2014). The role of mentalizing and epistemic trust in the therapeutic relationship. *Psychotherapy: Theory, Research, & Practice, 51*(3), 372–380. https://doi.org/10.1037/a0036505

Frankel, Z. E., & Levitt, H. M. (2009). Clients' experiences of disengaged moments in psychotherapy: A grounded theory analysis. *Journal of Contemporary Psychotherapy, 39*(3), 171–186. https://doi.org/10.1007/s10879-008-9087-z

Geller, J. D., & Farber, B. A. (2020). Ready when you are: Answering your questions about psychotherapy. *Journal of Clinical Psychology, 76*(8), 1438–1446. https://doi.org/10.1002/jclp.22996

Gendlin, E. T. (2003). *Focusing: How to gain direct access to your body's knowledge.* Rider.

Gordon, R. (2012). Where oh where are the clients? The use of client factors in counselling psychology. *Counselling Psychology Review, 27*(4), 8–17.

Göstas, M. W., Wiberg, B., Neander, K., & Kjellin, L. (2013). "Hard work" in a new context: Clients' experiences of psychotherapy. *Qualitative Social Work: Research and Practice, 12*(3), 340–357. https://doi.org/10.1177/1473325011431649

Grafanaki, S., & McLeod, J. (2002). Experiential congruence: Qualitative analysis of client and counsellor narrative accounts of significant events in time-limited person-centred therapy. *Counselling & Psychotherapy Research, 2*(1), 20–32. https://doi.org/10.1080/14733140212331384958

Henretty, J. R., Currier, J. M., Berman, J. S., & Levitt, H. M. (2014). The impact of counselor self-disclosure on clients: A meta-analytic review of experimental and quasi-experimental research. *Journal of Counseling Psychology, 61*(2), 191–207. https://doi.org/10.1037/a0036189

Henretty, J. R., & Levitt, H. M. (2010). The role of therapist self-disclosure in psychotherapy: A qualitative review. *Clinical Psychology Review, 30*(1), 63–77. https://doi.org/10.1016/j.cpr.2009.09.004

Henretty, J. R., Levitt, H. M., & Mathews, S. S. (2008). Clients' experiences of moments of sadness in psychotherapy: A grounded theory analysis. *Psychotherapy Research, 18*(3), 243–255. https://doi.org/10.1080/10503300701765831

Hill, C. E. (2009). *Helping skills: Facilitating, exploration, insight, and action* (3rd ed.). American Psychological Association.

Hill, C. E., Knox, S., & Pinto-Coelho, K. G. (2018). Therapist self-disclosure and immediacy: A qualitative meta-analysis. *Psychotherapy: Theory, Research, & Practice, 55*(4), 445–460. https://doi.org/10.1037/pst0000182

Hoener, C., Stiles, W. B., Luka, B. J., & Gordon, R. A. (2012). Client experiences of agency in therapy. *Person-Centered and Experiential Psychotherapies, 11*(1), 64–82. https://doi.org/10.1080/14779757.2011.639460

Hook, J. N., Davis, D. E., Owen, J., Worthington, E. L., Jr., & Utsey, S. O. (2013). Cultural humility: Measuring openness to culturally diverse clients. *Journal of Counseling Psychology, 60*(3), 353–366. https://doi.org/10.1037/a0032595

Hook, J. N., Farrell, J. E., Davis, D. E., DeBlaere, C., Van Tongeren, D. R., & Utsey, S. O. (2016). Cultural humility and racial microaggressions in counseling. *Journal of Counseling Psychology, 63*(3), 269–277. https://doi.org/10.1037/cou0000114

Kashdan, T. B., & Steger, M. F. (2007). Curiosity and pathways to well-being and meaning in life: Traits, states, and everyday behaviors. *Motivation and Emotion, 31*(3), 159–173. https://doi.org/10.1007/s11031-007-9068-7

Klein, M. H., Mathieu-Coughlan, P., & Kiesler, D. J. (1986). The experiencing scales. In L. S. Greenberg & W. M. Pinsof (Eds.), *The psychotherapeutic process: A research handbook* (pp. 21–71). Guilford Press.

Knox, R. (2008). Clients' experiences of relational depth in person-centred counselling. *Counselling & Psychotherapy Research, 8*(3), 182–188. https://doi.org/10.1080/14733140802035005

Kolden, G. G., Wang, C.-C., Austin, S. B., Chang, Y., & Klein, M. H. (2018). Congruence/genuineness: A meta-analysis. *Psychotherapy: Theory, Research, & Practice, 55*(4), 424–433. https://doi.org/10.1037/pst0000162

Kramer, U., & Stiles, W. B. (2015). The responsiveness problem in psychotherapy: A review of proposed solutions. *Clinical Psychology: Science and Practice, 22*(3), 277–295. https://doi.org/10.1111/cpsp.12107

Levitt, H. M. (2015). Qualitative psychotherapy research: The journey so far and future directions. *Psychotherapy: Theory, Research, & Practice, 52*(1), 31–37. https://doi.org/10.1037/a0037076

Levitt, H. M. (2016). How clients' experiences of therapy inform theories of psychotherapy integration: A meta-analysis. In H. M. Levitt (Chair), *Advancing the exploration of psychotherapy integration by using qualitative methods*. Paper presented at the Society of Psychotherapy Integration 32nd Annual Conference, Dublin, Ireland.

Levitt, H. M. (2021). *Essentials of critical-constructivist grounded theory*. American Psychological Association. https://doi.org/10.1037/0000231-000

Levitt, H. M., Butler, M., & Hill, T. (2006). What clients find helpful in psychotherapy: Developing principles for facilitating moment-to-moment change. *Journal of Counseling Psychology, 53*(3), 314–324. https://doi.org/10.1037/0022-0167.53.3.314

Levitt, H. M., Grabowski, L. M., Morrill, Z., & Minami, T. (2021). *The Clients' Experience of Therapy Scale (CETS): Broadening the view of outcome as symptom change to include therapy quality* [Unpublished manuscript]. University of Massachusetts Boston, Boston, MA.

Levitt, H. M., Minami, T., Greenspan, S. B., Puckett, J. A., Henretty, J. R., Reich, C. M., & Berman, J. S. (2016). How therapist self-disclosure relates to alliance and outcomes: A naturalistic study. *Counselling Psychology Quarterly, 29*(1), 7–28. https://doi.org/10.1080/09515070.2015.1090396

Levitt, H. M., & Morrill, Z. (2021). Measuring silence: The pausing inventory categorization system and a review of findings. In M. Buchholz & A. Dimitrijevic (Eds.), *Silence and silencing in psychoanalysis: Cultural, clinical and research perspectives* (pp. 233–250). Routledge.

Levitt, H. M., & Piazza-Bonin, E. (2017). The professionalization and training of psychologists: The place of clinical wisdom. *Psychotherapy Research, 27*(2), 127–142. https://doi.org/10.1080/10503307.2015.1090034

Levitt, H. M., Pomerville, A., & Surace, F. I. (2016). A qualitative meta-analysis examining clients' experiences of psychotherapy: A new agenda. *Psychological Bulletin, 142*(8), 801–830. https://doi.org/10.1037/bul0000057

Levitt, H. M., Surace, F. I., Wu, M. B., Chapin, B., Hargrove, J. G., Herbitter, C., Lu, E. C., Maroney, M. R., & Hochman, A. L. (2020). The meaning of scientific objectivity and subjectivity: From the perspective of methodologists. *Psychological Methods.* Advance online publication. https://doi.apa.org/doi/10.1037/met0000363

Levitt, H. M., & Williams, D. C. (2010). Facilitating client change: Principles based upon the experience of eminent psychotherapists. *Psychotherapy Research, 20*(3), 337–352. https://doi.org/10.1080/10503300903476708

Lilliengren, P., & Werbart, A. (2005). A model of therapeutic action grounded in the patients' view of curative and hindering factors in psychoanalytic psychotherapy. *Psychotherapy: Theory, Research, & Practice, 42*(3), 324–339. https://doi.org/10.1037/0033-3204.42.3.324

Mackrill, T. (2008). Exploring psychotherapy clients' independent strategies for change while in therapy. *British Journal of Guidance & Counselling, 36*(4), 441–453. https://doi.org/10.1080/03069880802343837

Mallinckrodt, B., & Jeong, J. (2015). Meta-analysis of client attachment to therapist: Associations with working alliance and client pretherapy attachment. *Psychotherapy: Theory, Research, & Practice, 52*(1), 134–139. https://doi.org/10.1037/a0036890

Miller-Bottome, M., Talia, A., Safran, J. D., & Muran, J. C. (2018). Resolving alliance ruptures from an attachment-informed perspective. *Psychoanalytic Psychology, 35*(2), 175–183. https://doi.org/10.1037/pap0000152

Muntigl, P., Knight, N., & Watkins, A. (2014). Empathic practices in client-centred psychotherapies: Displaying understanding and affiliation with clients. In E.-M. Graf, M. Sator, & T. Spranz-Fogasy (Eds.), *Discourses of helping professions* (pp. 33–57). John Benjamins. https://doi.org/10.1075/pbns.252.03mun

Muran, J. C., & Eubanks, C. F. (2020). *Therapist performance under pressure: Negotiating emotion, difference, and rupture.* American Psychological Association. https://doi.org/10.1037/0000182-000

Nienhuis, J. B., Owen, J., Valentine, J. C., Winkeljohn Black, S., Halford, T. C., Parazak, S. E., Budge, S., & Hilsenroth, M. (2018). Therapeutic alliance, empathy, and genuineness in individual adult psychotherapy: A meta-analytic review. *Psychotherapy Research, 28*(4), 593–605. https://doi.org/10.1080/10503307.2016.1204023

Norcross, J. C., & Wampold, B. E. (2018). A new therapy for each patient: Evidence-based relationships and responsiveness. *Journal of Clinical Psychology, 74*(11), 1889–1906. https://doi.org/10.1002/jclp.22678

Østlie, K., Stänicke, E., & Haavind, H. (2018). A listening perspective in psychotherapy with suicidal patients: Establishing convergence in therapists and patients private theories on suicidality and cure. *Psychotherapy Research, 28*(1), 150–163. https://doi.org/10.1080/10503307.2016.1174347

Owen, J., Tao, K. W., Drinane, J. M., Hook, J., Davis, D. E., & Kune, N. F. (2016). Client perceptions of therapists' multicultural orientation: Cultural (missed) opportunities and cultural humility. *Professional Psychology, Research and Practice, 47*(1), 30–37. https://doi.org/10.1037/pro0000046

Owen, J. J., Tao, K., Leach, M. M., & Rodolfa, E. (2011). Clients' perceptions of their psychotherapists' multicultural orientation. *Psychotherapy: Theory, Research, & Practice, 48*(3), 274–282. https://doi.org/10.1037/a0022065

Palmstierna, V., & Werbart, A. (2013). Successful psychotherapies with young adults: An explorative study of the participants' view. *Psychoanalytic Psychotherapy, 27*(1), 21–40. https://doi.org/10.1080/02668734.2012.760477

Pope-Davis, D. B., Toporek, R. L., Ortega-Villalobos, L., Ligiéro, D. P., Brittan-Powell, C. S., Liu, W. M., Bashshur, M. R., Codrington, J. N., & Liang, C. T. H. (2002). Client perspectives of multicultural counseling competence: A qualitative examination. *The Counseling Psychologist, 30*(3), 355–393. https://doi.org/10.1177/0011000002303001

Rennie, D. L. (1994). Clients' deference in psychotherapy. *Journal of Counseling Psychology, 41*(4), 427–437. https://doi.org/10.1037/0022-0167.41.4.427

Rennie, D. L. (2007). Reflexivity and its radical form: Implications for the practice of humanistic psychotherapies. *Journal of Contemporary Psychotherapy, 37*(1), 53–58. https://doi.org/10.1007/s10879-006-9035-8

Rogers, C. R. (1957). The necessary and sufficient conditions of therapeutic personality change. *Journal of Consulting Psychology, 21*(2), 95–103. https://doi.org/10.1037/h0045357

Rogers-Sirin, L., Melendez, F., Refano, C., & Zegarra, Y. (2015). Immigrant perceptions of therapists' cultural competence: A qualitative investigation. *Professional Psychology, Research and Practice, 46*(4), 258–269. https://doi.org/10.1037/pro0000033

Rousmaniere, T. (2017). *Deliberate practice for psychotherapists: A guide to improving clinical effectiveness.* Routledge/Taylor & Francis.

Saxon, D., Firth, N., & Barkham, M. (2017). The relationship between therapist effects and therapy delivery factors: Therapy modality, dosage, and non-completion. *Administration and Policy in Mental Health, 44*(5), 705–715. https://doi.org/10.1007/s10488-016-0750-5

Schnellbacher, J., & Leijssen, M. (2009). The significance of therapist genuineness from the client's perspective. *Journal of Humanistic Psychology, 49*(2), 207–228. https://doi.org/10.1177/0022167808323601

Shadish, W. R. (1986). Planned critical multiplism: Some elaborations. *Behavioral Assessment, 8*(1), 75–103.

Shine, L., & Westacott, M. (2010). Reformulation in cognitive analytic therapy: Effects on the working alliance and the client's perspective on change. *Psychology and Psychotherapy: Theory, Research and Practice, 83*(2), 161–177. https://doi.org/10.1348/147608309X471334

Spielberger, C. D., & Reheiser, E. C. (2009). Assessment of emotions: Anxiety, anger, depression, and curiosity. *Applied Psychology. Health and Well-Being, 1*(3), 271–302. https://doi.org/10.1111/j.1758-0854.2009.01017.x

Stiles, W. B., Honos-Webb, L., & Surko, M. (1998). Responsiveness in psychotherapy. *Clinical Psychology: Science and Practice, 5*(4), 439–458. https://doi.org/10.1111/j.1468-2850.1998.tb00166.x

Swift, J. K., Greenberg, R. P., Whipple, J. L., & Kominiak, N. (2012). Practice recommendations for reducing premature termination in therapy. *Professional Psychology, Research and Practice, 43*(4), 379–387. https://doi.org/10.1037/a0028291

Talia, A., Taubner, S., & Miller-Bottome, M. (2019). Advances in research on attachment-related psychotherapy processes: Seven teaching points for trainees and supervisors. *Research in Psychotherapy, 22*(3), 405. Advance online publication. https://doi.org/10.4081/ripppo.2019.405

Thompson, M. N., Nitzarim, R. S., Cole, O. D., Frost, N. D., Ramirez Stege, A., & Vue, P. T. (2015). Clinical experiences with clients who are low-income: Mental health practitioners' perspectives. *Qualitative Health Research, 25*(12), 1675–1688. https://doi.org/10.1177/1049732314566327

Timulák, L., & Lietaer, G. (2001). Moments of empowerment: A qualitative analysis of positively experienced episodes in brief person-centred counselling. *Counselling & Psychotherapy Research, 1*(1), 62–73. https://doi.org/10.1080/14733140112331385268

Waehler, C. A. (2013). Curiosity and biculturalism as key therapeutic change activities. *Psychotherapy: Theory, Research, & Practice, 50*(3), 351–355. https://doi.org/10.1037/a0033029

Wampold, B. E., & Imel, Z. E. (2015). *The great psychotherapy debate: The evidence for what makes psychotherapy work.* Routledge. https://doi.org/10.4324/9780203582015

Watson, J. C., & Greenberg, L. S. (2009). Empathic resonance: A neuroscience perspective. In J. Decety & W. Ickes (Eds.), *The social neuroscience of empathy* (pp. 125–138). MIT Press. https://doi.org/10.7551/mitpress/9780262012973.003.0011

Watson, J. C., McMullen, E. J., Rodrigues, A., & Prosser, M. C. (2019). Examining the role of therapists' empathy and clients' attachment styles on changes in clients' affect regulation and outcome in the treatment of depression. *Psychotherapy Research, 30*(6), 693–705. https://doi.org/10.1080/10503307.2019.1658912

Watson, J. C., & Wiseman, H. (Eds.). (2021). *The responsive psychotherapist: Attuning to clients in the moment.* American Psychological Association. https://doi.org/10.1037/0000240-000

Williams, D. C., & Levitt, H. M. (2007). Principles for facilitating agency in psychotherapy. *Psychotherapy Research, 17*(1), 66–82. https://doi.org/10.1080/10503300500469098

Wiseman, H., & Tishby, O. (2014). Client attachment, attachment to the therapist and client–therapist attachment match: How do they relate to change in psychodynamic psychotherapy? *Psychotherapy Research, 24*(3), 392–406. https://doi.org/10.1080/10503307.2014.892646

Wu, M. B., & Levitt, H. M. (2020). A qualitative meta-analytic review of the therapist responsiveness literature: Guidelines for practice and training. *Journal of Contemporary Psychotherapy, 50*(3), 161–175. https://doi.org/10.1007/s10879-020-09450-y

10

Clients' Influence on Psychotherapists and the Treatment They Provide

Rodney K. Goodyear and Hideko Sera

Mental health professionals' training and certification, as well as the ethical principles that guide them (e.g., American Psychological Association [APA], 2017), are all concerned with therapists' responsibilities to their clients. The weight of these responsibilities is perhaps even more pronounced for therapists who operate from variants of what Wampold and Imel (2015) would characterize as a medical model, in which it is assumed that the quality of particular kinds of technical interventions will predict anticipated outcomes (Lyon et al., 2018). But as Duncan and Miller (2000) observed, "The love affair with models blinds therapists to the roles clients play in bringing about change" (p. 170). All forms of psychotherapy occur in the context of a relationship in which the participants each bring characteristics that affect not only outcomes (Lambert, 2013) but each other as well. Clients are not passive recipients of therapists' services.

Clients appropriately expect their therapists to use skills that will help them meet their goals. But in the process of implementing their service, therapists inevitably respond to client behaviors and characteristics and to the feedback they provide. Some of those responses are intentional, such as when therapists adjust their interventions and how they respond to client feedback. Other therapist responses may be less intentional or elicited by clients' particular interpersonal behaviors, such as when therapists respond to nonverbal behaviors or when clients exhibit more withdrawn or reserved expressions or hostility toward the therapist than usual. Clients can also have more pervasive

https://doi.org/10.1037/0000303-011
The Other Side of Psychotherapy: Understanding Clients' Experiences and Contributions in Treatment, J. N. Fuertes (Editor)

and enduring impacts on therapists over time, particularly during frequent discussions of clients' profound traumatic experiences. Examples include the effects of vicarious trauma, such as when therapists work with particular client subpopulations (Branson, 2019) or the more personal effects that these cumulative client experiences have on therapists and their relationships (Råbu et al., 2016). In addition, therapists learn from clients and assimilate new values, beliefs, or behaviors as part of their lifelong professional development (Skovholt & Rønnestad, 1992; Swift & Parkin, 2017).

This chapter focuses on the effects that clients have on therapists (Fuertes & Williams, 2017) and is organized into two sections. First, we address clients' effects on therapists as they encounter each other in the therapy context. Second, we focus on the more enduring, cumulative effects that clients can have on therapists over time. We also address ways in which therapists can proactively seek client involvement and manage the unintentional influences that occur through countertransference (CT) and reactivity. Finally, we speak to issues of therapist self-care, which has been identified as an ethical imperative (Barnett et al., 2007).

EFFECTS OF INDIVIDUAL CLIENTS ON TREATMENT

Clients are active agents who influence their therapists (Bohart & Wade, 2013; see also Chapter 1, this volume) and, therefore, the nature and quality of the treatment they receive. Client influence can occur at multiple levels. For example, client influence occurs as therapists tailor treatment in response to particular client characteristics, including reactivity levels, culture, preferences, stage of change, and so on (Norcross & Wampold, 2018). At this level, the client's effects on the therapist are in how they conceptualize their work.

At least as important are the very specific and often moment-by-moment effects that clients have on their therapists and the work they do. This section is organized to first address the effects that arise from the interpersonal dynamics between client and therapist. Organic and nuanced interactions often have lingering effects on human relationships because implicit messaging can be as powerful as (if not more powerful than) thoughts and ideas that are explicitly stated and expressed. In addition, this section describes how the relational dynamics and exchanges that occur in a therapeutic relationship evolve frequently as the therapist and the client are participants in a fluid, ever-changing relationship.

Models Concerning Client–Therapist Interdependence

Gregory Bateson (1972), one of the founding members of the Palo Alto group of behavorial theorists (Ray, 2018), proposed a cybernetics perspective in which a psychotherapist can be understood as a member of the same system in which they are working to effect change. Therefore, the therapist simultaneously is influencing client behavior and is being influenced by it in turn.

Bateson's colleagues Watzlawick et al. (2011) focused on communication as the mechanism by which this influence occurs, famously proposing the axiom that "one cannot *not* communicate" (p. 49). Humans frequently use verbal and nonverbal channels to communicate with individuals with whom they interact, and they seek information about (a) a message's content and (b) the nature of their relationship with that person. A client who directly challenges something the therapist has said or done is communicating but so too is the client who has been responsive and engaged in the process but sits in "nonresponsive" silence. Each individual is communicating a message that will, in turn, affect the therapist's response.

Watzlawick et al. (2011) were interested in how the individual messages of people in a relationship are chained together as interactions. A substantial body of literature has been developed to confirm participants' mutual influence on each other's messages. For example, Lichtenberg and Hummel (1976) conceptualized therapy interactions as a stochastic process such that what one person in the dyad says during one utterance will affect the probability that the next person's utterance will be of a certain type. In a chain of interlocking utterances, any one utterance is simultaneously a "reinforcing stimulus" for the one immediately before it and a "discriminative stimulus" for the one that immediately follows. In this way, each person—whether the client or the therapist—is continually both being responsive to and affecting the other person.

While Bateson and other members of the Palo Alto group were developing this framework for understanding relational interactions, interpersonal theorists were developing a similar framework, influenced by Sullivan's (1953) notion that a therapist and a client interact in an interpersonal field. Both the Palo Alto group and interpersonal theorists used the concept of *complementarity*, which concerns the degree of interpersonal reciprocity of two people—that is, how well they "fit" with one another in the context of behavioral exchanges. Any behavior by one participant could simultaneously reward the most recent behavior by the other participant and constrain the other participant's next behavior.

In the Palo Alto group's conception, individuals in a relationship are constantly working to define their relationship to one another on a dimension of control. Any particular interchange with another person could be understood as having either an intention to be "one up" (assuming control) or "one down" (relinquishing control; Haley, 1963). Complementarity exists to the extent that the person who receives a one-up message follows it with a one-down message or vice versa. Symmetry, however, exists when a person delivers a message at one end of this control dimension, and the other person responds with a message that is on the same end of the dimension (specifically, a one-up message is followed by the other person's one-up message).

Interpersonal theorists retained this control dimension in mapping interchanges between two people. However, they added a second affiliative dimension so that any message from one person to another can be mapped in two-dimensional space in the degree to which it conveys both dominance and affiliation (i.e., a hostility-to-friendliness dimension). This dimension has been captured in the circumplex model that originates from Timothy Leary's (1957) extrapolation of Sullivan's work and that has occurred in several later variants (for a summary, see Wiggins, 1996). For example, the circumplex depicted in Figure 10.1 shows that a leading response would be coded as relatively high on dominance and somewhat high on friendliness. In contrast, a distrustful reaction would be coded as relatively high on hostility and somewhat submissive. Coding systems such as the Interpersonal Communication Rating Scale (Strong & Hills, 1986) more fully explicate how particular responses would be coded on a circumplex similar to Figure 10.1.

In the paradigm of the interpersonal theorists, a complementary response is one that responds to another person's message by (a) staying on the same side of the HOSTILE–FRIENDLY axis in Figure 10.1 but (b) responding from the opposite side of the DOMINANT–SUBMISSIVE axis. For example, a client might begin with the request "Please, just tell me what to do" (submissive

FIGURE 10.1. Spatial Arrangements of Antecedent Stimulus and Consequent Interpersonal Communication Rating Scale Octant Codes Representing Perfect Complementarity

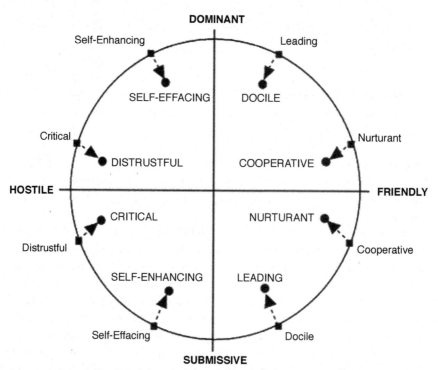

Note. The squares and lowercase terms represent the antecedent behavior, the circles and uppercase terms represent the consequence, and the dotted lines represent complementary responses. From "An Examination of the Complementarity of Interpersonal Behavior," by T. J. Tracey, 1994, *Journal of Personality and Social Psychology, 67*(5), p. 873 (https://doi.org/10.1037/0022-3514.67.5.864). Copyright 1994 by the American Psychological Association.

message). The therapist might respond, "I really wish I could, but that is not my role. Let's explore some options" (leading message). In this case, both responses are on the friendlier side of the circumplex, but each is on a different end of the DOMINANT–SUBMISSIVE axis.

Figure 10.1 depicts the expected responses to a range of possible behaviors. The squares and lowercase terms represent the antecedent behavior, the circles and uppercase terms represent the consequence, and the dotted lines represent complementary responses. To illustrate with an example of a multiple-interchange sequence from Tracey et al. (2012), a client presents with a problem in their life and seeks the therapist's advice (docile response); the therapist then responds by providing advice (leading response), which is complementary. The client, however, responds with a *yes, but* statement (distrustful), which is noncomplementary to the advice/leading response. Over several *yes, but* responses, the therapist's responses begin to shift to become subtly critical (e.g., as a complementary response to the distrust shown in the *yes, but* statements, the content of the therapist's responses may remain facilitative but exasperation begins to "leak" into their tone of voice).

From this framework, strong alliances are characterized by collaboration or mutuality, manifest as complementarity in client–therapist interactions, which Larsson et al. (2019) identified as one of the bond elements in an alliance. In fact, research has supported this link between alliance and complementarity (e.g., Friedlander, 1993; Kiesler & Watkins, 1989; Svartberg & Stiles, 1992). Friedlander (1993) provided an excellent literature review of the similarities and differences in the notion of complementarity as understood by the two models discussed earlier. The author concluded that complementarity, at least as assessed from the interpersonal theory framework, predicted client outcomes. However, this relationship between complementarity and alliance was more pronounced for earlier stages of therapy.

In fact, Tracey (1994) provided a rationale that might explain Friedlander's (1993) stage-related findings in his discussion of therapy as a three-stage process. There is an early stage in which the therapist and the client develop rapport, characterized by consistently high positive complementarity levels (i.e., therapist and client interactions would both be occurring primarily on the right-hand side of the circumplex depicted in Figure 10.1). As their work progresses, the client begins to replicate with the therapist relationship patterns from their everyday life; as a result, the pattern can shift to negative complementarity (i.e., interactions that would be mapped on the left side of the circumplex). It then becomes the therapist's task to identify the pattern and help the client modify it. The stress this causes on the therapeutic relationship can result in a period of relative instability with respect to the proportion of therapist–client interactions that are complementary (either positive or negative). The final stage of therapy is characterized by a return to greater complementarity. Using the client influence frame, Tracey's (1994) proposed model suggests that the extent and the type of client influence on the therapist vary by stage of therapy when influence is defined in terms of moment-to-moment effects on the other person's behavior.

It is also important to address parallel processes, a phenomenon described by supervision scholars (Gross Doehrman, 1976) as an example of how clients influence therapists. In this case, the therapist takes the role of the supervisee, and the dynamics occurring in their relationship with the client mirror the therapist's relationship with their supervisor. To date, research on parallel processes has consisted almost exclusively of case studies. One exception is from Tracey et al. (2012), who used the interpersonal psychotherapy framework to examine how the interactional patterns of the supervisee and the client are reflected in those of the supervisor–supervisee (and vice versa) in 17 supervisory triads (i.e., supervisor, supervisee, and client). From this framework, the authors concluded that there was clear evidence of parallel processes. Tracey et al. illustrated the kind of processes they documented as follows:

> So if a client tended to act in a distrustful and self-effacing manner (submissive-critical) in the prior session and the therapist complemented this by acting in a critical manner in therapy, then the therapist in the role of trainee would enact some of the distrustful client behavior in the subsequent supervision session. The supervisor would also demonstrate this parallel process by acting in a manner similar to how the therapist acted in the previous therapy session; in this example, the supervisor would become more critical than typical. (p. 339)

More Holistic Impacts of Clients on Therapists

Both the Palo Alto group and interactional theorists are concerned with the moment-to-moment influences that one person has on the other. There also are more holistic ways in which clients affect their therapists during their interactions. The actor–partner interdependence model is one framework in which this has been examined in the research. The concept of CT also relies on the more molar effects of the client on the therapist.

Actor–Partner Interdependence Model

The actor–partner interdependence model of dyadic relationships (Campbell & Stanton, 2014; Kenny, 2018) provides a method to test hypotheses about the effects that each member of a dyad has on the other. As Cook and Kenny (2005) observed,

> There is interdependence in a relationship when one person's emotion, cognition, or behaviour affects the emotion, cognition, or behaviour of a partner . . . A consequence of interdependence is that observations of two individuals are linked or correlated such that knowledge of one person's score provides information about the other person's score. (p. 101)

Much of this research has been focused on couples and families. However, a small body of research by Kivlighan and colleagues (Gelso et al., 2012; Kivlighan et al., 2014, 2015, 2016; Li et al., 2021), Salazar Kämpf et al. (2021), and Zilcha-Mano et al. (2016) has applied the actor–partner interdependence model in the context of psychotherapy. For example, researchers examined client–therapist mutual influence on variables such as ratings of the alliance, session depth or outcomes, and perceptions of the real relationship and outcomes. The results have not consistently demonstrated actor–partner effects. Regardless of the specific domains in which clients might influence therapists, research using the actor–partner interdependence model does support the broader thesis of this chapter: Clients do influence therapists. Whereas that client influence is immediate and specific when viewed through the lens of complementarity as discussed previously, here it concerns the influence of more molar constructs such as satisfaction, perceptions of relationships, and so on.

Furthermore, research indicates that factors such as the therapist's level of experience and the treatment setting influence the client's perception about the therapeutic relationship and the therapist (Kivlighan et al., 2014). Therefore, we are further intrigued by how the client's perception of the therapist indeed influences the ways in which the therapist responds to the client. For instance, if the client perceives the therapist as not as warm or relatable as they would wish a therapist to be, we would anticipate that the client would most likely behave, intentionally or unintentionally, to express their perceptions and experiences. For example, a client could passive-aggressively mention that their former therapist approached therapy "differently." When asked to elaborate more, the client would likely describe the former therapist's warmth and relatability but refrain from saying, "Therefore, I would like you also to be more relatable." Some clients could choose to shut down emotionally, hoping to draw the therapist in more to find out why emotional distancing has occurred—as a way to promote emotional engagement. In return, the therapist could easily hypothesize that the client may be disengaged and speculate that there is a level of disinterest in treatment. The therapist could also react to and be affected by the client's comparison with their former therapist and perhaps even sense the client's determination of or skepticism about the therapist's skill level or goodness of fit. These observations and inevitable emotional reactions to the client's words and actions affect the therapist. Furthermore, some of these reactions could not only foster ideas and thoughts about treatment modalities but could also substantively affect the therapist in terms of self-doubt and negative emotional reactions to the client.

Countertransference

Freud (1910/1959) conceptualized CT as a phenomenon that occurs for the psychotherapist "as a result of the patient's influence on his unconscious feelings" (p. 144). Hayes et al. (2018) observed that this is the classical conception of CT and that, in the decades since, two other concepts of CT developed: the *totalistic* (which encompasses all reactions a therapist might have to a client) and the *complementary* (which, as the name suggests, aligns with the notion of complementarity discussed earlier). In fact, Kiesler (2001) described CT as a "complementary response being pulled for so expertly and tenaciously by clients" (p. 1055). What all three conceptions of CT have in common is that the client is influencing the therapist, regardless of whether that is their intention.

Moreover, this form of client influence on the therapist is ubiquitous. Hayes et al. (1998) performed a meta-analytic review and found that therapists in their sample reported experiencing CT in approximately 80% of their cases. This finding is notable because Hayes et al. (2018) found that CT has deleterious effects on psychotherapy outcomes, and Tishby and Wiseman (2020) found that negative CT is associated with more relationship ruptures and less resolution of them.

However, Hayes et al. (2019) also found that managed CT is associated with better outcomes. This speaks to the importance of therapists being able to recognize when CT is affecting their work and to attending to the five elements that Gelso and Hayes (1998) identified as important to CT management: therapist self-insight, anxiety management, self-integration, empathy, and conceptualizing ability. Self-reflective practice is important and often will be sufficient in attending to these elements. But in some cases, consultation or supervision can be important. Although helping supervisees manage CT is an expected supervisory competence (APA, 2015), some supervisory models (e.g., Ladany et al., 2016) are especially explicit in articulating how supervisors might do that.

CUMULATIVE CLIENT IMPACTS

We have thus far addressed the effects that clients and therapists have on one another as they interact, but clients also can have critical cumulative effects on therapists. Clients can affect therapists' personal and interpersonal functioning, ranging from the therapeutic effects of providing therapy (e.g., those shown in the helper-therapy theory; Riessman, 1965; Skovholt, 1974) to more deleterious effects (e.g., the client's trauma affecting the therapist; Cohen & Collens, 2013). Longer term cumulative effects from working with clients can affect how therapists think about their work and clients' expectations (Rønnestad & Skovholt, 2003). We address each type of effect in turn.

Clients' Effects on Therapists' Personal and Interpersonal Functioning

S. L. Hatcher et al. (2012) found that virtually all psychotherapists they surveyed (95%) reported that their work with clients affected their own relationships. For example, one participant observed that "I think about my relationships more carefully, and more thoughtfully, and more lovingly than I used to" (p. 6). This kind of process might be observed, for example, when a male therapist who has not experienced gender discrimination begins questioning his role in perpetuating systemic sexism and gender biases after he has worked with female clients who present distress as a result of academic or work experiences where they have to navigate such issues frequently. Such a reflective change in this therapist could, in turn, shape his framework for therapeutic relationships and for all of his relationships with female individuals.

The Greek origin of the word "therapy" derives from *therapia*, which means healing (Cambridge Dictionary, 2011). From the small number of studies available on this topic (Riessman, 1965; Skovholt, 1974), it seems that healing can work in both directions, as therapists and clients interact with each other.

The flip side, however, is that for therapists working with some clients, there is a "cost to caring" (R. Hatcher & Noakes, 2010) that can be cumulative and result in burnout or secondary trauma stress (used here as a synonym for secondary or vicarious trauma; Cieslak et al., 2014; Schauben & Frazier, 1995). Secondary trauma stress manifests with reactions similar to posttraumatic stress disorder (Bride et al., 2004), including increased emotional arousal, avoidance of triggers and emotions, and intrusive and sometimes impulsive reactions.

In a qualitative study, Elias and Haj-Yahia (2019) interviewed social workers treating sex offenders and illustrated some of the personal and interpersonal consequences of working with this population. Participants reported, for example, a sense of overload and preoccupation with what their clients had reported: "It's very hard to go back to normal life and flip that switch, go home and everything is okay, it's hard, these are feelings that stick with you" (p. 857). Some reported having become hypervigilant when out at night alone. Respondents also reported interpersonal effects, including increased suspicion of others, heightened anxiety about their children's safety, and, in some cases, lowered sex drive or even aversion to sex.

Although some therapists are at high risk for vicarious trauma, which can set in when working with particular client subpopulations (Finklestein et al., 2015; Schauben & Frazier, 1995; Weitkamp et al., 2014), this risk increases when therapists do not engage in effective self-care. In fact, Barnett and colleagues (2005) identified self-care as an ethical imperative (APA, 2017); when self-care is neglected, it compromises ethical processes as well as clinical decision-making processes (Norcross, 2000). Therefore, we speculate that, perhaps, when the therapist does not attend well to their self-care, the type and level of the client's impact may be felt more harshly and negatively. Bender and Ingram (2018) noted the critical relationship among self-care, one's resilience, and self-efficacy. For instance, when therapists engage in ongoing self-care, they may retain their self-reflective practice without letting clients' negative feedback on their treatment modality turn into an emotionally devastating factor that casts intense self-doubt on their clinical skills and knowledge. With proper self-care, which promotes a sense of resilience and self-efficacy, the therapist may be able to appreciate elements of clients' critiques on therapy without deeply questioning their own effectiveness. With resilience, the therapist can receive clients' feedback and suggestions on improvements for therapy, objectively reflect on exactly how to implement improvements, and make the necessary changes without feeling as if they have somehow failed.

The prevailing assumption is that therapists with a history of traumas related to the ones being focused on in therapy are more vulnerable to vicarious trauma (or enactment of their own trauma); however, that kind of history is not a necessary precondition. For example, a female therapist who works with survivors of a sexual offense may experience vicarious trauma even if she has never experienced the same violation in her life. Therefore, one question to examine would be whether a therapist's level of empathy can moderate the impact clients have on them. In other words, could it be that a potent (R. L. Hatcher, 2015; Wampold, 2015) and perhaps necessary (Rogers,

1957) condition for effective therapy—that is, empathy—for therapists working with clients with trauma becomes a risk factor in therapists experiencing vicarious trauma? There seems to be a substantial difference between therapists whose empathy allows space for clients to affect them positively (e.g., they connect with their clients and use this connection to help them heal) and those whose empathy makes them vulnerable to reactions such as vicarious trauma, deep self-doubt, or heightened anxiety (Guy & Liaboe, 1986).

In addition to empathy, at least two other factors warrant mention as possible moderators of the extent to which client trauma can affect therapists. One factor is the therapist's level of ego strength (Bjorklund, 2000; see also Abdoulmaleki et al., 2020), and the other is the therapist's attachment style (e.g., Degnan et al., 2016). For example, the therapist's attachment style may have bearing on how the client expresses affect (Robinson et al., 2015) and then presumably on how the therapist, in turn, is affected by the client's material. In addition, the importance of self-care as an ethical imperative (Barnett et al., 2005) illustrates that the connection between therapists' well-being, when not carefully attended to, can be negatively affected by factors such as client trauma.

Clients' Cumulative Effects on Therapists' Development

Therapists credit working with clients as having been the most critical source of their professional development (Orlinsky et al., 2001). Skovholt (1974) and Skovholt and Rønnestad (1992) asserted that clients serve as primary teachers in the process of therapist development. Others have extended that argument to suggest that therapists' ideas about therapy are mostly shaped by particular clients who challenge them (Kottler & Hunter, 2010; Pargament et al., 2014). A similar parallel can be drawn when professors and teachers note that students who present hard-to-hear but thought-provoking questions contribute to their professional growth, as they are pushed to challenge their thinking or even the way they teach. However, it is important to make the distinction between therapists becoming more assured of their approach to therapy as they gain experience working with clients and becoming more effective, at least when effectiveness is measured by client outcomes. For example, Goldberg et al. (2016) found that the typical therapist does not increase their effectiveness over time simply by becoming more assured of their approach. One empirical question remains as to how some therapists are able to generate better outcomes with certain clients.

Earlier, we noted the effects that particular subpopulations of clients (e.g., sex offenders, trauma survivors) can have on therapists personally and interpersonally. Working with those clients also can affect therapists' implicit models of treatment, especially cognitive schema related to the clients they serve. In some cases, that can be positive. For example, R. Hatcher and Noakes (2010) found that upon further investigating the compassion fatigue of therapists working with challenging client subpopulations, therapists become aware of advocating for and creating a safe work environment for all staff and delineating clear boundaries and role definitions for their scope of work and clinical responsibilities. We specifically note here, therefore, that clients' impact could lead to structural or systemic improvements and/or changes for work conditions or environments for therapists to enhance their abilities further. For this reason, clients' impact on therapists could happen at an intrapersonal level, an interpersonal level, or even a systemic level—for example, how therapists reflect about themselves, their therapeutic relationships with clients (as well as others in the therapists' lives), or their work expectations and day-to-day operational processes at their workplace—all because of something the client said or did.

IMPLICATIONS FOR TREATMENT, TRAINING, AND RESEARCH

Based on the research described earlier, there are a number of implications for psychotherapists and for those who train and supervise them. In this section, we underscore several of these implications more directly and conclude with some observations about research concerning the influence that clients have on their therapists.

Treatment

The therapeutic alliances that so robustly predict treatment outcomes (Flückiger et al., 2018) require the client and therapist to work together as "allies" (Fuertes et al., 2019) who share consensus on the purposes and processes of their work together (Bordin, 1979; Duncan & Miller, 2000). But that consensus is possible only when clients have had a voice, and that requires therapists to solicit and respond to clients' expectations, perceptions, and experiences.

Therapists need to be intentional in soliciting client input, and they need to do so on an ongoing basis if they are to be prepared to minimize or address fluctuations in alliance strength and quality (Eubanks et al., 2018; Larsson et al., 2019). The importance of this is underscored by the data on how poorly therapists are able to judge when clients are at risk of treatment failure or are deteriorating (Hannan et al., 2005; Hatfield et al., 2010) or to identify what clients perceive to have been the most effective in a particular session (Bedi & Hayes, 2019).

Therapists begin seeking that feedback in their initial meetings with clients as they discuss their work together (Okiishi et al., 2003). This discussion also provides an important opportunity to set ground rules for the relationship, which should include the shared expectation that the client will bring to the therapist's attention instances of feeling misunderstood or worse and have that information received respectfully. This kind of encouragement is especially important with respect to differences related to race, gender, and other forms of diversity, including any instances of perceived microaggressions (Owen et al., 2014).

When clients then provide their perceptions of issues that they wish to be addressed, therapists must be receptive to that dialogue. This requires that therapists have both self-awareness and the willingness to be reflective about their work. It also is reasonable to speculate that one reason the very best therapists tend to be self-doubting (Nissen-Lie et al., 2013) or self-critical (Najavits & Strupp, 1994) is that these attitudes make them receptive to client input. It is important to acknowledge the role that consultation or supervision can play in facilitating self-reflection and attention to client input. The United Kingdom, Ireland, Australia, and New Zealand require therapists to participate in career-long supervision, which provides them with multiple benefits but particularly a reflective space (Nicholas & Goodyear, 2021). Although career-long supervision is not a regulatory requirement in the United States, Lichtenberg et al. (2014) found that more than half of a national sample of counseling psychologists (55%) reported regularly participating in some form of supervision. That this is true of so many is a strong testament to the perceived value of supervision.

Training and Supervision

The material we have covered highlights a number of areas that warrant attention from individuals supervising and training therapists. Examples include attention to therapist–client interaction sequences, management of CT, and parallel processes. Thus far, we also have underscored the importance of developing competence in self-care and reflective practice. In this section, we emphasize client feedback as a training focus and as a tool in supervision.

In reviewing studies on client disclosures in therapy, Farber (2003) observed that Freud's (1912/1958) *fundamental rule*—that clients would say whatever comes into their heads—is unfeasible. Shame is one factor, as is deference. Farber (2003) noted, for example, that shame "is an inexorable aspect of psychotherapeutic treatment . . . affecting the timing, focus, and depth of what is discussed" (p. 594). Rennie (1994) found that clients' most common way of expressing deference was to not disclose to their therapists their concerns about the therapy approach or the therapists' limitations, expectations, or frame of reference. In fact, Blanchard and Farber (2016) reported that more than 90% of adult clients in their study had lied to their therapists, and more than 70% admitted having lied about at least one aspect of therapy. The clients' rationale stemmed from wanting to be polite and not wanting to upset their therapists.

Gathering client feedback and inputs to "take the temperature" of the treatment and the therapeutic relationship may be commonsensical these days (Duncan et al., 2011; Heinonen & Nissen-Lie, 2020; Leibert et al., 2020). However, Alfred Adler introduced one of the earliest clinical tools for collecting and using client inputs to determine the direction of treatment. By collecting the client's early recollections—those memories with specific emotional reactions attached before age 10 years—and sharing clinical interpretations of what these memories meant for the client, Adler sought client reactions to gauge the accuracy of clinical impressions to set the expectations and tone of treatment (Kern et al., 2004). Adler also noted that clients might at times provide inputs that are contradictory to what has been discussed, decided, or even accomplished in therapy. For instance, the therapist might think that positive progress has been achieved, but the client could voice their frustration that nothing has been accomplished. However, that contradiction itself can serve as valuable clinical feedback of where clients are in their treatment. This feedback, in turn, could guide therapists to reflect on various aspects of therapy such as chosen interventions, approaches, and pace of therapy.

The systematic collection of information from clients using instruments with established psychometric properties is a relatively recent development. Since Howard et al. (1996) first proposed its use, routine outcome monitoring (ROM) quickly became established as an essential standard of care, owing to its positive influence on client outcomes and retention (Boswell et al., 2015; Lambert et al., 2018; see also Chapter 8, this volume). Central to the point of this chapter is that ROM provides an important mechanism for clients to have a say about the therapist and the treatment that they are receiving. Indeed, the very name for one of the two ROM systems that has been researched most to date (Lambert et al., 2018)—the Partners for Change Outcome Management System (Miller et al., 2005)—speaks to the client's role as a partner in treatment, framing clients as experts of their own being who are capable of noting when and how their reactions are provoked in therapy (Swift et al., 2017).

Most ROM systems provide the therapist with feedback on both (a) the client's level of functioning, which can provide a signal to action if the client is not progressing as expected or is deteriorating, and (b) the client's perception of the alliance. This is important, given the stark differences in the accuracy with which these systems can predict client deterioration (highly accurate) versus the accuracy of therapists' clinical judgment (highly inaccurate; Hannan et al., 2005; Hatfield et al., 2010). These scores do not provide information about why the treatment or the relationship is as it is, but they do provide the opportunity for conversations with the client, for analysis of session recordings, and for other actions that might be useful to consider in redirecting treatment.

Clinical supervisors can play an essential role in teaching supervisees both to seek this kind of client input and to use it in their professional development. In particular, Swift et al. (2015) suggested the following steps:

1. Supervisors train supervisees to obtain and use objective client feedback.

2. Supervisors use specific client data to inform work they are doing in supervision. For example, by watching for data that show that a particular client is either deteriorating or signaling a problem in the alliance, the supervisor and supervisee can know to take specific actions, including having conversations with the client and carefully reviewing videos or recordings of sessions with that client.

3. Supervisors use data to identify patterns of outcomes across clients to facilitate supervisee growth and development. For example, Swift et al. (2015) described using an Excel spreadsheet to break out data by client categories (gender, race, and so on) to see whether the supervisee is obtaining better results with particular groups. This is similar to a process described by Muir et al. (2019), who observed the following:

> [C]linicians who employ ROM can relatively easily generate statistics (e.g., by calculating a standardized, average pre- to posttreatment change rate) that objectively represent their overall efficacy and their outcome domain-specific efficacies, and then benchmark such data against the aforementioned established averages . . . a clinician might learn, for example, that although she is average with regard to her general effectiveness, she is above average in treating patients with anxiety problems and below average in treating patients with depression. (p. 6)

In the counseling foundational skills course of many graduate programs, educators often use the analogy of a client and a therapist walking side by side on a path. Both have to stop and assess where they stand from time to time to continue to walk on the same path, at a pace on which they mutually agree. Metaphorically speaking, one may have a compass, while the other has a map or a recollection of a similar path they have previously walked, which may guide the current endeavor. Again, the message is clear that without their inevitable interdependent collaboration and mutuality, the client and the therapist may not experience a therapeutic relationship where they constructively reflect on the impact that they have on each other.

Research

Active research programs exist for virtually all of the topics addressed in this chapter. This is true, for example, for the work on achieving complementarity, managing CT, and using ROM in treatment. Moreover, the actor–partner interdependence model is itself a method of research. In addition, there are emerging areas of research on the influence of clients that were not covered here but warrant watching. One example is the influence that clients have on therapists at a physiological level such as synchronized heart or respiratory rates (e.g., Stratford et al., 2012; Tschacher & Meier, 2020).

Rather than suggest new domains of research that affect the influence that clients have on therapists, we recommend that scholars engaged in this work ask more research questions that explicitly focus on the client. In doing so, we are reaffirming the argument Fuertes and Williams (2017) made. Their suggested research questions concerning clients' experiences of the therapy relationship, how better to tailor therapy to the client, and what engages and motivates clients provide a valuable roadmap for researchers. The chapters in this book are also a rich source of additional questions about the likely effects that clients have on their therapists and on therapy.

CONCLUSION

The thesis of this chapter is that clients are active agents who substantially affect not only the therapy they receive but their therapists as well. A client's impacts can range (a) from those that occur during moment-to-moment interactions to those that are cumulative and more enduring and (b) from those that facilitate therapy to those that impede it. Therapy is effective to the extent that therapists invite input, are attuned to the meaning of clients' messages, and are appropriately responsive. In addition, clients' longer term impact on therapists depends on their ability to be self-reflective and to engage in self-care.

持ちつ持たれつ (*mochitsu-motaretsu*) is a well-known Japanese concept that discusses the interdependence and mutuality between individuals in a relationship, with an understanding that no one person holds the whole truth and, for the relationship to foster and mature, it is incumbent on those in the relationship to contribute to their shared space. The underlying goal is for those in a relationship to share and contribute to the totality of that relationship, creating a fuller and more comprehensive understanding of one another as well as the space they share. Another way of highlighting an understanding of this concept is that the shared relational space does not become mutually beneficial without the other person(s) and their authentic inputs.

This framework seems to have a particular resonance when discussing clients' influences on therapists and the complementarity between the client and the therapist (Tracey, 2004). This saying is often translated to have a nuance of "because of you, I exist." However, we caution that this should not be misinterpreted as a form of psychological dependence between the client and therapist when applied to a therapeutic context as they cannot, in a quite literal sense, exist without each other. Rather, the saying highlights the inevitable process of the client and the therapist keenly observing one another, sharing their thoughts verbally or nonverbally with one another, and cocreating their therapeutic relationship.

The information we have presented is not new. But we hope that by framing it as we have, this will draw more attention to client effects. Those effects tend to be overshadowed by the field's emphasis on therapists' responsibilities for managing treatment. Occasionally shifting the lens to focus on clients and their powerful influence on therapy and therapists can help therapists be more intentional in seeking and attending to client messages and characteristics that affect them and their work.

REFERENCES

Abdoulmaleki, L., Amiri, A., Hosseini, S. S., Amirpor, B., & Afshariniya, K. (2020). The role of self-compassion and ego strength on secondary post-traumatic stress disorder in wives of war veterans. *Journal of Military Caring Sciences, 6*(4), 267–275. https://doi.org/10.29252/mcs.6.4.2

American Psychological Association. (2015). Guidelines for clinical supervision in health service psychology. *American Psychologist, 70*(1), 33–46. https://doi.org/10.1037/a0038112

American Psychological Association. (2017). *Ethical principles of psychologists and code of conduct* (2002, Amended June 1, 2010, and January 1, 2017). http://www.apa.org/ethics/code/index.html

Barnett, J. E., Baker, E. K., Elman, N. S., & Schoener, G. R. (2007). In pursuit of wellness: The self-care imperative. *Professional Psychology: Research and Practice, 38*(6), 603–612. https://doi.org/10.1037/0735-7028.38.6.603

Barnett, J. E., Johnston, L. C., & Hillard, D. (2005). Psychotherapist wellness as an ethical imperative. In L. VandeCreek & J. B. Allen (Eds.), *Innovations in clinical practice: Focus on health & wellness* (pp. 257–271). Professional Resource Press.

Bateson, G. (1972). *Steps to an ecology of mind.* Ballantine.

Bedi, R., & Hayes, S. (2019). Clients' perspectives on, experiences of, and contributions to the working alliance. In J. N. Fuertes (Ed.), *Working alliance skills for mental health professionals* (pp. 111–136). Oxford University Press. https://doi.org/10.1093/med-psych/9780190868529.003.0006

Bender, A., & Ingram, R. (2018). Connecting attachment styles to resilience: Contributions of self-care and self-efficacy. *Personality and Individual Differences, 130*(1), 18–20. https://doi.org/10.1016/j.paid.2018.03.038

Bjorklund, P. (2000). Assessing ego strength: Spinning straw into gold. *Perspectives in Psychiatric Care, 36*(1), 14–23. https://doi.org/10.1111/j.1744-6163.2000.tb00685.x

Blanchard, M., & Farber, B. A. (2016). Lying in psychotherapy: Why and what clients don't tell their therapists about therapy and their relationship. *Counselling Psychology Quarterly, 29*(1), 90–112. https://doi.org/10.1080/09515070.2015.1085365

Bohart, A. C., & Wade, A. G. (2013). The client in psychotherapy. In M. J. Lambert (Ed.), *Bergin and Garfield's handbook of psychotherapy and behavior change* (6th ed., pp. 219–257). John Wiley & Sons, Inc.

Bordin, E. S. (1979). The generalizability of the psychoanalytic concept of the working alliance. *Psychotherapy: Theory, Research, & Practice, 16*(3), 252–260. https://doi.org/10.1037/h0085885

Boswell, J. F., Kraus, D. R., Miller, S. D., & Lambert, M. J. (2015). Implementing routine outcome monitoring in clinical practice: Benefits, challenges, and solutions. *Psychotherapy Research, 25*(1), 6–19, corrigendum, iii. https://doi.org/10.1080/10503307.2013.817696

Branson, D. C. (2019). Vicarious trauma, themes in research, and terminology: A review of literature. *Traumatology, 25*(1), 2–10. https://doi.org/10.1037/trm0000161

Bride, B. E., Robinson, M. M., Yegidis, B., & Figley, C. R. (2004). Development and validation of the Secondary Traumatic Stress Scale. *Research on Social Work Practice, 14*(1), 27–35. https://doi.org/10.1177/1049731503254106

Cambridge Dictionary. (2011). *Cambridge business English dictionary.* Cambridge University Press.

Campbell, L., & Stanton, S. C. (2014). Actor–partner interdependence model. In R. L. Cautin & S. O. Lilienfeld (Eds.), *The encyclopedia of clinical psychology* (pp. 1–7). John Wiley & Sons.

Cieslak, R., Shoji, K., Douglas, A., Melville, E., Luszczynska, A., & Benight, C. C. (2014). A meta-analysis of the relationship between job burnout and secondary traumatic stress among workers with indirect exposure to trauma. *Psychological Services, 11*(1), 75–86. https://doi.org/10.1037/a0033798

Cohen, K., & Collens, P. (2013). The impact of trauma work on trauma workers: A metasynthesis on vicarious trauma and vicarious posttraumatic growth. *Psychological Trauma: Theory, Research, Practice, and Policy, 5*(6), 570–580. https://doi.org/10.1037/a0030388

Cook, W. L., & Kenny, D. A. (2005). The actor–partner interdependence model: A model of bidirectional effects in developmental studies. *International Journal of Behavioral Development, 29*(2), 101–109. https://doi.org/10.1080/01650250444000405

Degnan, A., Seymour-Hyde, A., Harris, A., & Berry, K. (2016). The role of therapist attachment in alliance and outcome: A systematic literature review. *Clinical Psychology & Psychotherapy, 23*(1), 47–65. https://doi.org/10.1002/cpp.1937

Duncan, B. L., & Miller, S. D. (2000). The client's theory of change: Consulting the client in the integrative process. *Journal of Psychotherapy Integration, 10*(2), 169–187. https://doi.org/10.1023/A:1009448200244

Duncan, B. L., Miller, S. D., & Sparks, J. A. (2011). *The heroic client: A revolutionary way to improve effectiveness through client-directed, outcome-informed therapy*. John Wiley & Sons.

Elias, H., & Haj-Yahia, M. M. (2019). On the lived experience of sex offenders' therapists: Their perceptions of intrapersonal and interpersonal consequences and patterns of coping. *Journal of Interpersonal Violence, 34*(4), 848–872. https://doi.org/10.1177/0886260516646090

Eubanks, C. F., Muran, J. C., & Safran, J. D. (2018). Alliance rupture repair: A meta-analysis. *Psychotherapy: Theory, Research, & Practice, 55*(4), 508–519. https://doi.org/10.1037/pst0000185

Farber, B. A. (2003). Patient self-disclosure: A review of the research. *Journal of Clinical Psychology, 59*(5), 589–600. https://doi.org/10.1002/jclp.10161

Finklestein, M., Stein, E., Greene, T., Bronstein, I., & Solomon, Z. (2015). Post-traumatic stress disorder and vicarious trauma in mental health professionals. *Health & Social Work, 40*(2), e25–e31. https://doi.org/10.1093/hsw/hlv026

Flückiger, C., Del Re, A. C., Wampold, B. E., & Horvath, A. O. (2018). The alliance in adult psychotherapy: A meta-analytic synthesis. *Psychotherapy: Theory, Research, & Practice, 55*(4), 316–340. https://doi.org/10.1037/pst0000172

Freud, S. (1958). Recommendations to physicians practicing psycho-analysis. In J. Strachey (Ed. & Trans.), *The standard edition of the complete psychological works of Sigmund Freud* (Vol. 12, pp. 109–120). Hogarth Press. (Original work published 1912)

Freud, S. (1959). Future prospects of psychoanalytic psychotherapy. In J. Strachey (Ed. & Trans.), *The standard edition of the complete psychological works of Sigmund Freud* (Vol. 11, pp. 139–151). Hogarth Press. (Original work published 1910)

Friedlander, M. L. (1993). Does complementarity promote or hinder client change in brief therapy? A review of the evidence from two theoretical perspectives. *The Counseling Psychologist, 21*(3), 457–486. https://doi.org/10.1177/0011000093213010

Fuertes, J. N., Moore, M. T., & Pagano-Stalzer, C. C. (2019). Consensus and collaboration in the working alliance. In J. N. Fuertes (Ed.), *Working alliance skills for mental health professionals* (pp. 91–110). Oxford University Press. https://doi.org/10.1093/med-psych/9780190868529.003.0005

Fuertes, J. N., & Williams, E. N. (2017). Client-focused psychotherapy research. *Journal of Counseling Psychology, 64*(4), 369–375. https://doi.org/10.1037/cou0000214

Gelso, C. J., & Hayes, J. A. (1998). *The psychotherapy relationship: Theory, research, and practice*. John Wiley & Sons.

Gelso, C. J., Kivlighan, D. M., Jr., Busa-Knepp, J., Spiegel, E. B., Ain, S., Hummel, A. M., Ma, Y. E., & Markin, R. D. (2012). The unfolding of the real relationship and the outcome of brief psychotherapy. *Journal of Counseling Psychology, 59*(4), 495–506. https://doi.org/10.1037/a0029838

Goldberg, S. B., Rousmaniere, T., Miller, S. D., Whipple, J., Nielsen, S. L., Hoyt, W. T., & Wampold, B. E. (2016). Do psychotherapists improve with time and experience? A longitudinal analysis of outcomes in a clinical setting. *Journal of Counseling Psychology, 63*(1), 1–11. https://doi.org/10.1037/cou0000131

Gross Doehrman, M. J. (1976). Parallel processes in supervision and psychotherapy. *Bulletin of the Menninger Clinic, 40*(1), 1–104.

Guy, J. D., & Liaboe, G. P. (1986). The impact of conducting psychotherapy on psychotherapists' interpersonal functioning. *Professional Psychology, Research and Practice, 17*(2), 111–114. https://doi.org/10.1037/0735-7028.17.2.111

Haley, J. (1963). *Strategies of psychotherapy*. Grune & Stratton. https://doi.org/10.1037/14324-000

Hannan, C., Lambert, M. J., Harmon, C., Nielsen, S. L., Smart, D. W., Shimokawa, K., & Sutton, S. W. (2005). A lab test and algorithms for identifying clients at risk for treatment failure. *Journal of Clinical Psychology, 61*(2), 155–163. https://doi.org/10.1002/jclp.20108

Hatcher, R., & Noakes, S. (2010). Working with sex offenders: The impact on Australian treatment providers. *Psychology, Crime & Law, 16*(1–2), 145–167. https://doi.org/10.1080/10683160802622030

Hatcher, R. L. (2015). Interpersonal competencies: Responsiveness, technique, and training in psychotherapy. *American Psychologist, 70*(8), 747–757. https://doi.org/10.1037/a0039803

Hatcher, S. L., Kipper-Smith, A., Waddell, M., Uhe, M., West, J. S., Boothe, J. H., . . . & Gingras, P. (2012). What therapists learn from psychotherapy clients: Effects on personal and professional lives. *Qualitative Report, 17*(48), 1–21. https://doi.org/10.46743/2160-3715/2012.1702

Hatfield, D., McCullough, L., Frantz, S. H., & Krieger, K. (2010). Do we know when our clients get worse? an investigation of therapists' ability to detect negative client change. *Clinical Psychology & Psychotherapy, 17*(1), 25–32. https://doi.org/10.1002/cpp.656

Hayes, J. A., Gelso, C. J., Goldberg, S., & Kivlighan, D. M. (2018). Countertransference management and effective psychotherapy: Meta-analytic findings. *Psychotherapy: Theory, Research, & Practice, 55*(4), 496–507. https://doi.org/10.1037/pst0000189

Hayes, J. A., Gelso, C. J., Kivlighan, D. M., & Goldberg, S. B. (2019). Managing countertransference. In J. Norcross and M. J. Lambert (Eds.), *Psychotherapy relationships that work. Vol. 1. Evidence-based therapist contribution* (pp. 533–547). Oxford University Press. https://doi.org/10.1093/med-psych/9780190843953.003.0015

Hayes, J. A., McCracken, J. E., McClanahan, M. K., Hill, C. E., Harp, J. S., & Carozzoni, P. (1998). Therapist perspectives on countertransference: Qualitative data in search of a theory. *Journal of Counseling Psychology, 45*(4), 468–482. https://doi.org/10.1037/0022-0167.45.4.468

Heinonen, E., & Nissen-Lie, H. A. (2020). The professional and personal characteristics of effective psychotherapists: A systematic review. *Psychotherapy Research, 30*(4), 417–432. https://doi.org/10.1080/10503307.2019.1620366

Howard, K. I., Moras, K., Brill, P. L., Martinovich, Z., & Lutz, W. (1996). Evaluation of psychotherapy. Efficacy, effectiveness, and patient progress. *American Psychologist, 51*(10), 1059–1064. https://doi.org/10.1037/0003-066X.51.10.1059

Kenny, D. A. (2018). Reflections on the actor–partner interdependence model. *Personal Relationships, 25*(2), 160–170. https://doi.org/10.1111/pere.12240

Kern, R. M., Belangee, S. E., & Eckstein, D. (2004). Early recollections: A guide for practitioners. *Journal of Individual Psychology, 60*(2), 132–140.

Kiesler, D. J. (2001). Therapist countertransference: In search of common themes and empirical referents. *Journal of Clinical Psychology, 57*(8), 1053–1063. https://doi.org/10.1002/jclp.1073

Kiesler, D. J., & Watkins, L. M. (1989). Interpersonal complementarity and the therapeutic alliance: A study of relationship in psychotherapy. *Psychotherapy: Theory, Research, & Practice, 26*(2), 183–194. https://doi.org/10.1037/h0085418

Kivlighan, D. M., Jr., Gelso, C. J., Ain, S., Hummel, A. M., & Markin, R. D. (2015). The therapist, the client, and the real relationship: An actor–partner interdependence analysis of treatment outcome. *Journal of Counseling Psychology, 62*(2), 314–320. https://doi.org/10.1037/cou0000012

Kivlighan, D. M., Jr., Hill, C. E., Gelso, C. J., & Baumann, E. (2016). Working alliance, real relationship, session quality, and client improvement in psychodynamic psychotherapy: A longitudinal actor partner interdependence model. *Journal of Counseling Psychology, 63*(2), 149–161. https://doi.org/10.1037/cou0000134

Kivlighan, D. M., Jr., Marmarosh, C. L., & Hilsenroth, M. J. (2014). Client and therapist therapeutic alliance, session evaluation, and client reliable change: A moderated actor–partner interdependence model. *Journal of Counseling Psychology, 61*(1), 15–23. https://doi.org/10.1037/a0034939

Kottler, J. A., & Hunter, S. V. (2010). Clients as teachers: Reciprocal influences in therapy relationships. *Australian and New Zealand Journal of Family Therapy, 31*(1), 4–12. https://doi.org/10.1375/anft.31.1.4

Ladany, N., Friedlander, M. L., & Nelson, M. L. (2016). *Supervision essentials for the critical events in psychotherapy supervision model.* American Psychological Association. https://doi.org/10.1037/14916-000

Lambert, M. J. (2013). Efficacy and effectiveness of psychotherapy. In M. J. Lambert (Ed.), *Bergin and Garfield's handbook of psychotherapy and behavior change* (6th ed., pp. 169–216). John Wiley & Sons.

Lambert, M. J., Whipple, J. L., & Kleinstäuber, M. (2018). Collecting and delivering progress feedback: A meta-analysis of routine outcome monitoring. *Psychotherapy: Theory, Research, & Practice, 55*(4), 520–537. https://doi.org/10.1037/pst0000167

Larsson, M. H., Björkman, K., Nilsson, K., Falkenström, F., & Holmqvist, R. (2019). The Alliance and Rupture Observation Scale (AROS): Development and validation of an alliance and rupture measure for repeated observations within psychotherapy sessions. *Journal of Clinical Psychology, 75*(3), 404–417. https://doi.org/10.1002/jclp.22704

Leary, T. (1957). *Interpersonal diagnosis of personality.* Ronald Press.

Leibert, T. W., Powell, R. N., & Fonseca, F. D. (2020). Client descriptions of outcomes compared with quantitative data: A mixed-methods investigation of a quantitative outcome measure. *Counselling & Psychotherapy Research, 20*(1), 9–18. https://doi.org/10.1002/capr.12260

Li, X., O'Connor, S., Kivlighan, D. M., Jr., & Hill, C. E. (2021). "Where is the relationship" revisited: Using actor–partner interdependence modeling and common fate model in examining dyadic working alliance and session quality. *Journal of Counseling Psychology, 68*(2), 194–207. https://doi.org/10.1037/cou0000515

Lichtenberg, J. W., Goodyear, R. K., Overland, E. A., & Hutman, H. B. (2014, March). *A snapshot of counseling psychology: Stability and change in the roles, identities and functions (2001–2014)* [Paper presentation]. Counseling Psychology National Conference, Atlanta, GA, United States.

Lichtenberg, J. W., & Hummel, T. J. (1976). Counseling as stochastic process: Fitting a Markov chain model to initial counseling interviews. *Journal of Counseling Psychology, 23*(4), 310–315. https://doi.org/10.1037/0022-0167.23.4.310

Lyon, A. R., Stanick, C., & Pullmann, M. D. (2018). Toward high-fidelity treatment as usual: Evidence-based intervention structures to improve usual care psychotherapy. *Clinical Psychology: Science and Practice, 25*(4), e12265. https://doi.org/10.1111/cpsp.12265

Miller, S. D., Duncan, B. L., Sorrell, R., & Brown, G. S. (2005). The Partners for Change Outcome Management System. *Journal of Clinical Psychology, 61*(2), 199–208. https://doi.org/10.1002/jclp.20111

Muir, H. J., Coyne, A. E., Morrison, N. R., Boswell, J. F., & Constantino, M. J. (2019). Ethical implications of routine outcomes monitoring for patients, psychotherapists, and mental health care systems. *Psychotherapy: Theory, Research, & Practice, 56*(4), 459–469. https://doi.org/10.1037/pst0000246

Najavits, L. M., & Strupp, H. H. (1994). Differences in the effectiveness of psychodynamic therapists: A process-outcome study. *Psychotherapy: Theory, Research, & Practice, 31*(1), 114–123. https://doi.org/10.1037/0033-3204.31.1.114

Nicholas, H., & Goodyear, R. K. (2021). Supervision of a sample of clinical and counselling psychologists in the UK: A descriptive study of their practices, processes and perceived benefits. *European Journal of Counselling Psychology*, *9*(1), 41–50. https://doi.org/10.46853/001c.22014

Nissen-Lie, H. A., Monsen, J. T., Ulleberg, P., & Rønnestad, M. H. (2013). Psychotherapists' self-reports of their interpersonal functioning and difficulties in practice as predictors of patient outcome. *Psychotherapy Research*, *23*(1), 86–104. https://doi.org/10.1080/10503307.2012.735775

Norcross, J. C. (2000). Psychotherapist self-care: Practitioner-tested, research-informed strategies. *Professional Psychology, Research and Practice*, *31*(6), 710–713. https://doi.org/10.1037/0735-7028.31.6.710

Norcross, J. C., & Wampold, B. E. (2018). A new therapy for each patient: Evidence-based relationships and responsiveness. *Journal of Clinical Psychology*, *74*(11), 1889–1906. https://doi.org/10.1002/jclp.22678

Okiishi, J., Lambert, M. J., Nielsen, S. L., & Ogles, B. M. (2003). Waiting for supershrink: An empirical analysis of therapist effects. *Clinical Psychology & Psychotherapy*, *10*(6), 361–373. https://doi.org/10.1002/cpp.383

Orlinsky, D. E., Botermans, J. F., & Rønnestad, M. H. (2001). Towards an empirically grounded model of psychotherapy training: Four thousand therapists rate influences on their development. *Australian Psychologist*, *36*(2), 139–148. https://doi.org/10.1080/00050060108259646

Owen, J., Tao, K. W., Imel, Z. E., Wampold, B. E., & Rodolfa, E. (2014). Addressing racial and ethnic microaggressions in therapy. *Professional Psychology, Research and Practice*, *45*(4), 283–290. https://doi.org/10.1037/a0037420

Pargament, K. I., Lomax, J. W., McGee, J. S., & Fang, Q. (2014). Sacred moments in psychotherapy from the perspectives of mental health providers and clients: Prevalence, predictors, and consequences. *Spirituality in Clinical Practice*, *1*(4), 248–262. https://doi.org/10.1037/scp0000043

Råbu, M., Moltu, C., Binder, P. E., & McLeod, J. (2016). How does practicing psychotherapy affect the personal life of the therapist? A qualitative inquiry of senior therapists' experiences. *Psychotherapy Research*, *26*(6), 737–749. https://doi.org/10.1080/10503307.2015.1065354

Ray, W. (2018). The Palo Alto group. In J. Lebow, A. Chambers, & D. Breunlin (Eds.), *Encyclopedia of couple and family therapy*. Springer International Publishing AG. https://doi.org/10.1007/978-3-319-15877-8_596-1

Rennie, D. L. (1994). Clients' deference in psychotherapy. *Journal of Counseling Psychology*, *41*(4), 427–437. https://doi.org/10.1037/0022-0167.41.4.427

Riessman, F. (1965). The "helper" therapy principle. *Social Work*, *10*(2), 27–32. https://doi.org/10.1093/sw/10.2.27

Robinson, N., Hill, C. E., & Kivlighan, D. M., Jr. (2015). Crying as communication in psychotherapy: The influence of client and therapist attachment dimensions and client attachment to therapist on amount and type of crying. *Journal of Counseling Psychology*, *62*(3), 379–392. https://doi.org/10.1037/cou0000090

Rogers, C. R. (1957). The necessary and sufficient conditions of therapeutic personality change. *Journal of Consulting Psychology*, *21*(2), 95–103. https://doi.org/10.1037/h0045357

Rønnestad, M. H., & Skovholt, T. M. (2003). The journey of the counselor and therapist: Research findings and perspectives on professional development. *Journal of Career Development*, *30*(1), 5–44. https://doi.org/10.1177/089484530303000102

Salazar Kämpf, M., Nestler, S., Hansmeier, J., Glombiewski, J., & Exner, C. (2021). Mimicry in psychotherapy—An actor partner model of therapists' and patients' non-verbal behavior and its effects on the working alliance. *Psychotherapy Research*, *31*(6), 752–764. https://doi.org/10.1080/10503307.2020.1849849

Schauben, L. J., & Frazier, P. A. (1995). Vicarious trauma the effects on female counselors of working with sexual violence survivors. *Psychology of Women Quarterly, 19*(1), 49–64. https://doi.org/10.1111/j.1471-6402.1995.tb00278.x

Skovholt, T. M. (1974). The client as helper: A means to promote psychological growth. *The Counseling Psychologist, 4*(3), 58–64. https://doi.org/10.1177/001100007400400308

Skovholt, T. M., & Rønnestad, M. H. (1992). Themes in therapist and counselor development. *Journal of Counseling and Development, 70*(4), 505–515. https://doi.org/10.1002/j.1556-6676.1992.tb01646.x

Stratford, T., Lal, S., & Meara, A. (2012). Neuroanalysis of therapeutic alliance in the symptomatically anxious: The physiological connection revealed between therapist and client. *American Journal of Psychotherapy, 66*(1), 1–21. https://doi.org/10.1176/appi.psychotherapy.2012.66.1.1

Strong, S. R., & Hills, H. I. (1986). *Interpersonal Communication Rating Scale.* Virginia Commonwealth University.

Sullivan, H. S. (1953). *The interpersonal theory of psychiatry.* Norton.

Svartberg, M., & Stiles, T. C. (1992). Predicting patient change from therapist competence and patient-therapist complementarity in short-term anxiety-provoking psychotherapy: A pilot study. *Journal of Consulting and Clinical Psychology, 60*(2), 304–307. https://doi.org/10.1037/0022-006X.60.2.304

Swift, J. K., Callahan, J. L., Rousmaniere, T. G., Whipple, J. L., Dexter, K., & Wrape, E. R. (2015). Using client outcome monitoring as a tool for supervision. *Psychotherapy: Theory, Research, & Practice, 52*(2), 180–184. https://doi.org/10.1037/a0037659

Swift, J. K., & Parkin, S. R. (2017). The client as the expert in psychotherapy: What clinicians and researchers can learn about treatment processes and outcomes from psychotherapy clients. *Journal of Clinical Psychology, 73*(11), 1486–1488. https://doi.org/10.1002/jclp.22528

Swift, J. K., Tompkins, K. A., & Parkin, S. R. (2017). Understanding the client's perspective of helpful and hindering events in psychotherapy sessions: A micro-process approach. *Journal of Clinical Psychology, 73*(11), 1543–1555. https://doi.org/10.1002/jclp.22531

Tishby, O., & Wiseman, H. (2020). Countertransference types and their relation to rupture and repair in the alliance. *Psychotherapy Research.* Advance online publication. https://doi.org/10.1080/10503307.2020.1862934

Tracey, T. J. (1994). An examination of the complementarity of interpersonal behavior. *Journal of Personality and Social Psychology, 67*(5), 864–878. https://doi.org/10.1037/0022-3514.67.5.864

Tracey, T. J. (2004). Levels of interpersonal complementarity: A simplex representation. *Personality and Social Psychology Bulletin, 30*(9), 1211–1225. https://doi.org/10.1177/0146167204264075

Tracey, T. J. G., Bludworth, J., & Glidden-Tracey, C. E. (2012). Are there parallel processes in psychotherapy supervision? An empirical examination. *Psychotherapy: Theory, Research, & Practice, 49*(3), 330–343. https://doi.org/10.1037/a0026246

Tschacher, W., & Meier, D. (2020). Physiological synchrony in psychotherapy sessions. *Psychotherapy Research, 30*(5), 558–573. https://doi.org/10.1080/10503307.2019.1612114

Wampold, B. E. (2015). How important are the common factors in psychotherapy? An update. *World Psychiatry, 14*(3), 270–277. https://doi.org/10.1002/wps.20238

Wampold, B. E., & Imel, Z. E. (2015). *The great psychotherapy debate: The evidence for what makes psychotherapy work.* Routledge. https://doi.org/10.4324/9780203582015

Watzlawick, P., Bavelas, J. B., & Jackson, D. D. (2011). *Pragmatics of human communication: A study of interactional patterns, pathologies and paradoxes.* W. W. Norton & Company.

Weitkamp, K., Daniels, J. K., & Klasen, F. (2014). Psychometric properties of the Questionnaire for Secondary Traumatization. *European Journal of Psychotraumatology, 5*(1), 21875. https://doi.org/10.3402/ejpt.v5.21875

Wiggins, J. S. (1996). An informal history of the interpersonal circumplex tradition. *Journal of Personality Assessment, 66*(2), 217–233. https://doi.org/10.1207/s15327752jpa6602_2

Zilcha-Mano, S., Muran, J. C., Hungr, C., Eubanks, C. F., Safran, J. D., & Winston, A. (2016). The relationship between alliance and outcome: Analysis of a two-person perspective on alliance and session outcome. *Journal of Consulting and Clinical Psychology, 84*(6), 484–496. https://doi.org/10.1037/ccp0000058

11

Clients' Own Perspectives on Psychotherapy Outcomes and Their Mechanisms

Michael J. Constantino, Averi N. Gaines, and Alice E. Coyne

Having read, lauded, and concurred with Fuertes and Williams's (2017) call for more client-focused psychotherapy research, we eagerly agreed to contribute this chapter on clients' own views of psychosocial treatment outcomes and their mechanisms. That said, we also appreciated the inherent challenge in identifying this chapter's unique and complementary scope within the overall volume. In its broadest sense, client-focused psychotherapy research could conceivably cover any outcome construct or variable that pertains to the client (whether defined by researchers, therapists, or clients), with data collected in any number of ways. After having recently contributed a comprehensive review of the research on the client, therapist, and relational factors to *Bergin and Garfield's Handbook of Psychotherapy and Behavior Change* (seventh ed.; Constantino, Boswell, & Coyne, 2021), we were acutely aware of how vast and unwieldy a review of "all things client related" could get!

However, to us, truly client-focused outcome research requires more than an examination of any inherently client-related factors that change or predict change. Rather, such research needs to explicitly draw out and privilege the client's voice or narrative to understand these primary outcome-related elements. To draw on McLeod et al.'s (2009) rubric of stakeholder positions, such focus reflects user-constructed outcomes and their mechanisms, as opposed to researcher- or therapist-constructed outcomes and mechanisms. Accordingly, we discuss herein research that has, in both content and method, directly asked adult clients (this age criterion is consistent with the volume's overall

https://doi.org/10.1037/0000303-012
The Other Side of Psychotherapy: Understanding Clients' Experiences and Contributions in Treatment, J. N. Fuertes (Editor)

focus) about their outlook before therapy, and/or their experiences during or after therapy, with the data produced clearly reflecting the client's agentically expressed internal frame of reference. Thus, we excluded studies (of which many exist) in which clients were solely asked to complete standardized, non-personalized outcome or outcome predictor measures. Although pertinent in that the client does the rating (in a way that presumably conveys their internal experience), these measures, arguably, privilege the researchers and/or the therapists' vantage points on what connotes good or poor outcomes and the mechanisms that influence them.

Accordingly, in this review, we spotlight clients' voices as the most important, as they are the consumers of mental health services and the ultimate arbiters of their utility. Moreover, we believe one could readily argue that these stakeholders' vantage point has been understudied and even undervalued in the history of psychotherapy research, theory, and training (Constantino, Morrison, et al., 2017; Heatherington et al., 2012; Hill et al., 2013; Valkonen et al., 2011). Therefore, we agree with Fuertes and Williams (2017) that "it seems valuable and potentially revealing to involve clients more directly and to make their perspective a primary lens by which process and outcome are examined. This can be achieved by asking clients directly about their experiences in psychotherapy" (p. 370). In many ways, this approach may lend itself best to qualitative methods, which is borne out in our following review. However, we also considered pertinent any quantitative approaches for which the data emanated from measures that clients notably shaped or from the coding of clients' unconstrained utterances or responses in a way that allowed for inferential statistics.

To further contextualize our present work, we can extend Fuertes and Williams's (2017) gym analogy, in which they referred to the therapist as a psychological trainer who works in a psychological gym—allowing the client to engage in a psychological workout. For our chapter, the key notion is that the client has the most important view on what they are trying to accomplish with their workouts, which needs to be honored (as opposed to simply accepting the idea that all workouts are aimed toward the same goal, whether it is strength-building, weight loss, and/or something else, for every person). Understandably, people use the gym in different ways and may expect, value, or prefer different things from their trainer. Hence, we can learn something about positive, neutral, and negative "workout" results (and determinants of them) by not only listening to the trainers and fitness gurus but also (and, perhaps, especially) to those engaging in the workout. This is the current review's unique focus (for which the research base remains relatively small but growing). It complements the other chapters in this volume, which center more broadly on client factors (with research initiated from various stakeholder positions) in therapy processes and outcomes (e.g., motivation, attachment) or on client–therapist interactions (e.g., clients' experience of the therapeutic relationship or a client's impact on their therapist).

In this vein, we cover three main areas, highlighting practice implications across all of them. First, we review research on clients' forward-looking perspectives on psychotherapy outcomes and/or their mechanisms, with such inquiry generally occurring before treatment (either a given course of treatment or, in some cases, before having ever experienced therapy). Second, we review research on clients' own operationalizations of acute and long-term psychotherapy outcomes (both positive and negative) as they engage in or look back on their treatment. Third, we review research on clients' own views on what contributes or contributed to their outcomes as they engage in or look back on their treatment, respectively. Importantly, we note that our review is not comprehensive. Rather, we highlight prominent examples of outcome-related research that is client stakeholder-centered in the sense that clients' outcome-related perspectives take center stage, produced from methods that allowed for agentic expression. Following the research review, we propose several future research directions and designs, discuss several teaching and training implications based on the current literature, and offer several summative concluding thoughts.

CLIENTS' FORWARD-LOOKING PSYCHOTHERAPY OUTCOME PERSPECTIVES

Unsurprisingly, clients arrive to therapy with their own ideas about it (Lloyd et al., 2019). Most relevant here is that clients likely have some idea about the outcomes they hope a course of therapy will influence and the ways in which such change can occur during their time in therapy. Although such research on clients' forward-looking perspectives on outcomes and their mechanisms remains rather limited, we provide some examples of both research threads.

How Do Clients Prospectively Operationalize Outcomes?

As previously noted, few studies have prospectively explored clients' freely generated operationalizations of outcome prior to the start of therapy. More commonly, studies have asked clients to retrospectively reflect on their pretherapy beliefs (including those related to outcomes) after they have initiated or completed treatment (e.g., De Smet et al., 2019), often in the service of illuminating confirmed or disconfirmed expectations. Such studies, some of which we review later, may not only suffer from the typical biases associated with retrospective recall but may also provide different information than truly prospective studies, given that clients' therapy perspectives can be shaped by the therapist or treatment (e.g., Rennie, 1994). Therefore, consistent with the main sections of this chapter, we separately review the results of studies that examined client outcome operationalizations at pretherapy versus during or after therapy.

Most pretherapy research in this area has focused on developing or employing idiographic quantitative measures of clients' freely defined treatment targets and problems or goals and objectives (Lloyd et al., 2019). Regarding targets and problems, one of the oldest and most well-known of these measures is the Target Complaints assessment, which relies on a clinical interview in which clients are asked to autonomously identify three issues they would like to address via therapy (Battle et al., 1966). Clients and therapists are typically both asked to rate the significance of the complaints and then rate improvement on them at some point during and/or after therapy. Other target/problem-focused measures tend to follow relatively similar procedures (e.g., Ashworth et al., 2005; Elliott et al., 2016). Regarding goals and objectives, a recent systematic review identified nine different idiographic measures (Lloyd et al., 2019). Of these, the most widely used is Goal Attainment Scaling (Kiresuk & Sherman, 1968; Kiresuk et al., 1994), which involves the guided (usually by a therapist) identification of a focal therapy issue, setting at least three goals with specific indicators (behavioral, affective, skill, or process), and, for each goal, defining expected, better-than-expected, and worse-than-expected posttreatment outcomes.

Although these personalized measures have much potential for revealing clients' pretherapy outcome definitions, researchers have more typically used them to quantify client improvement in an aggregated sense. That is, the scores generally inform global change indices, with little systematic focus on the thematic content of these forward-looking client perspectives. As notable exceptions, one study validated a simplified version of the Target Complaints assessment in a sample of 138 clients referred for cognitive behavior therapy (Deane et al., 1997). In doing so, the authors categorized the complaints, the most common of which were specific symptoms (e.g., anxiety, eating problems, depression), self-concept, general stress, career or life decisions, and interpersonal or family problems. Similarly, another study of 118 clients who were given a checklist of goal statements found that clients most commonly endorsed symptom or problem reductions, personal growth, existential clarity, improved well-being or functioning, and improved interpersonal relating (Ramnerö & Jansson, 2016).

In sum, research on how clients prospectively operationalize outcomes is in its relative infancy. At present, the most robust clinical implication is at the case level. That is, integrating ideographic measurement from baseline through treatment can be helpful in tracking clients' progress on personalized therapy foci (Lloyd et al., 2019). Regarding research implications, it is clear that more research is especially needed to understand explicit, generalizable themes in how clients prospectively define their own positive and negative psychotherapy outcomes, free from researcher-defined categories. It may be that these perspectives will largely align with researcher or therapist perspectives (e.g., a focus on symptom reduction), though nuanced differences could emerge that would bear importantly on case conceptualization, treatment selections, and therapist attunement to clients' own beliefs (looking forward) as to what would connote a successful or unsuccessful (or even harmful) course of treatment. With a better understanding of such client-generated nuances, for which more qualitative assessment is needed to complement measures such as the aforementioned Target Complaints Assessment and Goal Attainment Scaling, it is plausible that the field could improve upon outcome tracking, feedback, and related therapist responsiveness.

How Do Clients Prospectively Operationalize Outcome Mechanisms?

The most prominent focus in this limited research area is on what clients expect to work on in therapy. How patients conceptualize, or "story," their presenting problems prior to treatment can illuminate, at least indirectly, their expectations for what general treatment processes or foci will facilitate improvement in their personally pertinent mental health concerns. From this framework, one study included baseline interviews with 14 depressed clients who would ultimately be randomized to either short-term solution-focused therapy or long-term psychodynamic psychotherapy for depression (Valkonen et al., 2011). Thematic analyses of client responses revealed three main stories representing how they understood their pathology. First, some attributed their depression to historical and often traumatic life events (even if not immediately recalled), and they expected that therapy would need to address these events for recovery to occur. Second, some attributed their depression to their current life situation, viewing it to be a natural part of life. These clients expected that therapy would need to help them build resources to better cope with these normative (though, currently, more distressing than usual) mood issues. Third, other clients attributed their depression to the moral order, feeling as though they had fallen short of cultural standards for a good life. To recover, these clients expected that therapy would need to help them find culturally acceptable meaning and goals in their life.

These results indicate that people meeting diagnostic criteria for the same problem can, nonetheless, frame that problem differently and have diverse ideas about what therapy needs to accomplish in order to be successful. Clinically, this points to the importance of learning each client's story before assuming that one specific, or any general, therapy will benefit them. As Valkonen et al. (2011) astutely noted, "Persons are not a tabula rasa when they enter therapy (e.g., Miller, 2004). Nor are the outcomes of therapy drawn on a blank sheet of paper" (p. 238). Rather, clients have an inner narrative that might help in selecting a treatment frame and corresponding principles that align with this personal narrative.

Notably, Valkonen et al. (2011) also conducted posttreatment interviews with their sample, which allowed them to qualitatively examine whether the alignment of therapy approach to the presenting-problem story mattered for these clients' outcomes. Generally, such convergence was adaptive; long-term psychodynamic psychotherapy most notably helped address the life-history story, solution-focused therapy most notably addressed the current-situation story, and neither treatment was a particularly good fit to the moral story. Hence, these findings support the general benefits of pretreatment storying for treatment selection. That said, there were exceptions to these "match" results. In some cases, it appeared that a discrepancy between one's baseline narrative and the treatment they received was beneficial, predominantly in helping clients formulate a new story about themselves and their depression (unexpected outcome). These findings are consistent with other client-focused work (including for problems other than depression) that indicates the helpfulness of unmet expectancies in therapy processes or mechanisms (e.g., Nilsson et al., 2007; Westra et al., 2010) or self-narrative changes in the forms of unexpected outcome and discovery-oriented storytelling (e.g., Boritz et al., 2017; Carpenter et al., 2016; Khattra et al., 2017). Hence, before the clinical implications can be fully actionable, much more research is needed on the benefits of, strategies for, and potential moderators of matching treatment frameworks to clients' problem narratives and corresponding expectations for outcome-enhancing mechanisms. That said, the extant research indicates that we can have some current confidence that clients' narratives have a meaningful bearing on treatment processes and outcomes. Clinicians should be asking about and validating such narratives to be optimally collaborative, responsive, and client-focused in their work.

Clients can also express their prospective expectations for what specific treatment processes will work in psychotherapy. Although research in this area remains limited, some studies have addressed such expectancies both qualitatively and quantitatively. In one quantitative study of 381 participants (some of whom did or did not have prior therapy experience), the researchers reported on the psychometrics of a novel measure assessing clients' conceptualizations of theory-based active therapeutic ingredients—the Expectations of Active Processes in Psychotherapy Scale (EAPPS; Tzur Bitan et al., 2018). Through this work, clients' ideas did not necessarily map tightly onto our profession's theoretically well-established change constructs such as insight, hope, and transference management/interpretation. Rather, they identified the following treatment ingredients: experiencing positive client–therapist relations, processing the therapy relationship verbally, exploring previously unexpressed material, sharing personal material openly and safely, working through challenging emotions, fostering resilience, and providing tools for cognitive control.

A follow-up study (Tzur Bitan & Lazar, 2019) used both qualitative and quantitative methods to examine, respectively, a different sample of 174 participants' (again, some of whom did or did not have prior therapy experience) open expectations of therapy change mechanisms and their rank-ordering of the importance of the seven mechanisms of the EAPPS (Tzur Bitan et al., 2018). Qualitative analysis revealed some themes that were consistent with the seven EAPPS themes (e.g., exploring previously unexpressed material), whereas others were more novel (e.g., the client's belief in oneself or motivation to change). The most frequent theme was that clients expected therapy to work through emotional and verbal expressions during sessions. The quantitative analyses indicated that the ability to share personal material openly and safely was the highest ranked EAPPS-assessed mechanism expected to foster improvement (with the mean rank being significantly greater than five other factors). The second most important expected change mechanism (providing tools for cognitive control) was the only other one to be ranked significantly higher than any others (three in this case). Although there were no differences in rankings between participants who did or did not have therapy experience, younger individuals ranked exploring previously unexpressed material as being more important than older individuals (an important nod to examining moderators in client-focused research, as is necessarily done in other psychotherapy research methods).

Finally, Tzur Bitan and Lazar (2019) spotlighted that none of the top three perceived change mechanisms were related to the therapeutic relationship, despite this construct being rather ingrained in our field's consciousness of what drives therapeutic change. Obviously, although this does not render the construct of the alliance unimportant (as clients still point to elements of the relationship as being contributors to outcome), a perspective on change that integrates the client's internal frame of reference may somewhat deemphasize the relationship in terms of our most common definition of agreement on tasks or goals and bond (Bordin, 1979). Rather, an integrated perspective might emphasize the cultivation of a space where clients can emotionally, verbally, and safely express themselves (including their most sensitive narratives). Although this may still imply relational conditions, it is a slight, though potentially meaningful, deviation from our more typically accepted alliance aspects of collaborative working and emotional bonding.

Such deviation is consistent with another study in which the same research team examined differences in the importance of perceived change mechanisms among therapists ($n = 107$), clients ($n = 97$), and laypersons with no therapy experience ($n = 160$; Tzur Bitan & Abayed, 2020). In brief, and consistent with the alliance discussion earlier, therapists rated the alliance more highly than did clients and laypersons. Conversely, clients and laypersons rated cognitive and emotional reconstruction more highly than did therapists. Additionally, therapists, more than the other two groups, expected the exploration of unconscious material to be helpful, whereas the other two groups, more than therapists, expected cognitive control to be a driver of change.

Although research on the question of what clients prospectively expect to work in therapy (outcome mechanisms) remains in relative infancy, the themes that have emerged (including in a rigorous series of studies that integrated both qualitative and quantitative inquiry) can give us some growing confidence in how clients view change ingredients. At present, it seems that professionals can be pleased in that clients do express mechanisms in ways that are near to, or even overlapping with, some of the field's established ideas. Yet, professionals can also be humbled in that clients' ideas can add nuance and even challenge some existing ideas on the relative importance or established definitions of varied change mechanisms. In practice, then, such client-focused research is beginning to inform how therapists should behave to optimize the chance of meaningful client change as perceived by their clients themselves. As the research base grows, clinicians can prioritize such mechanisms or at least include them alongside other evidence-based actions deriving from other types of research.

CLIENTS' DURING- AND/OR POSTTREATMENT PERSPECTIVES ON PSYCHOTHERAPY OUTCOMES

In addition to having their own understanding of psychotherapy outcomes as they consider or arrive at treatment, clients also have their own ideas about outcomes as they participate in therapy or look back on it, which may or may not align with our field's theory-driven change concepts. To the extent that the notion of a treatment outcome is based on socially constructed knowledge (McLeod, 2001), the existence of such definitional plurality makes sense. In this vein, some research has focused on what clients "freely" consider to be good or poor outcomes when largely unencumbered by existing scholarly definitions. Other research has attempted to ascertain clients' take (user-constructed) on existing theoretical or scholarly (researcher- or therapist-constructed) outcome concepts. In this section, we provide some examples of both types of inquiry.

How Do Clients Freely Operationalize Treatment Outcomes?

In this section, we review prominent examples of studies that had a primary goal of understanding what clients autonomously consider to be good or positive or poor or negative outcomes. Regarding positive outcomes, a qualitative metasynthesis of 37 studies focused on clients' experiences in psychotherapies for depression. The following core outcome domains emerged: symptom improvement or reduction, improvement in relationships, increased empowerment, increased coping skills, and improvement in self-esteem or self-acceptance (McPherson et al., 2020). Similarly, in a mixed-methods study of 47 clients who were empirically classified (on a standard researcher-established measure) as having had a "good outcome" following cognitive behavior therapy or psychodynamic psychotherapy for depression, posttreatment interviews revealed that a client-defined good outcome included the core domains of empowerment (e.g., increased self-confidence, emancipation, coping skills) and finding a personal balance (e.g., increased insight or self-understanding, improvement in relationships, feeling calmer; De Smet, Meganck, De Geest, et al., 2020).

These themes have also largely been replicated in more heterogeneous client samples. For example, in a study of 10 clients with diverse presenting problems whose therapist classified them as having had a positive outcome after systemic therapy, the clients themselves endorsed positive outcome themes of improvement in self-esteem or self-confidence, boundary-setting or self-differentiation, resetting goals or directions in life, and changing or repairing relationships (Dourdouma et al., 2020). Similarly, in a sample of 17 former psychotherapy clients with diverse presenting problems, the most commonly identified positive outcome domains were interpersonal change, intrapersonal change, emotional change, and improved quality of life (Olivera et al., 2013). In a mixed-methods study of 17 clients who had reliably improved, deteriorated, or did not change after counseling, the authors identified the following categories of adaptive change: interpersonal (i.e., increased assertiveness and sociability), cognitive and behavioral (i.e., insight, realistic thinking, and self-regulation), affective change (i.e., less negative affect and more determination), and attitude change (i.e., increased acceptance of self and others; Leibert et al., 2020). Additionally, clients highlighted variable degrees of improvement in their self-confidence, happiness, and presenting problems, suggesting that these domains also represented valued (though not always achieved) components of a positive outcome (Leibert et al., 2020). Finally, in a sample of 16 clients who experienced standardized measurement-driven reliable improvement and were interviewed at termination and a long-term follow-up, they identified diverse positive outcomes. The most commonly endorsed outcomes included role engagement, cognitive changes (e.g., more understanding), affective change, enhanced autonomy, catharsis or relief, empowerment, and symptom reduction (Ekroll & Rønnestad, 2017).

Although client-focused definitions of a "poor outcome" are sometimes conflated with unhelpful experiences in therapy (an area reviewed later), they are conceptually distinct in that such negative outcomes are often the result of unhelpful experiences (or the lack of helpful ones). In the aforementioned qualitative metasynthesis of client experiences in psychotherapies for depression, client-endorsed negative outcomes included a lack of improvement in important contextual factors (e.g., family, social, health problems) and, specific to cognitive behavior therapy, a sense that therapy had not explored the causes of their depression (McPherson et al., 2020). Specific to studies that interviewed clients at a long-term follow-up to acute treatment, clients also described poor outcomes to be the loss of motivation to practice skills after treatment ended (especially in cognitive behavior therapy), a low sense of self-efficacy or control, feelings of loss or loneliness (specific to ending group therapy), and some persistence or return of symptoms or problems (McPherson et al., 2020).

In this area of client-focused research on poor outcomes, individual studies have commonly interviewed clients who failed to benefit from treatment (based on a variety of researcher-derived metrics). For example, in a study of 19 empirically nonimproved clients who received cognitive behavior therapy or PDT for depression, the authors identified an overall theme of clients feeling "stuck between knowing vs. doing" (De Smet et al., 2019, p. 7) or a sense of understanding the problem but feeling unable to change it (De Smet et al., 2019). Similarly, in a study of 20 patients who empirically deteriorated or did not improve after psychoanalytic therapy, the clients described a clear theme of "spinning one's wheels" (Werbart et al., 2015, p. 551). They also indicated that their core problems (not specified) remained unchanged and that their emotional well-being had deteriorated (Werbart et al., 2015). Another study of eight empirically nonimproved clients found that they tended to blame themselves for not improving, often believing they were too broken to be helped (Radcliffe et al., 2018). Other themes included a sense that they had to "make do" with what they could achieve, but they were unable to change the problems that were most important to them.

Although research on client operationalizations of their therapy outcomes has disproportionally focused on certain clinical presentations (e.g., depression), the volume and partial replicability of findings render it at least moderately established. Moreover, with depression being a common primary and comorbid presenting issue, we have moderate-to-high confidence in the emergent themes being generalizable to many clients. Regarding client-defined positive outcomes, studies have consistently pointed to primary symptom improvement or reduction, improved relationships, increased empowerment, enhanced agency or self-efficacy and confidence in coping skills or abilities, enhanced self-esteem or self-concept, and improved general functioning or well-being and quality of life. In contrast, client-defined poor or negative outcomes centered around a feeling of being stuck, a sense of low self-efficacy or even self-blame or indictment, and a simple lack of improvement on key problems or goals.

Clinically, these findings have several implications. First, in terms of good news, they suggest that, when freely asked, clients describe many of the same outcomes that were identified during the Society for Psychotherapy Research and the American Psychological Association's Core Battery Conference (Horowitz et al., 1997), such as general and domain-specific symptoms or distress, role functioning, and interpersonal functioning. However, the results also suggest that several client-valued outcomes may currently be absent from our field's typical assessment batteries. Namely, clients consistently valued improvements in what may be considered more classically social–psychological variables, such as empowerment, agency or self-efficacy, and improvements in self-esteem and self-concept. Therefore, if therapists and researchers wish to capture client-centered outcomes, they could incorporate well-validated social psychological measures, such as the Self-Liking/Self-Competence scale—a multidimensional measure of self-esteem (Tafarodi & Swann, 2001). Additionally, to the extent that some forms of psychotherapy may place relatively less emphasis on helping clients achieve self-growth or positive psychology outcomes (compared to reducing symptoms/problems), therapists may wish to seek additional training on specific growth-focused strategies or interventions (e.g., Guindon, 2010).

Second, despite the apparent overlap between client-defined outcomes and those that might be included in core outcome batteries, clients' definitions of these constructs sometimes differ from what is typically captured by existing measures. For example, although clients identified improvement in relationships as an important outcome, their operationalization seemed to be more about developing satisfying levels of intimacy and boundaries than about reducing one's interpersonal distress or the excesses and inhibitions captured by commonly used interpersonal outcome measures, such as the Inventory of Interpersonal Problems (Horowitz et al., 1988). In other words, when assessing client goals or targets, the extant research base suggests that we should not assume that clients' definitions of familiar-sounding constructs map onto our existing theories and measures. The results also point to the need to integrate measures from other disciplines (or even develop new measures) in order to adequately capture the outcomes that clients most value from their own internal narrative or frame of reference. For example, it seems pertinent for clinicians to assess clients' felt levels of agency or empowerment, personal balance, and enhanced elements of one's self-concept.

Finally, with specific regard to client-defined negative outcomes, the results suggest that therapists may wish to pay particular attention to clients' reports of feeling "stuck," as such feelings could represent a risk factor for varied poor outcomes. Additionally, therapists may also wish to closely attend to low or lowered self-efficacy, as this appears to be a common way that clients experience poor outcomes. Relatedly, given the unfortunate reality that not all outcomes will be positive, in cases where therapists notice that treatment may not be going well, it seems possible that simply helping clients recognize that they are not at fault for treatment failures could be one means for forestalling some of the worst outcomes that clients themselves identified.

Corrective Experiences: What Do Clients Say Gets Corrected?

As stated, we can also ask clients to help shape or refine how we understand existing concepts of change, including those that have persisted in the literature for some time. For example, theorists and clinicians have long discussed the pantheoretical concept of *corrective experience* (CE) in psychotherapy (Alexander & French, 1946; Wallerstein, 1990). Although varied definitions exist in the professional literature, most can be subsumed under the general idea of clients coming to understand or experience something (be it a relationship, event, or set of experiences) in a novel, unexpected, and often transformative manner (Castonguay & Hill, 2012). In this sense, theory highlights that CEs are more than positive or helpful occurrences in therapy; rather, they need to reach a level of being momentous vis-à-vis one's psychological functioning (Heatherington et al., 2012). That said, CE scholarship has historically failed to account for clients' own ideas about the construct and whether such conceptions would cohere with existing theory. As Heatherington and colleagues (2012) stated, "This lack is notable considering that CEs ultimately belong to the client and that a client's subjective sense of what is corrective represents a unique vantage point on therapy process and outcome" (p. 161). Embedded in this passage is the notion that CEs involve two elements—what it is that gets corrected (what we will refer to as a *CE outcome*) and those things that are corrective in that they contribute to the change (what we will refer to as a *CE mechanism*; Constantino & Westra, 2012). Most pertinent to this section, clients can help illuminate what gets corrected, revised, or transformed when engaging in mental health treatment—CE outcomes. (Note that later we discuss clients' perceptions of CE mechanisms.)

Addressing the aforementioned gap, Heatherington et al. (2012) conducted one of the first empirical analyses of clients' subjective, during-treatment perceptions of CEs. Across five diverse sites (including three university training clinics, one community mental health center, and one hospital-based practice),

76 clients completed a brief, open-ended questionnaire following one or more of their sessions (while still actively engaged in their current course of treatment). Participants were asked to describe in vivid detail any times since they began therapy when they became aware of an important or meaningful change, or changes, in their thinking, feeling, behavior, or relationships. Grounded theory analysis (Strauss & Corbin, 1990) of client responses indicated two major CE outcome themes. First, clients described having gained new experiential awareness of etiologic factors for their presenting problems. Second, they described having gained new cognitive perspectives on both their adaptive and maladaptive functioning. Thus, preliminarily at least, clients who were still actively engaged in treatment (in different contexts with therapists who had varied experience levels and theoretical backgrounds) expressed that their most transformative shifts came in the form of seeing their mental health problems in a novel light and better appreciating, at a cognitive level, aspects of functioning that benefit or detract from their well-being.

Complementing Heatherington et al.'s (2012) focus on clients' postsession CE accounts, a subsequent series of qualitative studies examined such accounts after clients' therapy had ended. Hypothesizing that it could be challenging for clients to fully understand or articulate CE outcomes that are still in progress, these studies employed a uniform posttreatment semistructured interview protocol (namely, the Patients' Perceptions of Corrective Experiences in Individual Therapy [PPCEIT]; see Constantino & Angus, 2017) to investigate CEs at a time when clients might be better equipped to reflect on, appreciate, and express them. Once again reflecting diverse clinical samples, cultural settings, and treatment types, one study involved interviews with 14 clients who received naturalistic psychotherapy in a training clinic located in the northeastern part of the United States (Constantino, Morrison, et al., 2017). A second study included interviews with eight clients who received naturalistic psychotherapy in Buenos Aires, Argentina (Roussos et al., 2017). A third study included interviews with eight clients with generalized anxiety disorder (GAD) who received cognitive behavior therapy with motivational interviewing responsively integrated to address a client's resistances (Macaulay et al., 2017). These treatments took place in Toronto, Ontario, Canada. Finally, in a fourth study, researchers interviewed 10 therapists who had recently completed their own psychoanalysis in Vienna, Austria (Moertl et al., 2017). Such treatment was a mandatory element of their training, and they completed the PPCEIT interview in this client role.

Summarizing the results—again, focusing on CE outcomes (what clients said got corrected)—clients in both the Roussos et al. (2017) and Moertl et al. (2017) samples highlighted having a new, positive experience of self (as we will discuss in more detail the CE mechanisms sections, this self-concept of "correction" was attributed to elements of the therapeutic relationship). Across all four studies in the series, clients also discussed other CE outcomes, such as new experiential awareness, a new understanding of problematic patterns, increased emotional openness, and increased relational effectiveness (e.g., being more adaptively connected to and assertive with others). Perhaps, unsurprisingly, participants in the GAD study discussed CE outcomes in relation to worry; namely, they expressed a heightened ability to tolerate and regulate difficult feelings, as well as having more agency over, versus being controlled by, the worry process (Macaulay et al., 2017). Notably, patients in Roussos et al.'s (2017) study, who had more diverse problems and treatments than GAD, also indicated having similar outcomes of increased agency, self-acceptance, and negative affect tolerance, as well as decreased symptoms of depression and anxiety. As a connecting CE outcome thread, many of the PPCEIT interview clients alluded to being better able to keep their psychological problems at bay (in contrast to prior experiences of feeling helpless to combat them), which resulted in a more empowered and hopeful self-conception (Angus & Constantino, 2017).

In terms of generalizability, it seems important to note that some of the CE outcome themes that emerged in the PPCEIT interview studies also converged with other qualitative posttreatment interview studies that endeavored to examine CEs. For example, in both a case study of short-term dynamic psychotherapy (Friedlander et al., 2012) and a small sample study of clients who were also therapists-in-training (Knox et al., 2012), adaptive shifts in self and self–other relations also emerged as key perceptions of what got corrected through therapy. With this modest burst of diverse and rigorous qualitative studies that focused on clients' own accounts of CEs, it is, arguably, safe to consider this circumscribed research base as being at least moderately established, and we have moderate-to-high confidence in the emergent themes.

Consequently, one straightforward practice implication is that therapists should make room for clients' ideas of CE outcomes. Assimilating the client vantage point into case formulations and treatment planning (especially when the goal is to cultivate CEs) can help therapists compellingly align the goals, tasks, and frame of treatment with clients' own conceptualizations of, and language for, the outcomes they would see as meaningfully transformative. Fortunately, this accommodation should not be too challenging, as a perusal of the aforementioned client-generated themes of what gets corrected in therapy are rather well-aligned with how major theoretical systems (and the therapists who deliver them) define CE outcomes—for example, a new experience of the self, improved relational abilities, a new understanding of mental health problems and the inputs into them, and so forth. Such alignment may underscore that clients are influenced by their therapists' theory-based descriptions of treatment aims and processes—that is, they appear capable of being socialized to think of treatment outcomes in the way that a given treatment calls for, which generally bodes well for therapists being able to credibly and persuasively discuss their methods. Importantly, though, in the CE mechanisms section, we will review how clients may have more unique or nuanced ideas on how the therapist and the therapy help them arrive at their theory-consistent CE outcomes. As a quick spoiler, they do not necessarily align with the idea that it is the theory-specified techniques that are the main corrective mechanisms.

Another practice implication of research on CE outcomes could be viewed as a positive side effect of the method—that is, for some clients, the process of "storying" their CE outcomes, whether through the PPCEIT or other interview protocols, appeared to have a therapeutic effect in itself (e.g., Roussos et al., 2017). As Angus and Constantino (2017) summarized,

> A shared story in the context of PPCEIT interviews, may represent an important processing step that provides clients with a memorable, coherent understanding of the relation between their personal experiences of transformative change in therapy (e.g., therapist actions/interventions, disconfirmation of expectations) and the emergence of a new, more agentic experience of self. (p. 194)

Hence, even if only for clinical reasons, clinicians could include a PPCEIT-style inquiry at termination or follow-up that allows clients to look back on their work, reflect on its impact, amplify through expression their experience of transformative shifts, and own their self-narrative identity change (Angus & Kagan, 2013). This notion is consistent with cognitive and developmental research, which demonstrates that the ability to tell a story about our most important and meaningful life events is paramount for developing more adaptive, differentiated, and flexible self-conceptions (Bruner, 2004; McAdams & Janis, 2004). Of course, with proper permissions, client responses to such interviews could also add to the client-focused research base on CEs (either in the form of case or aggregated studies), which would represent a true and exciting confounding of practice and science.

CLIENTS' DURING- AND/OR POSTTREATMENT PERSPECTIVES ON PSYCHOTHERAPY OUTCOME MECHANISMS

As noted, another key element of client-focused psychotherapy outcome research involves clients' own accounts of contributors to, or mechanisms of, their treatment outcomes as they participate in, or look back on, their therapy. And, similar to the outcome definitions, clients' ideas of how change comes about may or may not align with our field's theory-driven ideas of treatment-related change mechanisms. In this vein, some research has focused on clients' freely stated accounts of outcome mechanisms when largely unencumbered by existing scholarly definitions. In this section, we include client-focused studies of positive or helpful or negative or hindering events that, to date, encompass the largest research base fitting our present inclusion criteria. We also discuss work on client-focused studies of positively or negatively valenced culturally oriented experiences that occur through the course of psychotherapy. Similar to the prior section on outcome definitions, other research has attempted to ascertain clients' take (user-constructed) on the mechanisms of existing theoretical or scholarly (researcher- or therapist-constructed) outcome concepts. We include client-focused studies of CE- and hope-generating mechanisms.

What Do Clients Freely View as Salient or Significant Events in Therapy?

Client-focused research on treatment outcome mechanisms can be traced back to Elliott's (1985) pioneering work on client-identified significant events in therapy. This ample literature now encompasses a range of subgenres (e.g., helpful vs. hindering events or aspects or important moments), measurement occasions (e.g., postsession, posttreatment, long-term follow-up), and methodologies (e.g., quantitative measures, qualitative analysis of semistructured interviews, mixed methods), and it has culminated in a series of meta-analyses, metasyntheses, and thematic reviews (namely, Levitt et al., 2016; McPherson et al., 2020; Timulak, 2007, 2010; Timulak & Keogh, 2017). Consistent with much of the extant research, we organize our discussion of client-reported mechanism themes using the helpful or hindering events heuristic.

Helpful Events

Therapists can be confident in a number of well-established client perspectives on positive contributions to their therapy outcomes. Across multiple metasyntheses and subsequent studies, clients routinely highlighted the helpfulness of a therapeutic relationship that is safe, supportive, trusting, authentic, and nonjudgmental (e.g., Levitt et al., 2016; Sousa & Vaz, 2020; Timulak, 2007). With respect to related therapist actions, clients have indicated that they benefit when therapists listen, affirm, validate, empathize, reassure, demonstrate positive regard, and convey acceptance. Additionally, clients have expressed that therapists collaborating with them on the goals and tasks of therapy and granting them autonomy over the treatment's direction is helpful (e.g., Levitt et al., 2016; Morrison et al., 2017). These findings corroborate the robust quantitative literature that links similar researcher- or therapist-constructed factors, including the higher quality alliance (Flückiger et al., 2018) and goal consensus or collaboration (Tryon et al., 2018) with adaptive treatment outcomes. Accordingly, it seems clear that therapists should seek to both cultivate a supportive and genuine relationship and prioritize client agency by including clients in discussions about how best to shape (and adapt over time) the direction of their treatment (e.g., McPherson et al., 2020; Wucherpfennig et al., 2020).

Whereas many clients appear to find the moments in which therapists allow them to self-reflect and draw their own connections helpful (e.g., Jones et al., 2016; Levitt et al., 2016; Sousa & Vaz, 2020), they can also (and, in some instances, simultaneously) find it beneficial when therapists offer interpretations, provide guidance, and challenge their assumptions, beliefs, and perspectives to facilitate seeing things in a new way (e.g., Chui et al., 2020; Sousa & Vaz, 2020). As for additional prominent outcome mechanism themes, clients have stated that it is helpful when therapists (a) work with them to clarify and resolve specific problems (Castonguay et al., 2010; Timulak, 2010); (b) focus on specific strategies, skills, and techniques (e.g., Swift et al., 2017; Timulak, 2007; Timulak & Keogh, 2017); (c) empathically elicit, explore, and provide a space to feel difficult emotions (e.g., De Smet, Meganck, Truijens, et al., 2020;

Jones et al., 2016; Levitt et al., 2016); and (d) stimulate insight, awareness, or self-understanding (e.g., Castonguay et al., 2010; McPherson et al., 2020; Timulak, 2007). Notably, in Levitt and colleagues' qualitative meta-analysis of 109 studies, clients highlighted instances in which therapists helped them to recognize and address multiple kinds of patterns in their lives (e.g., cognitive, behavioral, interpersonal, and emotional), not just those that traditionally align with a single school of therapy. Thus, taken with the previous findings, clients may see more traditionally classified theory-common factors as most contributing to their improvement. Coming directly from the client stakeholder's collective mouth, this speaks to the therapeutic importance of therapists working nimbly within or across schools while always attending to the relational climate (Castonguay et al., 2010; Constantino & Bernecker, 2014).

Moreover, clients' emphasis on the helpfulness of the seemingly contradictory themes of personal agency and a therapist's directiveness may point to the utility of ongoing therapist attunement and corresponding responsiveness to clients' momentary needs and preferences (which, fittingly, also has moderate support as being helpful from the client perspective; Jones et al., 2016; Levitt et al., 2016). In managing these competing pulls, it is important that therapists sensitively shift toward directiveness at the "right" time so that they do not eclipse the autonomy-granting stance that clients also feel contributes to their improvement (Chui et al., 2020). Indeed, this frame on therapist responsivity also jibes with client perspectives on metacommunication. More specifically, clients have indicated that it is helpful when therapists invite an open conversation about the therapeutic process and provide them with opportunities for disagreement, as resolving such tensions can promote a deeper, more genuine relationship and be restorative in and of itself (Chui et al., 2020; Levitt et al., 2016; Swift et al., 2017). These metacommunication findings are further supported by related research indicating that clients often wished that therapists were more responsive to and communicative about how well the treatment aligned with the client's own preferences and goals (e.g., Levitt et al., 2016). Thus, in addition to striving for greater responsivity (or as a central part of it), we recommend that therapists metacommunicate with their clients frequently. Doing so would be a clear evidence-based practice (outcome mechanism) that emanates from client-focused outcome research.

Hindering Events

A relatively smaller literature on hindering events or aspects of psychotherapy requires more cautious interpretation and implementation. Nonetheless, the existing research points to a handful of key themes that center on client disappointment. For example, one study provided preliminary evidence that clients find some of the logistics of therapy (e.g., fee reminders, an inflexible cancellation policy, pressure to schedule additional sessions) to disrupt its benefits (Burton & Thériault, 2020). Moreover, supporting the earlier discussion of therapist responsivity, clients have also expressed general disappointment with (and a negative impact of) the perceived absence of a personally good treatment fit (e.g., Chui et al., 2020; De Smet, Meganck, Truijens, et al.,

2020). For example, some clients receiving psychodynamic therapies have commented on a lack of structure and strategies, while some clients receiving cognitive behavior therapy have said that treatment was too structured and focused too heavily on the present day. In addition, whereas clients acknowledged the role of their own agency, motivation, and internal obstacles in impeding (or facilitating) their improvement (e.g., De Smet, Meganck, Truijens, et al., 2020; Nilsson et al., 2007), they also highlighted a number of hindering therapist actions, such as when therapists seem inattentive or distracted; make clients feel disrespected, misunderstood, unheard, judged, or stigmatized; and/or fail to address such transgressions (Burton & Thériault, 2020; Levitt et al., 2016; Timulak, 2010; Timulak & Keogh, 2017). Clients also believe their progress is hindered when they perceive clinical mistakes or therapist misdirection; this can happen when therapists engage core therapy elements unskillfully (e.g., ineffective reflective listening or inauthentic empathy), when therapists are more directive than the client would like (e.g., structuring the session without client input, inserting too much of their own perspective, disguising advice as a question), or even when clients perceive therapist mistreatment, negligence, or incompetence (e.g., asking inappropriate questions, assessing clients inaccurately, pushing clients into action before they are ready; Burton & Thériault, 2020; Swift et al., 2017; Timulak, 2010).

Notably, the variability in client-reported significant events suggests that (a) what one client sees as helpful may be seen as hindering by another (e.g., Timulak, 2010) and (b) the degree to which therapists' actions are deemed helpful or hindering may depend on a combination of when and how they act (e.g., Morrison et al., 2017). Given that clients can experience helpful and hindering events on a moment-by-moment basis (Swift et al., 2017), therapists need to attune to subtle (often nonverbal) reactions, especially those that suggest disappointment or misunderstanding (Timulak, 2010). While the aspiration is to avoid making mistakes, the inevitability of missteps underscores the importance of how therapists respond after they occur, especially given that leaving them unresolved can contribute to client perceptions of poorer outcomes (Burton & Thériault, 2020; Swift et al., 2017; Wucherpfennig et al., 2020). Therefore, because clients may be hesitant to raise these issues themselves, therapists should explicitly address possible ruptures, openly solicit feedback, and metacommunicate about possible negative therapy process (and their own contributions to it).

WHAT DO CLIENTS FREELY VIEW AS CULTURALLY ORIENTED COMPETENCIES OR EXPERIENCES IN THERAPY?

Though the association between a therapist's multicultural competence (MCC) and a client's treatment outcomes has accumulated to the level of meta-analytic study (e.g., Tao et al., 2015), the literature on freely reported client perspectives of therapists' MCC and cultural experiences in therapy, and how they may influence their outcomes, remains relatively limited (Plumb, 2019; Tao et al.,

2015). However, from the small qualitative literature, we can glean a handful of preliminary client-reported themes to inform clinical practice. For example, across several studies, clients have highlighted the benefit of when therapists (a) express openness toward engaging in cultural discussions and do so with sensitivity and humility, (b) display comfort with metacommunicating about cultural differences and cultural and professional power differentials, (c) demonstrate accurate cultural knowledge and understanding of clients' experiences, (d) exhibit a willingness to help with practical issues in clients' lives (particularly when working with traditionally marginalized populations), and (e) conceptualize clients as multifaceted cultural beings (i.e., intersectionality) whose problems are situated within particular cultural contexts (e.g., Levitt et al., 2016; McPherson et al., 2020; Plumb, 2019; Pope-Davis et al., 2002). Notably, when such experiences have been absent from their past experiences in therapy, clients report that these would have been helpful components of their treatment (Plumb, 2019).

Additionally, there has a growing interest in exploring clients' perspectives on strengths-based approaches, as emphasized in the American Psychological Association's (2017) Multicultural Guidelines. In one study, clients of color who worked with White therapists reported that therapists' skillful exploration and leveraging of clients' culture-based strengths stimulated and increased both clients' self-understanding and the therapist's understanding of the client, as well as improved symptoms, well-being, and functioning (Plumb, 2019). Clients in this study also highlighted that adopting a cultural strengths-based approach is most appropriate when clients feel strongly (positively) connected to specific cultures or identities. Conversely, when therapists overly emphasize or make assumptions about cultural strengths or vulnerabilities based on identities that clients actually experience as peripheral or unimportant, it could induce a misunderstanding (a client-reported hindering event, as noted in the previous section). These findings corroborate those of an earlier landmark study, which also found that clients' perceptions of therapists' MCC largely resulted from therapists meeting clients' unique and personally salient cultural needs (Pope-Davis et al., 2002). These findings are reminiscent of quantitative research, which suggests that therapists' MCC ratings are more dependent on a particular client or unique dyad than they are on a therapist-level threshold (e.g., Owen et al., 2011).

Taken together, these preliminary findings support a shift away from seeking the "achievement" of MCC toward the adoption of a multicultural orientation (see Davis et al., 2018; Owen et al., 2011, 2016). Accordingly, therapists may be wise to heed these authors' recommendations for adopting a therapeutic stance that emphasizes cultural humility, cultural comfort, and an appreciation of cultural opportunities. Moreover, the qualitative findings presented earlier suggest that therapists should embrace an intersectional lens that allows them to appreciate the unique strengths of each client. Therapists should also attune themselves to the salience of cultural identities for specific clients, grant autonomy to clients so they may identify their own cultural strengths or vulnerabilities, and avoid oversimplifying differences or relying on stereotypes.

Moreover, given the role that power and privilege play in the therapeutic relationship (with respect to therapist and client identities), therapists should also work to "level the playing field" within the therapeutic relationship by openly exploring cultural and professional power dynamics (Levitt et al., 2016). Doing so may decrease the likelihood of premature termination and increase client comfort with metacommunicating in the face of cultural misunderstandings or ruptures (e.g., Pope-Davis et al., 2002). Finally, as this area of study begins to mature, therapists should stay apprised of additional guidance that emerges from the client-focused research literature.

CORRECTIVE EXPERIENCES: WHAT DO CLIENTS SAY IS CORRECTIVE?

The aforementioned series of client-focused CE studies also yielded information on CE mechanisms; in other words, what do clients say is corrective in therapy that promotes their CE outcomes? From Heatherington et al.'s (2012) during-treatment assessment, clients articulated diverse corrective mechanisms, with the more prominent ones reflecting their own actions (e.g., engaged in self-reflection or engaged in exposures) or something the therapist did (e.g., provided empathy, demonstrated acceptance, supported clients' agency). Across the posttreatment interview studies (e.g., Constantino et al., 2017; Moertl et al., 2017; Roussos et al., 2017), one prominent theme centered again on the therapist. Notably, clients highlighted the unexpected experience of therapists being responsive and flexible with session structure and timing as contributing to their aforementioned CE outcome of gaining a new, positive experience of the self.

Clients also identified a therapist's authentic engagement (including making prudent personal disclosures and delivering treatment-related feedback) as contributing to a transformative in-session relational experience that was a component of the aforementioned ultimate CE outcome of increased relational effectiveness. This focus on the clinician more than the treatment as being the corrective mechanism was also revealed in Friedlander et al.'s (2012) psychodynamic case study. Specifically, the client partially attributed their CE outcomes to the therapist's making them feel safe and accepted. Similarly, in Knox et al.'s (2012) study of clients who were also therapists-in-training, the participants pointed to the therapist's reassurance and rescuing (from acute emotional distress) as CE mechanisms of both self-related (e.g., increased self-assurance) and interpersonally related (e.g., relational effectiveness) CE outcomes. Finally, clients in some of the PPCEIT interview studies (e.g., Constantino et al., 2017) also indicated that dyadic collaboration and engagement were key CE mechanisms. This relationship component also shined through in Knox et al.'s (2012) study; namely, clients articulated that alliance rupture–repair resolutions were a CE mechanism. Similar to our previous discussion of client-focused CE outcomes research, the CE mechanisms research base is at least moderately established, and we have moderate-to-high confidence in the emergent themes.

Accordingly, we can derive some current practice implications. Most notably, although clients' ideas of CE outcomes are remarkably consistent with how therapists, theorists, and researchers often articulate therapeutic change (e.g., improved self-concept, improved relationships, reduced symptoms), clients' ideas of how they arrive at these outcomes seem to point more to their own actions, the therapist's actions, or their experiences of the therapeutic relationship than they do to a given treatment's theory-prescribed interventions (Angus & Constantino, 2017). Regarding their own actions as CE mechanisms, it is notable that clients were far more likely to identify them when reflecting back on their completed therapy in a posttreatment interview (e.g., Constantino et al., 2017) than when writing about such mechanisms while still in therapy (Heatherington et al., 2012). One implication of this trend is that therapists could use their knowledge of such CE-mechanism findings to help heighten clients' current sense that treatment can be helpful (heightened hope/outcome expectancy) and their sense of how it can work (heightened perceptions of treatment credibility)—both client factors that, in traditional psychotherapy research, associate positively (and meta-analytically) with client improvement (Constantino, Coyne, et al., 2018; Constantino, Vîslă, et al., 2018). For example, a clinician treating a relatively demoralized client might say,

> I know it seems bleak at the moment, but when clients are interviewed after therapy about what contributed to meaningful change, they often point to their own active engagement in the work, such as pushing themselves to discuss painful topics or reflecting deeply on their childhood and other important relationships.

Regarding therapist actions as CE mechanisms, we noted previously how it appears that clinicians can socialize their clients to appreciate a certain therapeutic "angle" that guides the work, and clients can even somewhat "speak our language" when describing CE outcomes. Yet, if therapists translated these results to mean, in a medical model sense, that they can simply administer and persist with uniformly sequenced treatment "prescriptions," they would be missing the mark, so to speak, from clients' vantage point on CE mechanisms. Despite what may be a natural pull to defer to their therapist's direction (Rennie, 1994), what seems most corrective for clients is their experience of some agency vis-à-vis their therapist (which not only manifests in their own behavior, as previously discussed, but also interpersonally in the therapist's responsiveness to their momentary state and needs). At a minimum, clinically, this suggests that therapists should appreciate that the course of therapy is more often dynamic than fixed and allow for regular metacommunicative check-ins with their clients to see if a given session focus or structure needs revision—in a way that genuinely supports the client's agency (Levitt et al., 2016). At a maximum, therapists can consume and apply the burgeoning literature on evidence-based responsivity to specific clinical markers that can help guide important clinical "departures" (from whatever foundational treatment they are administering) in salient moments that call for them—what has been referred to as *context-responsive psychotherapy integration* (Constantino, Goodwin, et al., 2021; Constantino et al., 2020). As just one example, therapists can become more client centered and autonomy granting in the face of client resistance to the therapist's direction (Westra et al., 2016).

Regarding their experiences of the therapeutic relationship as a CE mechanism, the extant client-focused research points to the therapist being relationally engaged in certain ways. Notably, clients find it corrective when therapists provide empathy, convey acceptance, cultivate safety, use personal disclosures authentically, and convey reassurance (e.g., Friedlander et al., 2012; Heatherington et al., 2012; Knox et al., 2012). Clients also see dyadic experiences of collaboration and alliance rupture repair as transformational mechanisms. Clinically, such results further support that the delivery of named treatment strategies are notably less corrective to clients than the manifestation of therapists' facilitative interpersonal skill (Anderson et al., 2016). Thus, to heed clients' crucially important internal reference point on CEs, therapists should be sharpening their theoretically common relational skills, such as verbal fluency, empathy, hope inspiration, and rupture repair, as a complement to (or even more centrally than) theory-specific treatment techniques (Constantino et al., 2017; Gaines et al., 2021; Laska et al., 2014).

WHAT DO CLIENTS SAY GENERATES HOPE?

As another well-established psychological construct, hope is a robust contributor to beneficial life outcomes, including mental health (Cheavens et al., 2005). Specific to psychotherapy and counseling, one theory suggests that hope can combat demoralization by helping people see a meaningful future and possible pathways to it, often via the receipt of a persuasive treatment rationale and engagement with related techniques (Larsen & Stege, 2010a, 2010b; Snyder, 2002). Like many existing constructs, though, we have limited information on what clients themselves see as hope-generating aspects of their treatment. Addressing this gap, one study (Larsen & Stege, 2012) used interpersonal process recall (IPR; Elliott & Shapiro, 1988), a video-assisted interview method, with 10 clients within 48 hours of completing an early therapy session. Specifically, these clients, who were working with therapists well versed in the hope literature, were asked what influenced their hope and how, as they reviewed the session video with minimal interviewer prompts. Three main themes emerged.

First, clients discussed a hope-fostering relationship that included feeling safe and supported, with the therapist demonstrating nonjudgmental investment in and understanding of the client. In this sense, the climate instilled hope. Second, clients pointed to supportive identity change through interventions that either encouraged positive self-reflection or through which therapists conveyed support for positive aspects of the client's self. Elaborating on this perspective, clients expressed feeling more agency, self-awareness, and worth, some of which were achieved simply by explicitly talking about hope and through the therapist being an "appreciative mirror" (Larsen & Stege,

2012, p. 49). In this sense, the dyad found hope. Third, clients identified perspective change as hope-inspiring through actionable therapist behaviors of highlighting strengths, focusing on the future, recognizing possibilities, making hope intentional, and reframing. In this sense, therapists created hope. Across these themes, it is clear that clients see hope as stemming from their contributions to and receipt of a hope-generating therapeutic relationship.

This dyadic or relational understanding of what contributes to hope as an outcome mechanism was extended in a subsequent study of 18 counseling clients who, in this case, saw therapists who had not received specialized training on the hope literature and self-identified largely as integrative and humanistic (Chamodraka et al., 2017). Through grounded theory analysis of interviews that occurred in the session after clients first demonstrated reliable change and increased hope from baseline (ranging from Sessions 3 to 9), client responses shaped what the authors referred to as the "hope as empowerment model." This model includes client and therapist contributions and interactions to clients' increased sense of control and direction (which map onto Snyder's, 2002, hope theory elements of agency-thinking and pathways-thinking, respectively), as well as faith in the treatment. For example, when clients possessed more flexible role preferences and moderate or positive outcome expectations, the alignment between client preferences and therapist actions was of less importance for clients' experience of higher control, direction, and faith. In these conditions, clients derived hope from experiencing the therapist as a neutral, objective listener and using direct hope-inspiring strategies. However, under the conditions of having more rigid role preferences and negative or moderate outcome expectations, high compatibility between client preferences and therapist actions was important for clients' experience of higher control and faith in the treatment. Conversely, when therapists failed to meet these rigid preferences, clients experienced all aspects of hope and faith as being lower.

In the Chamodraka et al. (2017) study, clients also experienced the greatest hope increase when their therapist was nondirective and their own contributions to therapy were strong. When therapists were more directive and clients' contributions were strong, clients experienced a stronger sense of control (agency) but a lower sense of direction (pathways). Finally, when therapists were more directive and clients' contributions were less influential, clients experienced a more tenuous sense of control (agency) and a lower sense of direction (pathways). These interactions provide valuable nuance to a client-focused understanding of what generates hope, and they connect directly and empirically to our prior discussion of understanding clients' prospective treatment preferences. That is, from a fully client-focused vantage point, we have some evidence as to the conditions under which meeting client preferences is especially important (versus those where it seems less important) for influencing the outcome mechanism of hope. Although more of this kind of research is needed before we have high confidence in the results, enough work has been done to draw some tentative practice implications. Rather, straightforwardly, clinicians should engage in hope-inspiring actions that appear important in all contexts (e.g., explicitly discuss hope or be an accepting, non-judgmental listener). Therapists should also keep in mind important inter-actions with other pantheoretical variables, such as preferences and outcome expectations, which can influence the degree to which therapists need to match clients' preferred therapy actions or processes in order to positively affect hope.

FUTURE RESEARCH DIRECTIONS AND DESIGNS

As the field considers future research directions and designs, it seems centrally important to accept (for the moment, anyway) that, despite knowing that psychotherapy generally works, we have a notably incomplete understanding of how it works and the "reach" of its outcomes. This makes sense considering we are a relatively young field, and the present review underscores that clients themselves are well-positioned not only to help us nurture and grow the research base but also to colead the endeavor as the key psychotherapy stakeholder. Accordingly, the most important (and, hopefully, most obvious) future direction is to continue to measure clients' freely stated conceptualizations of important therapy outcomes and outcome mechanisms (across the time span of looking forward to therapy, actively engaging in it, and looking back on it). Such client-focused outcome research—what has been termed an emic (client or insider) perspective (Larsen & Stege, 2012)—will contribute immensely to a fuller and more ecologically representative empirical foundation.

However, even as we emphasize clients' freely stated perspectives, it is important not to throw the baby out with the bathwater, so to speak. It also seems important to assess clients' perspectives on and experiences of existing (researcher- or therapist-constructed) theoretical constructs. To this end, as just one example, future outcomes-relevant research could adapt methods such as the PPCEIT interview (Constantino & Angus, 2017) for other constructs (beyond CEs) that represent clinical change, whether it is in the form of problem reduction (e.g., maladaptive transaction cycles in relationships), functional improvement (e.g., vocational skills), or even more social psychological (e.g., self-competence), wellness (e.g., empowerment), and thriving-related (e.g., flourishing) constructs that may currently take a back seat in our understanding of psychotherapeutic benefits.

We can also use clients' perspectives to redefine existing therapist constructs, such as treatment adherence and competence. For example, these concepts can be respectively reengineered toward being faithful to and effectively admin-istering the actions that clients themselves expect to help them (and for which they might become demoralized if they were not included), even if these con-cepts are not part of your preferred theoretical approach or any theoretical brand (Wucherpfennig et al., 2020). Perhaps, through capitalizing on placebo and/or attuning to client-focused theories or narratives on change (within per-sonally salient cultural contexts), such revised conceptualizations of adher-ence and competence may have a greater likelihood of explaining significant variance in client outcomes (Constantino & Bernecker, 2014). If so, this could relaunch a potentially important research focus, with adapted measurements, in our ongoing quest to explain outcome variance from inherently intersecting client-, therapist-, and treatment-level predictors.

As another future direction or design, researchers might consider capitalizing further on the, arguably, underutilized IPR method for understanding clients' "still fresh" internal frame of reference while actively engaged in therapy (whether focused on their current understandings of personally relevant therapy outcomes or the contributors to them). McLeod (2001) touted IPR as "a jewel in the crown of qualitative psychotherapy research" (p. 81), and we reiterate that such qualitative designs may be the most useful for meeting our present inclusion criteria for client-focused research. However, by no means do we see this as the only method to contribute to this research base. For example, researchers could use information from the research reviewed herein to develop or refine quantitative measures that clients will inherently value and that clinicians can easily implement, as it is certainly not feasible to use IPR or conduct a Change Interview (Elliott et al., 2001) with every client. With these refined or adapted measures, quantitative research can examine whether results from client-focused outcome and outcome mechanism research (which often derive from smaller samples) generalize to larger samples (Timulak & Keogh, 2017).

Future client-focused research should also include more underrepresented and marginalized populations (Levitt, 2015), with a focus on how the intersection of power and privilege can influence a client's perceptions of what works or harms in therapy and how this happens (Levitt et al., 2016). Relatedly, future client-focused research can address social justice in psychotherapy, such as by complementing existing research on therapists' perspectives on important social justice competencies (e.g., Brown et al., 2019). For too long, the field has failed to adequately address or study social justice issues (Paquin et al., 2019), and the client perspective can help to better define outcomes and outcome mechanisms that are respectful of diversity and inclusion. Also, future client-focused research should focus more on conceptions of poor outcomes and improvement-hindering events or actions in therapy. Not only has more research to date understandably focused on positive outcomes and improvement-facilitating mechanisms, but we also know that clients are more likely to underreport negative events and outcomes (Burton & Thériault, 2020). Finally, client-focused research, just like any form, will have to contend with discrepancies that may emerge across studies versus only building a type of "thick description" from which we can derive relatively few representative themes or directions. As one example from the research we reviewed here, recall that while clients can help us understand hope as a pantheoretical change mechanism (Chamodraka et al., 2017; Larsen & Stege, 2012), they did not freely identify hope as a top expected change mechanism (Tzur Bitan & Lazar, 2019). Thus, more work is needed to reconcile the fact that clients may view hope as relatively less important (to other mechanisms) than theorists, clinicians, or researchers; yet, when asked to help us understand it, they provide very useful information, and it is clearly not insignificant to them. As client-focused research increases, we need to keep building on prior work to establish core principles on which many or most agree, which will be a marker for heightened scientific maturity (Gaines et al., 2021).

TRAINING AND TEACHING IMPLICATIONS

As we learn from the client's vantage point, a primary implication is to teach it early and often. Starting with the didactic curriculum, trainees should be well aware of the growing, rich, and even multidisciplinary literature on client-perceived values, preferences, good or poor outcomes, CEs, significant in-session events, hope, and so forth. Failing to include such information in courses and colloquia would be a glaring oversight at best and, to the extent that a curriculum stays willfully constrained to researcher- or therapist-constructed content only, a form of empirical imperialism at worst (Castonguay et al., 2019).

Moving from didactics and knowledge development to practice, it seems important to train clinicians to assess the clients (users) or stakeholders' vantage point, including when people are just considering therapy and trying to make treatment or provider decisions. On the basis of the data reviewed here, clients should be involved in the selection process by addressing their presenting-problem story or narrative, understanding their values, and appreciating their most salient cultural contexts, identities, and preferences—all in the service of helping fit the treatment frame or principles to the client. This integrative focus has a chance to improve effectiveness through varied mechanisms that still need to be empirically confirmed; however, from client-focused research to date, these could reasonably involve a sense of agency in decision making, an experience of good personal fit of treatment to the narrative, and an experience of the therapist as invested, caring, and responsive.

Assimilating the client's perspective into early assessment and responding accordingly would require trainees to be conversational in different therapies and principles so that they can offer the best-fitting therapy rationales (myths) and related strategies (rituals; Frank, 1961). In this sense, treatment selection and therapist behavior would become less about the professionals' view of strict adherence to single treatment packages and more about clinicians privileging clients' perceptions of therapists behaving in ways that match the client's story (by drawing flexibly on those conversational understandings of existing theories or even by trying on new variants with client feedback). Although it might require a rewiring of sorts from how we traditionally train, the key idea is that it is not so much what therapists do, or whether those behaviors strictly replicate from client to client, but rather that there is an optimal, personal fit of therapist behavior (within each therapeutic relationship) to a rationale that a given client finds compelling (which can, of course, differ from other clients, thereby necessitating constant therapist responsivity at the emic level; Constantino, Coyne, et al., 2018). In fact, we might go so far as to suggest doing away with specialized training and credentialing for becoming so-called experts in a specific named treatment, as that may only mean "expert" from our restricted professional perspective. Or, at a minimum, there could be some alternative or complementary credentialing for demonstrating an ability to be optimally and ethically fluid and client-focused in one's work—including orienting toward the outcomes that clients say are most valued and engaging the mechanisms that clients say are most helpful for achieving these outcomes.

In fact, as we continue to engage in the great psychotherapy debate (Wampold & Imel, 2015)—a version of a "horse race" focused on the therapeutic merits of the so-called theory-common versus therapy-specific factors—some research reviewed here tells us that clients do not really see mechanisms of change in a way that neatly aligns with either camp (e.g., Tzur Bitan & Lazar, 2019). Tentatively, at least, it appears that clients mostly want to disclose in therapy (about themselves and the therapeutic relationship), which is neither specific to any talk therapy nor perfectly related to relationship variables that predominate the common factors' focus (e.g., alliance as goal or task agreement and bond). As one implication of this client-focused theme on outcome mechanisms, training programs (whether at the graduate or continuing education level) could focus heavily on teaching clinicians to invite and engage in metacommunication regularly with their clients. Metacommunication is an ever-available, client-valued therapeutic activity that we would guess is rarely at the center of training paradigms. To us, though, such a focus on disclosure and ongoing metacommunication is a good reminder that people ultimately treat people in psychotherapy, and clients are telling us that the talking in the "talking cure" is still paramount! Again, though, this does not mean we should abandon all ideas of clinical expertise as we know them. Rather, this is a call to integrate our ideas with clients' perspectives, self-knowledge, and expertise in a way that might promote updated training molds and innovations that are optimally disruptive to our historically limited professional perspectives (Rotheram-Borus et al., 2012).

CONCLUSION

This chapter spotlights the importance of asking, involving, and metacommunicating with the most important stakeholder of all—the consumer. Just like a hairstylist would not assume how a person wants their hair styled, we should not assume that our researcher- or therapist-constructed ideas of expertise or of specific name-brand treatments (and all of their largely scripted elements) are what a client wants or needs. Instead, we can be a listener, consultant, and collaborator, as needed, in defining and determining clients' personally relevant treatment targets while then engaging as just one element of the instruments of said change. We would suggest moving even further beyond Sullivan's (1953) notion of the therapist as participant–observer to an identity that also includes listener–collaborator. And with this fuller identity, therapists can better appreciate that the ultimate form of tailoring is involving the person you are tailoring to—a good tailor neither assumes they know, nor do they simply guess (yet, they do still collaborate and offer potentially useful options).

REFERENCES

Alexander, F., & French, T. M. (1946). *Psychoanalytic therapy; principles and application.* Ronald Press.

American Psychological Association. (2017). *Multicultural guidelines: An ecological approach to context, identity, and intersectionality, 2017.* https://www.apa.org/about/policy/multicultural-guidelines.pdf

Anderson, T., McClintock, A. S., Himawan, L., Song, X., & Patterson, C. L. (2016). A prospective study of therapist facilitative interpersonal skills as a predictor of treatment outcome. *Journal of Consulting and Clinical Psychology, 84*(1), 57–66. https://doi.org/10.1037/ccp0000060

Angus, L., & Constantino, M. J. (2017). Client accounts of corrective experiences in psychotherapy: Implications for clinical practice. *Journal of Clinical Psychology, 73*(2), 192–195. https://doi.org/10.1002/jclp.22432

Angus, L. E., & Kagan, F. (2013). Assessing client self-narrative change in emotion-focused therapy of depression: An intensive single case analysis. *Psychotherapy, 50*(4), 525–534. https://doi.org/10.1037/a0033358

Ashworth, M., Robinson, S. I., Godfrey, E., Shepherd, M., Evans, C., Seed, P., Parmentier, H., & Tylee, A. (2005). Measuring mental health outcomes in primary care: The psychometric properties of a new patient-generated outcome measure, "PSYCHLOPS" ("psychological outcome profiles"). *Primary Care Mental Health, 3*(4), 261–270.

Battle, C. C., Imber, S. D., Hoehn-Saric, R., Nash, E. R., & Frank, J. D. (1966). Target complaints as criteria of improvement. *American Journal of Psychotherapy, 20*(1), 184–192. https://doi.org/10.1176/appi.psychotherapy.1966.20.1.184

Bordin, E. S. (1979). The generalizability of the psychoanalytic concept of the working alliance. *Psychotherapy, 16*(3), 252–260. https://doi.org/10.1037/h0085885

Boritz, T., Barnhart, R., Angus, L., & Constantino, M. J. (2017). Narrative flexibility in brief psychotherapy for depression. *Psychotherapy Research, 27*(6), 666–676. https://doi.org/10.1080/10503307.2016.1152410

Brown, J., Wiendels, S., & Eyre, V. (2019). Social justice competencies for counselling and psychotherapy: Perceptions of experienced practitioners and implications for contemporary practice. *Counselling & Psychotherapy Research, 19*(4), 533–543. https://doi.org/10.1002/capr.12247

Bruner, J. (2004). The narrative creation of self. In L. E. Angus & J. McLeod (Eds.), *The handbook of narrative and psychotherapy: Practice, theory, and research* (pp. 3–14). Sage Publications, Inc. https://doi.org/10.4135/9781412973496.d3

Burton, L., & Thériault, A. (2020). Hindering events in psychotherapy: A retrospective account from the client's perspective. *Counselling & Psychotherapy Research, 20*(1), 116–127. https://doi.org/10.1002/capr.12268

Carpenter, N., Angus, L., Paivio, S., & Bryntwick, E. (2016). Narrative and emotion integration processes in emotion-focused therapy for complex trauma: An exploratory process-outcome analysis. *Person-Centered and Experiential Psychotherapies, 15*(2), 67–94. https://doi.org/10.1080/14779757.2015.1132756

Castonguay, L. G., Boswell, J. F., Zack, S. E., Baker, S., Boutselis, M. A., Chiswick, N. R., Damer, D. D., Hemmelstein, N. A., Jackson, J. S., Morford, M., Ragusea, S. A., Roper, J. G., Spayd, C., Weiszer, T., Borkovec, T. D., & Holtforth, M. G. (2010). Helpful and hindering events in psychotherapy: A practice research network study. *Psychotherapy, 47*(3), 327–344. https://doi.org/10.1037/a0021164

Castonguay, L. G., Constantino, M. J., & Beutler, L. E. (Eds.). (2019). *Principles of change: How psychotherapists implement research in practice.* Oxford University Press. https://doi.org/10.1093/med-psych/9780199324729.001.0001

Castonguay, L. G., & Hill, C. E. (Eds.). (2012). *Transformation in psychotherapy: Corrective experiences across cognitive behavioral, humanistic, and psychodynamic approaches.* American Psychological Association. https://doi.org/10.1037/13747-000

Chamodraka, M., Fitzpatrick, M. R., & Janzen, J. I. (2017). Hope as empowerment model: A client-based perspective on the process of hope development. *The Journal of Positive Psychology, 12*(3), 232–245. https://doi.org/10.1080/17439760.2016.1225115

Cheavens, J. S., Michael, S. T., & Snyder, C. R. (2005). The correlates of hope: Psychological and physiological benefits. In J. A. Eliott (Ed.), *Interdisciplinary perspectives on hope* (pp. 119–132). Nova Science Publishers.

Chui, H., Palma, B., Jackson, J. L., & Hill, C. E. (2020). Therapist–client agreement on helpful and wished-for experiences in psychotherapy: Associations with outcome. *Journal of Counseling Psychology, 67*(3), 349–360. https://doi.org/10.1037/cou0000393

Constantino, M. J., & Angus, L. (2017). Clients' retrospective accounts of corrective experiences in psychotherapy: An international, multisite collaboration. *Journal of Clinical Psychology, 73*(2), 131–138. https://doi.org/10.1002/jclp.22427

Constantino, M. J., & Bernecker, S. L. (2014). Bridging the common factors and empirically supported treatment camps: Comment on Laska, Gurman, and Wampold. *Psychotherapy, 51*(4), 505–509. https://doi.org/10.1037/a0036604

Constantino, M. J., Boswell, F. J., & Coyne, A. E. (2021). Patient, therapist, and relational factors. In M. Barkham, W. Lutz, & L. G. Castonguay (Eds.), *Bergin and Garfield's handbook of psychotherapy and behavior change* (7th ed., pp. 225–262). Wiley.

Constantino, M. J., Coyne, A. E., Boswell, J. F., Iles, B. R., & Vîslă, A. (2018). A meta-analysis of the association between patients' early perception of treatment credibility and their posttreatment outcomes. *Psychotherapy, 55*(4), 486–495. https://doi.org/10.1037/pst0000168

Constantino, M. J., Coyne, A. E., & Muir, H. J. (2020). Evidence-based therapist responsivity to disruptive clinical process. *Cognitive and Behavioral Practice, 27*(4), 405–416. https://doi.org/10.1016/j.cbpra.2020.01.003

Constantino, M. J., Goodwin, B. J., Muir, H. J., Coyne, A. E., & Boswell, J. F. (2021). Context-responsive psychotherapy integration as applied to cognitive-behavioral therapy. In J. C. Watson & H. Wiseman (Eds.), *The responsive psychotherapist: Attuning to clients in the moment* (pp. 151–169). American Psychological Association. https://doi.org/10.1037/0000240-008

Constantino, M. J., Morrison, N. R., Coyne, A. E., Goodwin, B. J., Santorelli, G. D., & Angus, L. (2017). Patients' perceptions of corrective experiences in naturalistically delivered psychotherapy. *Journal of Clinical Psychology, 73*(2), 139–152. https://doi.org/10.1002/jclp.22428

Constantino, M. J., Vîslă, A., Coyne, A. E., & Boswell, J. F. (2018). A meta-analysis of the association between patients' early treatment outcome expectation and their posttreatment outcomes. *Psychotherapy, 55*(4), 473–485. https://doi.org/10.1037/pst0000169

Constantino, M. J., & Westra, H. A. (2012). An expectancy-based approach to facilitating corrective experiences in psychotherapy. In L. G. Castonguay & C. E. Hill (Eds.), *Transformation in psychotherapy: Corrective experiences across cognitive behavioral, humanistic, and psychodynamic approaches* (pp. 121–139). American Psychological Association. https://doi.org/10.1037/13747-008

Davis, D. E., DeBlaere, C., Owen, J., Hook, J. N., Rivera, D. P., Choe, E., Van Tongeren, D. R., Worthington, E. L., & Placeres, V. (2018). The multicultural orientation framework: A narrative review. *Psychotherapy, 55*(1), 89–100. https://doi.org/10.1037/pst0000160

Deane, F. P., Spicer, J., & Todd, D. M. (1997). Validity of a simplified target complaints measure. *Assessment, 4*(2), 119–130. https://doi.org/10.1177/107319119700400202

De Smet, M. M., Meganck, R., De Geest, R., Norman, U. A., Truijens, F., & Desmet, M. (2020). What "good outcome" means to patients: Understanding recovery and improvement in psychotherapy for major depression from a mixed-methods perspective. *Journal of Counseling Psychology, 67*(1), 25–39. https://doi.org/10.1037/cou0000362

De Smet, M. M., Meganck, R., Truijens, F., De Geest, R., Cornelis, S., Norman, U. A., & Desmet, M. (2020). Change processes underlying "good outcome": A qualitative study on recovered and improved patients' experiences in psychotherapy for major depression. *Psychotherapy Research, 30*(7), 948–964. https://doi.org/10.1080/10503307.2020.1722329

De Smet, M. M., Meganck, R., Van Nieuwenhove, K., Truijens, F. L., & Desmet, M. (2019). No change? A grounded theory analysis of depressed patients' perspectives on non-improvement in psychotherapy. *Frontiers in Psychology, 10*, 1–17. https://doi.org/10.3389/fpsyg.2019.00588

Dourdouma, A., Gelo, O. C. G., & Moertl, K. (2020). Change process in systemic therapy: A qualitative investigation. *Counselling & Psychotherapy Research, 20*(2), 235–249. https://doi.org/10.1002/capr.12278

Ekroll, V. B., & Rønnestad, M. H. (2017). Processes and changes experienced by clients during and after naturalistic good-outcome therapies conducted by experienced psychotherapists. *Psychotherapy Research, 27*(4), 450–468. https://doi.org/10.1080/10503307.2015.1119326

Elliott, R. (1985). Helpful and nonhelpful events in brief counseling interviews: An empirical taxonomy. *Journal of Counseling Psychology, 32*(3), 307–322. https://doi.org/10.1037/0022-0167.32.3.307

Elliott, R., & Shapiro, D. A. (1988). Brief Structured Recall: A more efficient method for studying significant therapy events. *The British Journal of Medical Psychology, 61*(2), 141–153. https://doi.org/10.1111/j.2044-8341.1988.tb02773.x

Elliott, R., Slatick, E., & Urman, M. (2001). Qualitative change process research on psychotherapy: Alternative strategies. *Psychologische Beiträge, 43*(3), 69–111.

Elliott, R., Wagner, J., Sales, C. M. D., Rodgers, B., Alves, P., & Café, M. J. (2016). Psychometrics of the Personal Questionnaire: A client-generated outcome measure. *Psychological Assessment, 28*(3), 263–278. https://doi.org/10.1037/pas0000174

Flückiger, C., Del Re, A. C., Wampold, B. E., & Horvath, A. O. (2018). The alliance in adult psychotherapy: A meta-analytic synthesis. *Psychotherapy, 55*(4), 316–340. https://doi.org/10.1037/pst0000172

Frank, J. D. (1961). *Persuasion and healing: A comparative study of psychotherapy.* Johns Hopkins University Press.

Friedlander, M. L., Sutherland, O., Sandler, S., Kortz, L., Bernardi, S., Lee, H.-H., & Drozd, A. (2012). Exploring corrective experiences in a successful case of short-term dynamic psychotherapy. *Psychotherapy, 49*(3), 349–363. https://doi.org/10.1037/a0023447

Fuertes, J. N., & Williams, E. N. (2017). Client-focused psychotherapy research. *Journal of Consulting Psychology, 64*(4), 369–375. https://doi.org/10.1037/cou0000214

Gaines, A. N., Goldfried, M. R., & Constantino, M. J. (2021). Revived call for consensus in the future of psychotherapy. *Evidence-Based Mental Health, 24*, 2–4. https://doi.org/10.1136/ebmental-2020-300208

Guindon, M. H. (2010). What do we know about self-esteem interventions? In M. H. Guindon (Ed.), *Self-esteem across the lifespan: Issues and interventions* (pp. 25–44). Routledge.

Heatherington, L., Constantino, M. J., Angus, L., Friedlander, M., & Messer, S. (2012). Clients' perspectives on corrective experiences in psychotherapy. In L. G. Castonguay & C. E. Hill (Eds.), *Transformation in psychotherapy: Corrective experiences across cognitive behavioral, humanistic, and psychodynamic approaches* (pp. 161–190). American Psychological Association. https://doi.org/10.1037/13747-010

Hill, C. E., Chui, H., & Baumann, E. (2013). Revisiting and reenvisioning the outcome problem in psychotherapy: An argument to include individualized and qualitative measurement. *Psychotherapy, 50*(1), 68–76. https://doi.org/10.1037/a0030571

Horowitz, L. M., Rosenberg, S. E., Baer, B. A., Ureño, G., & Villaseñor, V. S. (1988). Inventory of interpersonal problems: Psychometric properties and clinical applications.

Journal of Consulting and Clinical Psychology, 56(6), 885–892. https://doi.org/10.1037/0022-006X.56.6.885

Horowitz, L. M., Strupp, H. H., Lambert, M. J., & Elkin, I. (1997). Overview and summary of the Core Battery Conference. In H. H. Strupp, L. M. Horowitz, & M. J. Lambert (Eds.), *Measuring patient changes in mood, anxiety, and personality disorders: Toward a core battery* (pp. 11–54). American Psychological Association. https://doi.org/10.1037/10232-001

Jones, S. A., Latchford, G., & Tober, G. (2016). Client experiences of motivational interviewing: An interpersonal process recall study. *Psychology and Psychotherapy, 89*(1), 97–114. https://doi.org/10.1111/papt.12061

Khattra, J., Angus, L., Westra, H., Macaulay, C., Moertl, K., & Constantino, M. (2017). Client perceptions of corrective experiences in cognitive behavioral therapy and motivational interviewing for generalized anxiety disorder: An exploratory pilot study. *Journal of Psychotherapy Integration, 27*(1), 23–34. https://doi.org/10.1037/int0000053

Kiresuk, T. J., & Sherman, R. E. (1968). Goal attainment scaling: A general method for evaluating comprehensive community mental health programs. *Community Mental Health Journal, 4*(6), 443–453. https://doi.org/10.1007/BF01530764

Kiresuk, T. J., Smith, A., & Cardillo, J. E. (Eds.). (1994). *Goal attainment scaling.* Lawrence Erlbaum Associates.

Knox, S., Hess, S. A., Hill, C. E., Burkard, A. W., & Crook-Lyon, R. E. (2012). Corrective relational experiences: Client perspectives. In L. G. Castonguay & C. E. Hill (Eds.), *Transformation in psychotherapy: Corrective experiences across cognitive behavioral, humanistic, and psychodynamic approaches* (pp. 191–213). American Psychological Association. https://doi.org/10.1037/13747-011

Larsen, D. J., & Stege, R. (2010a). Hope-focused practices during early psychotherapy sessions: Part I: Implicit approaches. *Journal of Psychotherapy Integration, 20*(3), 271–292. https://doi.org/10.1037/a0020820

Larsen, D. J., & Stege, R. (2010b). Hope-focused practices during early psychotherapy sessions: Part II: Explicit approaches. *Journal of Psychotherapy Integration, 20*(3), 293–311. https://doi.org/10.1037/a0020821

Larsen, D. J., & Stege, R. (2012). Client accounts of hope in early counseling sessions: A qualitative study. *Journal of Counseling and Development, 90*(1), 45–54. https://doi.org/10.1111/j.1556-6676.2012.00007.x

Laska, K. M., Gurman, A. S., & Wampold, B. E. (2014). Expanding the lens of evidence-based practice in psychotherapy: A common factors perspective. *Psychotherapy, 51*(4), 467–481. https://doi.org/10.1037/a0034332

Leibert, T. W., Powell, R. N., & Fonseca, F. D. (2020). Client descriptions of outcomes compared with quantitative data: A mixed-methods investigation of a quantitative outcome measure. *Counselling & Psychotherapy Research, 20*(1), 9–18. https://doi.org/10.1002/capr.12260

Levitt, H. M. (2015). Qualitative psychotherapy research: The journey so far and future directions. *Psychotherapy, 52*(1), 31–37. https://doi.org/10.1037/a0037076

Levitt, H. M., Pomerville, A., & Surace, F. I. (2016). A qualitative meta-analysis examining clients' experiences of psychotherapy: A new agenda. *Psychological Bulletin, 142*(8), 801–830. https://doi.org/10.1037/bul0000057

Lloyd, C. E. M., Duncan, C., & Cooper, M. (2019). Goal measures for psychotherapy: A systematic review of self-report, idiographic instruments. *Clinical Psychology: Science and Practice, 26*(3), Article e12281. https://doi.org/10.1111/cpsp.12281

Macaulay, C., Angus, L., Khattra, J., Westra, H., & Ip, J. (2017). Client retrospective accounts of corrective experiences in motivational interviewing integrated with cognitive behavioral therapy for generalized anxiety disorder. *Journal of Clinical Psychology, 73*(2), 168–181. https://doi.org/10.1002/jclp.22430

McAdams, D. P., & Janis, L. (2004). Narrative identity and narrative therapy. In L. E. Angus & J. McLeod (Eds.), *The handbook of narrative and psychotherapy: Practice, theory, and research* (pp. 159–173). Sage Publications. https://doi.org/10.4135/9781412973496.d13

McLeod, J. (2001). *Qualitative research in counseling and psychotherapy.* Sage Publications. https://doi.org/10.4135/9781849209663

McLeod, J., McLeod, J., Shoemark, A., & Cooper, M. (2009, February). *User constructed outcomes: Therapy and everyday life* [Paper presentation]. Psychotherapy Research Conference, University of Jyväskylä, Jyväskylä, Finland.

McPherson, S., Wicks, C., & Tercelli, I. (2020). Patient experiences of psychological therapy for depression: A qualitative metasynthesis. *BMC Psychiatry, 20.* Advance online publication. https://doi.org/10.1186/s12888-020-02682-1

Miller, R. B. (2004). *Facing human suffering: Psychology and psychotherapy as moral engagement.* American Psychological Association. https://doi.org/10.1037/10691-000

Moertl, K., Giri, H., Angus, L., & Constantino, M. J. (2017). Corrective experiences of psychotherapists in training. *Journal of Clinical Psychology, 73*(2), 182–191. https://doi.org/10.1002/jclp.22431

Morrison, N. R., Constantino, M. J., Westra, H. A., Kertes, A., Goodwin, B. J., & Antony, M. M. (2017). Using interpersonal process recall to compare patients' accounts of resistance in two psychotherapies for generalized anxiety disorder. *Journal of Clinical Psychology, 73*(11), 1523–1533. https://doi.org/10.1002/jclp.22527

Nilsson, T., Svensson, M., Sandell, R., & Clinton, D. (2007). Patients' experiences of change in cognitive–behavioral therapy and psychodynamic therapy: A qualitative comparative study. *Psychotherapy Research, 17*(5), 553–566. https://doi.org/10.1080/10503300601139988

Olivera, J., Braun, M., Gómez Penedo, J. M., & Roussos, A. (2013). A qualitative investigation of former clients' perception of change, reasons for consultation, therapeutic relationship, and termination. *Psychotherapy, 50*(4), 505–516. https://doi.org/10.1037/a0033359

Owen, J. J., Tao, K., Leach, M. M., & Rodolfa, E. (2011). Clients' perceptions of their psychotherapists' multicultural orientation. *Psychotherapy, 48*(3), 274–282. https://doi.org/10.1037/a0022065

Owen, J. J., Tao, K. W., Drinane, J. M., Hook, J., Davis, D. E., & Kune, N. F. (2016). Client perceptions of therapists' multicultural orientation: Cultural (missed) opportunities and cultural humility. *Professional Psychology: Research and Practice, 47*(1), 30–37. https://doi.org/10.1037/pro0000046

Paquin, J. D., Tao, K. W., & Budge, S. L. (2019). Toward a psychotherapy science for all: Conducting ethical and socially just research. *Psychotherapy, 56*(4), 491–502. https://doi.org/10.1037/pst0000271

Plumb, E. I. (2019). *Client perspectives on clinician multicultural competence in racially and/or ethically cross-cultural, strengths-based psychotherapy* (Publication No. 22623779) [Doctoral dissertation, University of California Santa Barbara]. ProQuest Dissertations and Theses Global.

Pope-Davis, D. B., Toporek, R. L., Ortega-Villalobos, L., Ligiéro, D. P., Brittan-Powell, C. S., Liu, W. M., Bashshur, M. R., Codrington, J. N., & Liang, C. T. H. (2002). Client perspectives of multicultural counseling competence: A qualitative examination. *The Counseling Psychologist, 30*(3), 355–393. https://doi.org/10.1177/0011000002303001

Radcliffe, K., Masterson, C., & Martin, C. (2018). Clients' experience of non-response to psychological therapy: A qualitative analysis. *Counselling & Psychotherapy Research, 18*(2), 220–229. https://doi.org/10.1002/capr.12161

Ramnerö, J., & Jansson, B. (2016). Treatment goals and their attainment: A structured approach to assessment and evaluation. *Cognitive Behaviour Therapy, 9*, 1–11. https://doi.org/10.1017/S1754470X15000756

Rennie, D. L. (1994). Clients' deference in psychotherapy. *Journal of Counseling Psychology,* *41*(4), 427–437. https://doi.org/10.1037/0022-0167.41.4.427

Rotheram-Borus, M. J., Swendeman, D., & Chorpita, B. F. (2012). Disruptive innovations for designing and diffusing evidence-based interventions. *American Psychologist, 67*(6), 463–476. https://doi.org/10.1037/a0028180

Roussos, A., Braun, M., & Olivera, J. (2017). *"For me it was a key moment of therapy"*: Corrective experience from the client's perspective. *Journal of Clinical Psychology, 73*(2), 153–167. https://doi.org/10.1002/jclp.22429

Snyder, C. R. (2002). Hope theory: Rainbows in the mind. *Psychological Inquiry, 13*(4), 249–275. https://doi.org/10.1207/S15327965PLI1304_01

Sousa, D., & Vaz, A. (2020). Significant events identified by clients engaged in existential psychotherapy: A descriptive phenomenological exploration. *Journal of Humanistic Psychology, 60*(6), 829–848. https://doi.org/10.1177/0022167817716304

Strauss, A., & Corbin, J. M. (1990). *Basics of qualitative research: Grounded theory procedures and techniques.* Sage Publications.

Sullivan, H. S. (1953). *The interpersonal theory of psychiatry.* W. W. Norton & Co.

Swift, J. K., Tompkins, K. A., & Parkin, S. R. (2017). Understanding the client's perspective of helpful and hindering events in psychotherapy sessions: A micro-process approach. *Journal of Clinical Psychology, 73*(11), 1543–1555. https://doi.org/10.1002/jclp.22531

Tafarodi, R. W., & Swann, W. B., Jr. (2001). Two-dimensional self-esteem: Theory and measurement. *Personality and Individual Differences, 31*(5), 653–673. https://doi.org/10.1016/S0191-8869(00)00169-0

Tao, K. W., Owen, J., Pace, B. T., & Imel, Z. E. (2015). A meta-analysis of multicultural competencies and psychotherapy process and outcome. *Journal of Counseling Psychology, 62*(3), 337–350. https://doi.org/10.1037/cou0000086

Timulak, L. (2007). Identifying core categories of client-identified impact of helpful events in psychotherapy: A qualitative meta-analysis. *Psychotherapy Research, 17*(3), 305–314. https://doi.org/10.1080/10503300600608116

Timulak, L. (2010). Significant events in psychotherapy: An update of research findings. *Psychology and Psychotherapy, 83*(4), 421–447. https://doi.org/10.1348/147608310X499404

Timulak, L., & Keogh, D. (2017). The client's perspective on (experiences of) psychotherapy: A practice friendly review. *Journal of Clinical Psychology, 73*(11), 1556–1567. https://doi.org/10.1002/jclp.22532

Tryon, G. S., Birch, S. E., & Verkuilen, J. (2018). Meta-analyses of the relation of goal consensus and collaboration to psychotherapy outcome. *Psychotherapy, 55*(4), 372–383. https://doi.org/10.1037/pst0000170

Tzur Bitan, D., & Abayed, S. (2020). Process expectations: Differences between therapists, patients, and lay individuals in their views of what works in psychotherapy. *Journal of Clinical Psychology, 76*(1), 20–30. https://doi.org/10.1002/jclp.22872

Tzur Bitan, D., & Lazar, A. (2019). What do people think works in psychotherapy: A qualitative and quantitative assessment of process expectations. *Professional Psychology: Research and Practice, 50*(4), 272–277. https://doi.org/10.1037/pro0000241

Tzur Bitan, D., Lazar, A., & Siton, B. (2018). Development of a scale quantifying expectations regarding active processes in therapy: The Expectations of Active Processes in Psychotherapy Scale (EAPPS). *Psychiatry Research, 267,* 131–139. https://doi.org/10.1016/j.psychres.2018.05.040

Valkonen, J., Hänninen, V., & Lindfors, O. (2011). Outcomes of psychotherapy from the perspective of the users. *Psychotherapy Research, 21*(2), 227–240. https://doi.org/10.1080/10503307.2010.548346

Wallerstein, R. S. (1990). The corrective emotional experience: Is reconsideration due? *Psychoanalytic Inquiry, 10*(3), 288–324. https://doi.org/10.1080/07351690.1990.10399609

Wampold, B. E., & Imel, Z. E. (2015). *The great psychotherapy debate: The evidence for what makes psychotherapy work* (2nd ed.). Routledge.

Werbart, A., von Below, C., Brun, J., & Gunnarsdottir, H. (2015). "Spinning one's wheels": Nonimproved patients view their psychotherapy. *Psychotherapy Research*, *25*(5), 546–564. https://doi.org/10.1080/10503307.2014.989291

Westra, H. A., Aviram, A., Barnes, M., & Angus, L. (2010). Therapy was not what I expected: A preliminary qualitative analysis of concordance between client expectations and experience of cognitive-behavioural therapy. *Psychotherapy Research*, *20*(4), 436–446. https://doi.org/10.1080/10503301003657395

Westra, H. A., Constantino, M. J., & Antony, M. M. (2016). Integrating motivational interviewing with cognitive-behavioral therapy for severe generalized anxiety disorder: An allegiance-controlled randomized clinical trial. *Journal of Consulting and Clinical Psychology*, *84*(9), 768–782. https://doi.org/10.1037/ccp0000098

Wucherpfennig, F., Boyle, K., Rubel, J. A., Weinmann-Lutz, B., & Lutz, W. (2020). What sticks? Patients' perspectives on treatment three years after psychotherapy: A mixed-methods approach. *Psychotherapy Research*, *30*(6), 739–752. https://doi.org/10.1080/10503307.2019.1671630

12

Clients' Experiences of Therapy Ending

Cheri Marmarosh

Although the psychotherapy literature has much to say about therapy relationship, process, and outcome (Flückiger et al., 2018) and the importance of therapists repairing ruptures to strengthen the relationship (Eubanks
et al., 2018; Safran & Muran, 2000), much less attention has been paid to the
end/ending of treatment (Swift & Greenberg, 2015; Wachtel, 2002). We all
know there is going to be a time when therapy will end, but the literature
seems to overlook that aspect of the work. Ending therapy can foster gratitude
toward a therapist, pride in achieving goals, hope for a positive future, and an
internal representation of a positive experience with the therapist. Therapists
have the opportunity to help clients end therapy and take the therapy experience with them so that it can provide hope and guidance in future psychological and emotional development and in other relationships (Marmarosh,
2017). Unfortunately, not all therapy ends this way. Many clients leave therapy
early in the treatment, contrary to clinical indications, and some fail to attend
the last sessions (Swift & Greenberg, 2012, 2015). Understanding how clients
experience therapy ending is critical as we try to help clients navigate this
important part of treatment.

There are many ways that clients experience the end of therapy. Some will
want to end as soon as therapy begins, some will drop out before they can say
goodbye, some will avoid ending at all costs, and some will experience gratitude and closeness at the end. One way to understand clients' experiences is
to explore the complexity of therapy relationships, starting with the different
types of endings. Certainly, terminations that are mutual and agreed on are

https://doi.org/10.1037/0000303-013
The Other Side of Psychotherapy: Understanding Clients' Experiences and Contributions in Treatment, J. N. Fuertes (Editor)

likely to be experienced differently than terminations that are unexpected and unilateral in nature. However, even clients who drop out can have different motivations for ending therapy. In addition to types of endings, the type of therapy treatment is likely to influence how a client experiences termination. We would expect that ending therapy by focusing on symptom relief would be quite different compared to ending therapy after a relational process. Adding to the complexity of termination are individual client factors that, when unattended to, can influence therapy and unwanted endings, such as a client's race, sexual orientation/identity, and ethnicity (Fuertes et al., 2005). The experiences of trauma/loss and attachment style also influence how clients cope with loss. Similarly, therapist characteristics influence how a client may experience termination (Zimmermann et al., 2017). Therapists with more empathy, tolerance for intimacy, and comfort with loss may facilitate a different process of ending compared to therapists with less capacity for empathy or with more difficulties coping with their own grief (Boyer & Hoffman, 1993).

This chapter aims to examine the different ways that clients experience the end of treatment, including unwanted endings. Theory and research will provide the background to understand how clients think and feel during termination, and clinical examples will shed light on the different ways clients can experience the ending of therapy.[1] The conclusion of the chapter focuses on future research and clinical implications.

TYPES OF THERAPY ENDINGS AND THEIR EFFECT ON TERMINATION

Not all therapy ends with a mutually agreed-on date, and sometimes clients end therapy for different reasons. Researchers have found that some clients go to the last scheduled session of the therapy and say goodbye to the therapist, which is what many refer to as a mutual termination. This type of ending is mutual because both therapist and client agree to the ending together. Although therapists would agree that mutual endings are preferred, many clients leave therapy without saying goodbye to the therapist or before the therapy is subjectively perceived as over from the therapist's perspective. These endings are unilateral endings (Swift & Greenberg, 2012). Unilateral endings can occur for different reasons, and they are the focus of many research studies because up to 50% of clients discontinue psychological services prematurely (Barrett et al., 2008; Swift et al., 2009).

In addition to unilateral and mutual terminations, there are endings based on therapists leaving the treatment when the client is still engaged in the therapy process. These transfer endings can occur when therapists need to leave their clinical role due to illness, pregnancy, their rotations ending, or a

---

[1]The identities of the individuals in this chapter's case examples have been properly disguised to protect client confidentiality.

need to relocate. All of these different types of endings influence the client's experience of ending therapy. While some are saying goodbye and feeling gratitude, some are feeling frustrated because they have not experienced symptom relief, and some are feeling misunderstood and abandoned. The type of ending influences the way a client thinks and feels.

When Clients Drop Out of Therapy

One of the best ways to understand how clients think and feel when they drop out of treatment is to ask them. O'Keeffe and colleagues (2019) used a multimethod analysis to understand why adolescents in treatment for depression left therapy prematurely. Out of 99 adolescents in their study, 32 dropped out of treatment. These clients who dropped out participated in a posttherapy interview about their experiences of therapy. After the interviews, the authors identified three different types of dropout: "dissatisfied" dropouts, "troubled" dropouts, and "got-what-they-needed" dropouts (O'Keeffe et al., 2019, p. 1). Eighteen were classified as "dissatisfied" dropouts and reported ending therapy because they did not find it useful to them anymore. Ten were classified as "got-what-they-needed" dropouts and reported ending therapy because they felt better and had benefited from therapy. Four were classified as "troubled" dropouts and reported ending therapy because of the stress in their lives. They reported feeling too overwhelmed to continue prioritizing their therapy sessions. These findings replicated earlier research that found that clients often drop out for these different reasons (Pekarik, 1992).

Dissatisfied Clients Dropping Out of Therapy

It is not hard to imagine the experience of clients who drop out of therapy when they feel that the therapy is not helping them. Why schedule sessions, drive to appointments, and deal with insurance reimbursement if you think therapy is not helping you resolve the issues that brought you to treatment? These clients are likely to feel relieved after they end with their therapist. Instead of confronting the therapist with their negative feelings or thoughts, they avoid them by withdrawing and ending the relationship. One can imagine that they often feel angry, disappointed, hopeless, and unable to voice these concerns to their therapist. Hummelen et al. (2007) interviewed eight female group members who dropped out of group therapy. While this is not the same as individual treatment, there are some possible parallels to client experiences of dropping out of individual treatment. They found that many of the members who dropped out felt as though the group made them feel worse, that the leaders did not notice how badly they felt, and that they could not share their experiences. Leaving therapy was the only way to feel better and resolve the painful situation.

What is even more concerning is that therapists can be unaware of how unhappy or frustrated with treatment their clients are feeling as they end therapy. According to Hunsley et al. (1999), therapists and clients made different attributions about failed therapy. These researchers compared training clinic therapists' reasons for their clients' termination written in their final reports with reasons reported directly from interviews with 87 clients. Their results suggested that therapists were not aware of their clients' reasons for ending and did not often indicate that their clients' reason for termination was their frustration with therapy. Clients reported leaving therapy because of their dissatisfaction with therapy around 12% of the time, while therapists did not describe a single client who ended therapy because they were dissatisfied with therapy.

Westmacott et al. (2010) presented similar findings in individual therapy. Specifically, they found that when clients terminated therapy unilaterally, compared with their therapists, they rated four reasons for termination as significantly more important to their decision to leave. Compared to the therapists, these clients ascribed higher importance to all of the reasons related to a dislike of therapy or the therapist. For example, they rated "Felt therapy was going nowhere so ended therapy," "Felt therapy was making things worse," "Weren't confident in therapist's ability to help," and "Therapy did not fit with ideas about what would be helpful." The researchers noted that clients and therapists are more similar when rating the other barriers to therapy such as schedule, transportation, and finances, but they are not similar when it comes to more personal reasons that include therapist skill or therapist helpfulness.

Clinical Example. Manny was a 25-year-old gay, African American, male client. He started therapy after the COVID-19 pandemic moved everything in his life online, including his job, relationship with his family, and social group. Manny met the criteria for a major depressive episode, but he was anxious about seeking therapy. For him, needing treatment was a weakness, and he felt ashamed that he "needed to be seen" by a therapist. He agreed to try online therapy when his partner suggested it to him. At the third session, the therapist recommended medication, and Manny felt humiliated. He did not think his symptoms were "that bad." He did not reveal his feelings to the therapist, a White, cisgender man. Manny wondered if the therapist referred him for medication because he was gay and Black. Manny started to not show up for sessions and said that he was "busy at work." The therapist did not explore the missed appointments in depth, and Manny stopped attending sessions. When the therapist finally called, Manny did not return the call. Manny later revealed that he did not think that the therapy was helping him, and he did not feel comfortable challenging the therapist's recommendation for medication. When asked, he said he felt misunderstood, intimidated, and frustrated during the therapy sessions.

As is evident from the case of Manny, clients can experience a rupture in the alliance when their therapists make treatment recommendations that they disagree with (e.g., recommending medication). This experience led Manny to feel dissatisfied and frustrated with the treatment. Manny expressed a safer issue, being busy at work, to explain his withdrawal from therapy. If his therapist had raised other possibilities for the missed sessions, the therapist and Manny could have possibly explored the rupture together. In this case, Manny relied on his internal explanation for the rupture. Manny, a gay Black man who has experienced oppression and discrimination, wondered if the therapist was influenced by the color of his skin or sexual orientation. This only increased Manny's sense of anger, hurt, and mistrust. Because Manny did not feel safe to say what he thought and/or felt with the therapist, he avoided challenging the therapist and left the treatment.

Troubled Dropouts: When Life Is Too Stressful for Therapy

It is common to hear clients say that they could not attend sessions because they do not have the finances, transportation, child care, or time away from work. This is what Manny said when he wanted to leave the treatment. These barriers to treatment include practical obstacles (e.g., losing a job) and they are associated with a greater risk of dropout (Kazdin & Wassell, 2000; O'Keeffe et al., 2019). According to Westmacott et al. (2010), therapists are often accurate when assessing these dropout risks, and clients are often more comfortable sharing these reasons for leaving therapy. Some therapists would argue that even though these are actual obstacles for therapy, they may mask underlying ambivalence to treatment related to more complex issues that are out of awareness or more difficult to talk about (Marmarosh, 2017). Clients who are fearful of intimacy and have a history of self-reliance may not feel comfortable depending on a therapist. They may prefer to depend on themselves, and often their work is a priority over their relationships. Through work, they can find meaning and stability. Relying on people makes them more anxious and uncomfortable. They may blame ending therapy on not being able to get time away from work, but it may actually be due to fears of intimacy and the increasing dependency on the therapist, an avoidant attachment style (Marmarosh, 2017). It is critical for therapists to explore the possibility of underlying issues so that clients can begin to work on some of the relationship issues they struggle with outside of therapy. Exploring these barriers may be helpful and illuminate exactly why a client wants to leave therapy.

Clinical Example. Kelly was a 50-year-old, single, White, cisgender woman. She came to therapy after getting divorced and struggling with feelings of anxiety and depression. She saw her therapist for a year in once-a-week psychotherapy. Over time, Kelly revealed more and more about her struggles to be alone and about her unhappiness that stemmed from a history of feeling unloved as a child. Kelly learned that she was always trying to please others and struggled to discover her own desires and needs. After her divorce, Kelly felt alone and betrayed after sacrificing her needs for her husband, who left her for another woman. During therapy, Kelly started to feel better about herself, felt less depressed, and started dating a man she met at work. Kelly revealed that she wanted to end therapy and said it was due to her finances. The therapist explored Kelly's desire to end treatment and wondered if it had anything to do with feeling better or being in a new relationship. At first, Kelly denied that these had anything to do with her feelings and focused on her financial demands. After a few sessions and gentle curiosity on the part of her therapist, she revealed that she did feel better and wanted to see if she could be OK on her own. The therapist wondered with Kelly about her desire to leave but praised her for asserting her needs/desires in the therapy relationship. The discussion led to her exploration of being fearful the therapist would be angry if Kelly wanted to end therapy, and she could never come back if she needed therapy in the future. She also revealed that she thinks that her husband left the marriage because she started to focus more on herself. Both Kelly and the therapist agreed that ending therapy was a good idea as long as they explored these emerging feelings. They agreed to continue to work together for another 3 months and then terminated. During the last session, Kelly revealed never having this type of close relationship with a caregiver who believed in her and was supportive, even when she was "being selfish." She always felt that she had to make others happy to get what she needed. Kelly felt some sadness during the last session but also pride, gratitude, and love.

It is helpful to understand the "troubled dropouts" and ensure that clients are leaving for the reasons they initially share. As we see from the clinical examples, Manny presented with work demands, instead of the hurt and frustration that he felt with his therapist's recommendation. Kelly initially said she wanted to end due to finances, but it was also because she felt better and wanted to end therapy. She was afraid to tell the therapist the truth because of her core fear of losing her caregiver if she prioritized her needs. Although it is common to have multiple reasons for termination as we described, it can be due to finances, work, and changing demands alone. It is important to try to understand all the possible motivations by being curious with clients, regardless of the reason they initially describe.

Got What They Needed: Clients Ending After Achieving Their Treatment Goals

Many researchers have found no difference in clinical outcomes between dropouts and completers (Kazdin et al., 1994; O'Keeffe et al., 2019). After interviewing and assessing adolescents who dropped out of therapy, O'Keeffe et al. (2019) did not find any strong evidence that there were poorer outcomes for those adolescents who dropped out of treatment compared to those who completed treatment. These findings suggest that dropping out of therapy may not always indicate worse clinical outcomes. Clients may end treatment because they are dissatisfied with therapy, but sometimes they end because they have achieved their goals. Those who have achieved their goals may perceive therapy to be a medical intervention where one leaves the treatment when one has fewer symptoms. The relational component of "saying goodbye" may not be expected. This may be due to a lack of information about psychotherapy expectations, interpersonal/attachment style, age, ethnicity, or cultural expectations. We will examine these client factors later in the chapter; they contribute significantly to how clients experience endings in therapy.

Clinical Example. Amal was a 27-year-old, cisgender, male graduate student who started therapy to cope with anxiety about his dissertation. He was an international student from Egypt and was hesitant to seek therapy services. He spoke about not being familiar with therapy and worrying about what his family would say if they knew he started treatment. Despite his fears, he said that he benefited from the relaxation techniques and said that the homework was helpful. After he defended his dissertation, Amal started to cancel sessions. When the therapist called him, he apologized and said he did not want to take up more time since he was feeling better and completed his research work. He wanted to make sure other people could have the opportunity to take his time slot. The therapist asked if he wanted to come in to say goodbye, and Amal said he preferred not to. He thanked the therapist and referred a friend to the clinic. Amal said he felt supported during the treatment and left the therapy when he achieved his goals. He said that he did not feel the need to say goodbye given his "professional" relationship with his therapist. He said he would definitely go back if he needed to in the future.

In this example, Amal revealed a positive alliance with his therapist and a desire to end therapy when his symptoms resolved. His Egyptian background influenced his comfort with therapy, and he compared the relationship with his therapist to a relationship with a medical doctor. For him, there is no need to continue therapy when the problems are addressed. Amal valued the structure of the therapy, felt good about the treatment, and left treatment when he felt better. It is common for clients to feel better and begin focusing on ending therapy during this time. The therapist may know that "feeling better" may not mean that there is nothing important to work on in therapy. Oftentimes, the issues that led to "feeling bad" initially are due to existing issues that remain and are risk factors for future struggles. It is helpful to explore this with clients if the therapist can. If they cannot explore this because the client dropped out, at least the clients leave the therapy feeling positive about the outcome of the treatment, and they feel able to return to therapy if/when they need to.

When Therapists End Therapy: The Impact of Therapist Transfer on Clients

Although there is not a lot of literature focused on how clients cope with therapists leaving them, this happens frequently. In many training clinics, therapists go on internship, externship, or postdoctoral training. When therapists leave, their clients are referred to new therapists entering the training program. In private practice, clients are referred to new therapists when clinicians leave due to maternity, health issues, life changes, and retirement. These therapy endings are different compared to any other, and research has shown that transfer is an important juncture in the therapy process (Marmarosh & Salamon, 2020; Schen et al., 2013). Clients are ending a relationship with one therapist while planning to begin another. One would expect this ending to feel different from one where both the client and the therapist feel ready to end the treatment.

Keith (1966) described a "transfer syndrome" that clients experience when treatment with one therapist ends and they begin treatment with another therapist. This syndrome includes feelings of rejection, depression, anger, grief, and anxiety. Researchers and clinicians have also described clients' feeling a sense of abandonment, grief, and loss (Clark et al., 2014); anger toward the transfer and the new therapist (Penn, 1990); and feelings of unworthiness (Penn, 1990). Clark and colleagues (2014) interviewed 11 clients about their personal experiences of being transferred at some time during their treatment. Most clients indicated that they felt some anxiety, fear, sadness, and anger about the transfer. Baum (2005) studied clients' reactions to terminations and found significant correlations between hurt/anger with the abruptness of the termination, the therapy relationship, and whether clients had a choice in treatment ending. The more abrupt the termination, the more important the relationship had been as perceived by the client, and the less choice that the client had in ending, the more hurt/anger the clients reported. It is no wonder that transfer can lead to clients dropping out of therapy; some studies report a dropout rate as high as 69% after a transfer (Tantam & Klerman, 1979; Wapner et al., 1986).

Clinical Example

Amy was a 50-year-old, White, female cisgender client who had been in treatment at the community mental health clinic for 5 years. The clinic is housed within a graduate training program, and Amy had gone through four transfers when her therapists left for advanced training. Each year, her therapists tried to refer her out of the clinic, but Amy said she did not have the financial resources to pay for therapy. She was often unemployed. Amy had a long history of trauma, and she was diagnosed with bipolar I disorder and borderline personality disorder. After the first transfer, Amy was depressed and angry. As the ending approached, Amy started cutting herself and missing sessions. She did not show up to the last session with her therapist, and she canceled several sessions with her new therapist. It took 3 months of "testing" her new therapist before Amy started to attend regularly. After years of multiple transfers, Amy's therapists became knowledgeable of her issues of abandonment and worked with her to increase her emotional regulation. They focused a significant amount of time on termination and transfer. During the last transfer, 5 years into treatment, the therapist took a significant amount of time helping Amy cope with her separation anxiety. She also referred Amy to group therapy so that she would feel less isolated. Amy was able to attend the last session and, although she still felt angry and abandoned, was able to talk about these feelings with the therapist. The therapist was able to empathize with Amy's experience and helped her adjust to the transition to the new therapist. Although the last session was not easy, Amy attended the session, felt like she was less alone, and felt capable of enduring the painful feelings of abandonment and loss. She said she felt less self-blame and felt hopeful because she had survived this before and developed more coping resources to help manage her distress.

The example of Amy demonstrates how clients feel when therapy ends because the therapist has to leave the treatment. After the first transfer, Amy felt abandoned and angry, and she channeled her rage into self-destructive behaviors. Over time, we see how Amy learned to cope with feelings of repeated loss and to remain engaged in therapy and tolerate the endings. Although transfers in therapy can be challenging, clients can have a variety of reactions to them that can evolve from negative to positive.

Mutual Terminations: Agreed-On Endings

All therapy approaches describe the process of termination, and most therapists would agree that ideally a mutually agreed-on ending to therapy is the best option. The experience of ending therapy from the clients' perspective is likely related to how the therapist addresses the treatment and the ending. There is much diversity with regards to how therapists end therapy. Different theoretical models influence how clients may experience the ending of treatment.

Existential therapists generally recommend focusing on ending from the beginning of the therapy treatment and continually looking for opportunities to explore mortality, loss, grief, and endings throughout the clinical work (Yalom, 2020). Psychoanalytic/dynamic therapists generally recommend allowing the client to determine the timing of termination, discussing the client's coping, reviewing gains and future goals, discussing the helpful and unhelpful aspects of therapy, and inviting the client to call with updates at a future point (Joyce et al., 2007). Emotion-focused therapists also suggest letting the client determine the termination date, helping the client work through feelings of loss and grief, empowering the client, setting realistic expectations for future challenges, and offering the possibility of future appointments (Greenberg, 2002). Cognitive behavioral therapists (Beck, 1995; Goldfried, 2002) argue that the therapist should focus less on the feelings of loss or the therapy relationship during the termination process. They argue that the therapist should help the client maintain the gains made during treatment by setting a termination date, gradually tapering sessions, focusing on the new skills learned, and allowing the client to work through their problems independently. A major principle of cognitive behavior therapy involves helping clients become their own therapists, so from the first session the therapist prepares the client for the end of therapy when they learn to take the skills they learned in treatment and apply them independently (Beck, 1995).

Two special issues dedicated to termination in the journal *Psychotherapy* (2017 and 2020) included papers devoted to different perspectives on termination. These papers explored termination in short-term, psychodynamic treatment (16 sessions; Harrison, 2020), cognitive behavioral dynamic therapy (Shahar & Ziv-Beiman, 2020), and cognitive behavior therapy (Vidair et al., 2017). Norcross et al. (2017) studied the commonalities in termination across these theoretical orientations and found that there were some things that all therapists did when helping their clients end therapy. These authors asked 65 experts from diverse theoretical orientations to indicate the frequency with which they used 80 tasks in a planned, mutually agreed-on termination of individual treatment. Principal components analyses of all behaviors/tasks identified eight unique factors:

> process feelings of patient and therapist, discuss patient's future functioning and coping, help patient use new skills beyond therapy, frame personal development as invariably unfinished, anticipate post-therapy growth, prepare explicitly for termination, reflect on patient gains and consolidation, and express pride in patient's progress and mutual relationship. (Norcross et al., 2017, p. 66)

When looking at the breakdown of the percentage of therapists who actually said goodbye to their clients, only 73% said they did that routinely. Only 50% said they validate clients' negative reactions to terminating, 50% said they frequently explore clients' feelings of loss, and 50% said they address what did not go well in therapy and negative reactions. Only 33% endorsed acknowledging termination as a real loss of a relationship, and half of the clinicians explored the possible negative aspects of the therapy relationship during termination.

When looking at the different approaches to ending therapy, it appears that some therapists believe there is a significant amount of growth that can occur at termination in addition to consolidating prior work (Quintana, 1993) and that ending therapy can have a significant impact on a client (Harrison, 2020; Marmarosh, 2017). Marmarosh (2017) described how therapists can be emotionally present and provide clients a different experience when they share painful emotions and intimate feelings that often are stirred during times of loss. Instead of being alone, abandoned, or rejected, clients can feel understood and valued, challenging earlier internal schemas of self and others. Harrison (2020) described accelerated experiential dynamic psychotherapy (AEDP), a short-term dynamic model that emphasizes attachment theory and emotional attunement during termination.

Both Marmarosh (2017) and Harrison (2020) argued that facilitating endings in therapy allows the therapist to address clients' underlying relational needs, foster emotion regulation, and facilitate a new relational experience that can be transformative for clients. Harrison described how clients feel relieved when they can express their loss, fear, and sadness with the therapist during termination. Experiencing the sadness with a caring therapist who is present and empathic facilitates an adaptive relational experience, one that is different from the interactions most clients have historically or outside of therapy. Many describe this as a corrective emotional experience (Alexander & French, 1946; Bridges, 2006) because clients have a new relational experience of empathic attunement, compassion, and curiosity during distress that is restorative and likely to engender feelings of closeness, hope, sadness, and gratitude. These positive reactions to termination are not new. Marx and Gelso (1987) asked clients about their experience with termination and found that half or more of the clients reported positive feelings about ending therapy that included feeling calm, happy, and healthy. Harrison described how AEDP therapists help clients "take in the good" and embrace positive emotional reactions during the ending of therapy. The therapist is encouraged to disclose personal thoughts, feelings, and reactions to the client that also deepen the emotional experience between them. Successful endings can provide new responses to loss and the ability to rely on attachment figures to downregulate distress and upregulate gratitude and hope (Wallin, 2007). According to neuroscientists, the therapist who acts as a secure figure for clients is able to facilitate emotion regulation and challenge automatic fight-or-flight responses that were adaptive early in life but inhibit closeness and intimacy (Porges, 2011, 2017; Schore, 2000, 2019). In essence, relational experiences where clients can be present and engaged, versus withdrawing or picking a fight, can facilitate changes in automatic interpersonal behaviors and impact future relationships.

When clients drop out of treatment, even if they feel better and have made important gains in therapy, they do not have the opportunity to say goodbye to their therapists. Some clinicians believe that this is an important component of the therapy treatment, regardless of whether the therapy is successful at reducing symptoms or facilitating change. A client can drop out of treatment, like Amal, while still having a strong working alliance and meeting treatment goals. What they may miss when they drop out includes learning how their therapist feels about them, how they experience the relationship, how it feels to end therapy, and how it feels when saying goodbye. More importantly, they get to share their vulnerability with their therapists and are able to rely on their therapists to cope with any feelings that come up when saying goodbye. They are not alone.

What Do Clients Say? Qualitative Data on Different Terminations

As we know, not all terminations end well. Knox et al. (2011) interviewed 12 clients who had experienced therapy and different types of terminations. They asked the clients about their experience ending their therapies and found that most had positive endings, while some had negative ones. Their findings are similar to those previously described. Those who had positive endings indicated that therapy ended because of logistical or financial reasons and sometimes because they felt good enough to end therapy. They reported that they expressed a variety of emotions and felt the therapy was helpful. For those who had negative endings, termination occurred because of unresolved ruptures in the therapy, although logistical or financial reasons also existed. The termination process was sometimes an abrupt and unilateral decision made by the client. These clients also said that the termination typically led to a decline in the therapy relationship. Knox et al. described one example of a client named Bonnie, who was furious with her therapist during the ending and dropped out. Bonnie described her therapist as "self-righteous and smug." Bonnie wanted to "slap [her] upside the head . . . and say 'What do you think you're doing?'" Bonnie stated that she felt "devastated" by the last session and cried after. She described feeling abandoned, and she noted that the therapy was a "major traumatic relationship that . . . caused damage similar to what she experienced as a child" (Knox et al., 2011, p. 162). Clearly, this is not how we plan for therapy to end, but unfortunately in this case, and others, it can happen. There are many reasons why endings, despite strong theory and good intentions, are painful and even destructive to the client. Many client and therapist factors influence how clients experience the ending of therapy.

CLIENT FACTORS THAT INFLUENCE CLIENTS' EXPERIENCE OF ENDINGS IN THERAPY

Many client factors influence how therapy will end, but one of the most important factors is how the client experiences the therapy relationship. The empirical literature on termination highlights the importance of the working alliance during the termination phase of treatment (Tryon & Kane, 1993; Westmacott et al., 2010). The *alliance* is defined as the relationship between the client and therapist that facilitates safety and trust. It includes the bond between them, the agreement on the goals of the work, and a shared commitment to the tasks of therapy (Bordin, 1979; Gelso & Hayes, 1998).

Anything that facilitates or engenders ruptures in the alliance is also likely to influence the experience of ending (Tryon & Kane, 1993; Westmacott et al., 2010). For example, microaggressions, which are subtle offensive comments that devalue clients based on their different identities, can occur during therapy, and these ruptures can lead to deteriorations in the alliance (Sue, 2010; Sue et al., 2007) and end in unilateral terminations (Vasquez, 2007). Client attachment style (Marmarosh, 2017; Marmarosh & Salamon, 2020; Zilberstein, 2008), personality (Ben David-Sela et al., 2020), and history of loss (Marx & Gelso, 1987) also influence the alliance and termination. Client self-esteem, self-blame, and sense of failure in treatment can impact the experience of ending as well (Baum, 2005). These factors are discussed next, primarily within the context of client attachment styles, following a review of how the working alliance affects clients' experiences of termination and how therapist microaggressions toward the client can impact the alliance.

Working Alliance: Impacting How Clients Feel as They End Treatment

The working alliance, the client and the therapist's agreement on the task, goal, and bond in therapy, is the most important component of the therapy process, regardless of orientation or approach to treatment (Wampold & Imel, 2015). Many studies have shown that the alliance relates to the overall success of therapy (Flückiger et al., 2018), and repairing ruptures in the alliance improves the treatment process (Safran & Muran, 2000) and facilitates positive outcomes (Eubanks et al., 2018). When it comes to ending therapy and how clients experience ending, the alliance between the client and therapist is what has the most impact (Tryon & Kane, 1993).

Westmacott et al. (2010) studied how the early treatment alliance related to premature termination. They found that the client–therapist dyads who made mutual decisions to end therapy reported a stronger working alliance early in treatment compared with the dyads where the client terminated unilaterally. In addition, they found that clients who unilaterally terminated reported lower quality alliances with their therapists and had worse therapy outcomes, perhaps indicating that the end of treatment was unplanned or premature. The authors suggested that when termination was a unilateral decision made by the client, therapists appeared to be unaware of the extent to which their clients perceived failure in therapy. The authors stated that therapists were largely aware of clients' dissatisfaction, but they rated the importance of clients' dissatisfaction as less important to staying in therapy. It appears that clients may be unlikely to share the extent of their negative perceptions of therapy and the therapist. Clients who struggle with the goals of therapy, disagree with the tasks of therapy, or do not feel a bond with the therapist are at an increased risk of dropping out and ending the therapy frustrated and disappointed.

On the other hand, Knox et al. (2011) found that clients who described positive termination experiences reported strong positive alliances with their therapists. They recalled the helpful effects from therapy, and they said that they terminated largely because of extratherapy issues that included finances or moving. They described planning and discussing the termination process together during sessions, clients reviewed the course of therapy and their related growth, and both the clients and therapists shared their feelings about termination. In essence, the better the alliance in therapy, the better the ending of therapy, where clients felt satisfied and positive about their treatment.

Ruptures in the Alliance: Microaggressions and Ending Therapy

What leads to these ruptures in the therapy alliance? Often ruptures are caused by therapists saying or doing offensive things based on their bias, insensitivity, or lack of knowledge regarding diversity (Constantine, 2007; Sue et al., 2007; Vasquez, 2007). We know that racial/ethnic minority clients receive fewer services and drop out more often compared with White clients (Whaley & Davis, 2007). People of color also underuse services and often terminate prematurely. Fifty percent of the time, when people of color enter treatment, they terminate after one session, in contrast to 30% of White clients who terminate after one session (Sue et al., 2007). It is likely that there are challenges that minority clients face that White clients do not.

Various studies have found that racial microaggressions negatively influence the alliance as well as satisfaction with therapy (Owen et al., 2014). Constantine (2007) described how well-intentioned therapists can unconsciously have biases that covertly communicate racist and prejudiced attitudes toward minority clients. These microaggressions cause ruptures in the alliance and are toxic to the therapy treatment. Owen et al. (2012) studied therapists' racial/ethnic disparities in clients' unilateral termination and found that some therapists have greater dropout rates when working with minority clients. Hook et al. (2016) examined 2,212 participants with both same and mixed dyads, and they found that 81% of clients reported at least one perceived microaggression in therapy, mostly consisting of denial or a lack of awareness of cultural stereotypes. Okosi (2018) relied on semistructured interviews to study racial microaggressions, their impact, barriers to repair, and attitudes toward therapy. The results revealed that clients of color reported microaggressions that hindered therapy and led to dropout. One example was a Black female client being treated by a White therapist. When the therapist suggested the client not be so hard on herself, the client said,

> You can't tell me that I can't be intense about my experience, or my education, or my expectations . . . when I am the only woman of color in my program. . . . It does stress me out, it does spike my anxiety, but I can't just not be a Black woman in a PhD program. So asking me blanket statements does not help me in therapy sessions because it's not coming from a place of understanding myself and my identity in relation to . . . my experiences in education. (Okosi, 2018, pp. 75–76)

It is important to note that this client did not tell the White therapist this is how she felt.

In another example, an Asian American client described a rupture when the therapist suggested that the client's deep concerns with her family were equivalent to being codependent (Okosi, 2018, p. 88). This client felt misunderstood and shamed by the therapist's pathologizing of her cultural values. These types of microaggressions, if not repaired, can erode the alliance and lead to premature terminations. Okosi (2018) described different kinds of microaggressions in therapy that shed light on why some clients drop out of therapy and do not feel a sense of gratitude or hope as they end therapy. Lee et al. (2018) demonstrated how therapists can address microaggressive enactments in psychotherapy and how therapists can address these ruptures in treatment. Therapists can empathize with the client, apologize for saying something offensive, and be curious about the impact of the microaggression on the client. When these enactments are addressed and repaired, clients can experience a positive alliance with their therapists and endings can be healing.

Client Attachment: Impacting How Clients End Therapy

Several theorists have applied attachment theory to understand the ending of psychotherapy treatment (Bowlby, 1980; Harrison, 2020; Holmes, 1997; Marmarosh, 2017; Zilberstein, 2008). The theory explains why some individuals struggle during the ending of therapy, some withdraw, and some have a meaningful termination. According to Bowlby (1988), clients develop an attachment to their therapists, and then the therapist can become a secure base for clients, similar to early development and the reliance on the caregiver for support. The therapist becomes a "secure base" that allows clients to open up and vulnerably explore various issues (Holmes, 2009; Wallin, 2007). Zilberstein (2008) described how therapy activates the attachment system because it replicates many of the characteristics of the early parent–child relationship. Research has shown that attachment styles influence how people leave relationships in general and handle issues of loss (Mikulincer & Shaver, 2016). Ending therapy certainly activates the attachment system and triggers automatic internal representations of the self and the other (Wallin, 2007; Zilberstein, 2008).

According to Bowlby (1988), adults with anxious attachment styles, and those with histories of insecurity, inconsistent care, and experiences of abandonment, are more vulnerable to prolonged or chronic grief, whereas individuals who have avoidant attachment styles, those with histories of being self-reliant, are more likely to express few overt signs of grief. Adults with secure attachment styles are the ones who are able to grieve and seek comfort from others. They tend to have a greater capacity to express emotions, a greater ability to forgive others, and an increased ability to trust those taking care of them (Mikulincer & Shaver, 2016).

Secure Attachment and Ending Therapy

According to Holmes (1997, 2009), securely attached clients have a stronger capacity for intimate engagement, and they cope better with the termination of therapy. They tend to approach the ending of treatment with an appreciation of both the gains and losses of treatment, are able to regulate their feelings, and have a larger repertoire of coping mechanisms when dealing with stress (Fraley & Shaver, 1999). Secure individuals are also better at seeking social support outside of treatment and have more resources to rely on when losing a secure base, such as a therapist. Shulman and Gold (1999) found that secure clients experienced more positive affect and less anxiety and depressive affect in response to termination. They had more of a capacity to cope with the loss. More importantly, secure individuals can rely on internal memories of attachment figures that allow them to remain connected to the individual despite them being physically alone (Bowlby, 1980). This internal bond with the therapist allows secure individuals to re-create their relationship from one that was real to one that is now representational.

Clinical Example: Secure Clients Ending Therapy. Robert, a transgender, 22-year-old, Black client who uses the pronouns they/their, was ending therapy at a university counseling center after seeking treatment due to anxiety and depression related to being a victim of discrimination and bullying on campus. Robert came from a close family who embraced their gender identity. Robert said they were supportive of them and that Robert did not experience this level of hatred until college. During treatment, Robert was able to open up to the therapist, took risks, and built a strong working alliance. At termination, they felt a sense of loss but also a sense of gratitude for the support they received. They revealed that therapy provided a safe place to express their anger and frustration. They also felt that they could feel safe with someone who valued their minority identities.

In this example, Robert was a secure client who was coping with systemic racism and cissexism, the devaluation of those who are not cisgender. Robert was able to seek out therapy services to cope with their anxiety and depression and was able to establish a strong therapeutic alliance. Therapy can provide a secure base for them where they feel understood, and Robert ended therapy feeling gratitude toward the therapist.

Anxious Adult Attachment and Ending Therapy

Pistole (1999) described how anxiously attached clients often display protest behaviors (e.g., missing appointments, the reemergence of symptoms, increased anger, anxiety) in response to termination. Because anxious patients have more painful experiences and less of a capacity to self-soothe, they have more difficulty downregulating their distress (Schore, 2000) and they are more easily stuck in their fight-or-flight response, which inhibits their engagement (Porges, 2011). As Bowlby (1980) described, they are more inclined to engage in hyper-activating attachment strategies in therapy (e.g., calling more, requesting more help, having more symptoms), they struggle to tolerate separations and being alone, and they continue to seek out the attachment figure years after that figure is gone. They struggle to accept a loss because they have trouble relying on a secure internal representation of someone who comforts them. These clients are likely to be more activated at termination and require emotional support during the ending. They may express more symptoms, perceive abandonment, and are often critical of themselves (Marmarosh, 2017). If the therapist is aware of their experience, they can help prepare them for the upcoming ending. There is hope that instead of experiencing their pain alone and feeling abandoned, they may feel a deep sense of connection and hope for future relationships (Harrison, 2020). The ending of therapy can be experienced differently depending on how the therapist facilitates the treatment, is able to explore and repair ruptures, and engages with the client during the termination process.

Clinical Example: Anxiously Attached Clients Ending Therapy. Serena was a 60-year-old, White, female, cisgender client referred to therapy by her primary care provider. She was experiencing many symptoms that included anxiety, weight gain, increased sleep, difficulty concentrating, and mood swings. Her primary care provider said that she often called the practice for emotional support and was never satisfied. She has a history of unsatisfying relationships and low self-esteem. In therapy, Serena initially deferred to the therapist and avoided any conflict. Over time, she became more open and revealed her fears that the therapist did not care about her. Serena revealed a history of abandonment by her parents who were struggling with her sister's mental health concerns. The only time she recalled getting attention was when she took care of others in her home. The therapist worked with Serena for 3 years to help her address her underlying depression and low self-esteem and to challenge her automatic perceptions of herself as unlovable and others as rejecting. The therapist worked with Serena for months to prepare her for termination. During the ending of treatment, Serena revealed more depression and grief. Despite the increase in symptoms, she was able to rely on the therapist to cope with these feelings instead of being overwhelmed by them. She ended treatment relying on the positive experience with a therapist who was very different from her early caregivers.

As we can see, Serena has a difficult time relying on relationships for support due to the impact of her early life experiences. This is different from

Robert, who had a more secure attachment style and did not struggle to develop a strong therapeutic alliance. Like others with elevated attachment anxiety, Serena has a negative internal representation of herself as needy/unlovable and others as more powerful and rejecting. When she is in distress, she demonstrates hyperactivating strategies that include calling frequently for help and becoming flooded with emotions. Termination triggered her feelings of emotional abandonment, and the therapist worked with Serena for many sessions to help her cope with the ending. Despite feeling some increased distress, she was able to end therapy by relying on the positive relational experience she had with her therapist. It is important to note that if the therapist ended suddenly or was not aware of how endings could trigger painful feelings for Serena, the ending could have been more challenging with many opportunities for ruptures.

Avoidant Adult Attachment and Ending Therapy

Unlike anxious clients, there are clients who do not express any significant signs of grief after a loss (Fraley & Shaver, 1999). Fraley and Bonanno (2004) studied how attachment styles related to different grief patterns for individuals experiencing the death of a loved one. They found that more avoidant individuals revealed less grief initially and even years later. Fraley and Shaver (1997) argued that these individuals did not allow themselves to become as attached in relationships to begin with, and that is why they experienced less grief when relationships ended. According to these authors, more avoidant-attached individuals do not overtly express sadness, anger, or distress. They also seek little solace from friends and often cope as if nothing ended or changed. Bowlby (1980) argued that those clients with avoidant attachment styles have learned early on how to deactivate their distress responses and engage defenses that protect them from feelings of longing and despair. Bowlby described this process as defensive exclusion. Fraley and Shaver (1999) contended that defensive exclusion is an adaptive strategy because it diverts attention away from painful experiences that threaten self-sufficiency, and it facilitates emotion regulation during times of loss. It is safe to say that clients with more attachment avoidance will end therapy feeling less distressed and may even feel more relief. These may be clients who terminate therapy prematurely because they are less attached to the group. They are also likely to provide vague reasons for ending, such as changes in their work schedule, and are more likely to fail to return the therapists' calls.

Clinical Example: Avoidantly Attached Clients Ending Therapy. Jose was a 57-year-old, cisgender, heterosexual, Latino man. He was referred by his wife, who threatened to divorce him if he did not go to therapy. Jose had multiple affairs and was detached from the relationship. Jose did not believe he needed treatment and only attended five sessions. During the treatment, it became clear that Jose did not have many memories from his childhood. When asked, he described being happy as a child, but he recalled few happy memories and spent much of his time alone. As an adult, he described a history of relationships that ended abruptly when he was no longer "interested." He had a hard time identifying his feelings in the sessions and externalized his problems. He often no-showed for sessions or came late to therapy. His therapist often felt like an object who was there to listen to him complain about others. When the therapist gave him feedback, he denied responsibility for his attendance and had trouble identifying his own issues to work on. He appeared relieved to end the therapy and denied any feelings of anger, loss, or grief.

As we can see, Jose presents differently from Serena. Jose denies feelings of distress and does not look for relational support. Much like those higher on attachment avoidance, Jose engages in deactivating strategies. He detaches from his wife, engages in affairs to get physical needs for intimacy met, ends relationships frequently when he is bored, and does not form a meaningful alliance with the therapist. When he ends the treatment after five sessions, he feels relieved because the therapy was stressful for him. He was not able to see how he was responsible for many of the issues in his marriage. He often felt frustrated in therapy and blamed his wife for their difficulties. Leaving relationships alleviates the distress he feels when challenged. The hardest thing for Jose is to stay in the relationship and work on reducing his avoidance.

Endings and the Client's Past: History of Loss, Trauma, and Personality Disorder

Similar to client attachment, client history of loss and trauma and client personality also influence how they experience ending therapy. Marx and Gelso (1987) found that a client's loss history predicted the importance they placed on discussing their reactions during termination. Ben David-Sela et al. (2020) examined how clients end treatment and found that the majority of clients felt regulated with a sense of gratitude except for clients who suffered from Cluster B personality disorders (PD). These personality disorders include borderline PD, narcissistic PD, and antisocial PD. The authors said that many of these clients could not manage the feelings at the end of the therapy and expressed their dissatisfaction or disagreement with the therapist at the end of treatment. They gave an example of a client who waited until the end of the last session to tell the therapist how bad she felt and how therapy did not help her at all. Baum (2005) studied therapists' perceptions of clients' feelings at termination and found that the more clients attained their therapeutic goals, the less they believed therapy failed, and the more they wanted the termination, the more positive self-feelings they had at the end of therapy. They also found significant correlations between sadness, attainment of therapeutic goals, and a sense of failure. The less the therapeutic goals were achieved, the higher the clients' sense of failure was, and the more sadness the therapists reported the clients had. Their findings were based on therapists' perspectives and not the clients', but they shed light on how clients' feelings of failure may relate to the clients' sadness/disappointment when ending therapy.

THERAPIST FACTORS THAT INFLUENCE CLIENTS' EXPERIENCES OF ENDINGS IN THERAPY

Just as client factors influence clients' experiences in the ending of therapy, there are therapist factors that also influence how clients feel when ending treatment. A therapist who is able to help a client say goodbye or address problems in the relationship is more likely to have a client who has a positive therapy experience and termination compared to a therapist who cannot.

Del Re and colleagues (2012) studied therapist effects and found that the therapist's contribution to the alliance was a statistically significant predictor of outcome, even when accounting for a number of factors. Their results suggest that some therapists are better at developing the therapeutic alliance than other therapists and that the clients of these therapists tend to achieve better outcomes. In addition to outcome, 6% to 7% of the variance in dropout was attributed to the therapist (Owen et al., 2012; Xiao et al., 2017; Zimmermann et al., 2017); therapists have the most important contribution to if clients may experience positive gains from treatment (Baldwin et al., 2007). Although not empirically studied, we will explore how therapists can influence clients' experiences of ending.

Therapists' Factors Hindering Clients' Termination

A review of unhelpful therapist qualities revealed that being rigid, uncertain, critical, distant, tense, and distracted contributed negatively to the alliance. Techniques such as overstructuring the therapy, inappropriate self-disclosure, overwhelming use of transference interpretation, and inappropriate use of silence also contributed negatively to the alliance (Ackerman & Hilsenroth, 2001). O'Keeffe et al. (2020) compared the alliance and ruptures with adolescents who ended treatment in different ways. They found that dissatisfied dropouts had poorer therapy alliances, more ruptures, more unresolved ruptures, and greater therapist-induced ruptures compared with those who dropped out and were satisfied as well as those who did not drop out. The results suggest that unresolved ruptures, caused by the therapists' intervention, often lead to unilateral terminations and poor experiences of the ending therapy.

One type of rupture occurs when therapists have a difficult time working with diverse clients and are unable to identify or repair these ruptures. Owen et al. (2012) studied unilateral termination rates for therapists and compared racial/ethnic minority client dropout to White client dropout rates. They found that for some therapists, unilateral termination rates were the same regardless of the race/ethnicity of the client. For other therapists, they had greater dropout rates for minority clients. The authors suggested that it is likely that some therapists are less multiculturally competent or have less of an ability to detect microaggressions or ruptures related to client diversity. Clients working with these therapists are more likely to drop out and feel bad about the therapy experience. We can imagine clients leaving therapy feeling discriminated against, attacked, and misunderstood.

Clinical Example

Paul is a 42-year-old, bisexual, White, Catholic man who came to therapy to address his feelings of attraction for a male colleague. He has been married to a woman for 10 years and has three children. Paul says that he has had relationships with both men and women in the past, and he loves his wife. When asked, Paul said that he did not want to end his marriage, but his attraction to his colleague was painful and disruptive at work. The therapist is a female, White, heterosexual therapist who is also a practicing Catholic. She struggles to empathize with Paul's extramarital attraction to his colleague and his bisexuality. Despite trying to be empathic, she has a hard time exploring Paul's feelings. She avoids talking about his sexual attraction, and Paul can sense her discomfort with his bisexuality. Without knowing it, she breaks eye contact, shifts back in her seat, and grimaces when he talks about his sexual longings for his colleague. Paul feels ashamed, and this mirrors his experience in his family, where they could not accept his attraction to men. He ends up automatically following his therapist's lead, avoiding conflict with the therapist and minimizing his feelings. He started to question the therapy. Rather than raising his concerns, though, Paul started to cancel sessions. The therapist did not address Paul's withdrawal, and he eventually stopped attending therapy. He tells the therapist that he is too busy with work now and will call later to return to treatment. Paul is relieved that therapy ends, but he feels a sense of sadness, hopelessness, and disappointment in the treatment. Paul's therapist feels a sense of relief since she was not comfortable with his bisexuality or his extramarital sexual feelings. The therapy was causing her anxiety as well. Although she feels relieved, she feels bad that he dropped out of treatment.

The case of Paul demonstrates how important therapist factors are when addressing ruptures, diversity, and termination in therapy. The rupture between Paul and his therapist may have felt subtle to her, but it felt awful to Paul and led to his withdrawal and eventual dropping out of therapy. We can see how his therapist avoided talking directly with Paul about his sexuality and his sexual feelings. Her avoidance and nonverbal behaviors led to his feelings of shame. If the therapist was able to reengage and repair this rupture, Paul may have had a corrective emotional experience. He might have felt understood and been able to share his feelings of anger and hurt with the therapist, feelings he may not have been able to share with his parents. Instead, the treatment became an enactment where he experienced the same discrimination, shame, and devaluation he felt outside of therapy. As we can see, avoidance, lack of empathy, and a lack of multicultural competence have a negative influence on termination. However, there are positive therapist factors that could have led to a repair of the rupture, a helpful therapy experience, and a positive termination.

Helpful Therapist Factors That Cause Positive Client Experiences of Termination

Therapists who are flexible, honest, respectful, trustworthy, confident, warm, interested, and open were found to have greater therapy alliances (Ackerman & Hilsenroth, 2003). In addition to personality qualities, therapists who use techniques such as exploration, reflection, accurate interpretation, facilitating the expression of affect, and attending to the client's experience had greater client alliances as well. Therapists who can identify ruptures and repair them using openness, active listening, and empathy will have better treatment outcomes and better endings with their clients (Safran & Muran, 2000). It makes sense that if these qualities influence the alliance and help in repairing ruptures, they are likely to enhance clients' experiences of the ending of therapy.

Clinical Example

Imagine if Paul's therapist seeks out supervision after Paul ends therapy. She explores her countertransference, avoidance of anxiety, and stereotypes and attitudes about bisexuality. Her supervisor gently confronts her on her nonverbal behaviors (i.e., eye-rolling, shifting in her seat, and her colder tone of voice) that are noticed when she talks about Paul's sexuality. In supervision, she becomes more aware of her negative attitudes and discomfort with sexuality in general and especially same-sex intimacy. She decides to start therapy to understand the roots of her disgust toward homosexuality and uncomfortableness with conversations about sexual intimacy. After reading more literature and working on herself in therapy and supervision, she becomes more empathic with the painful experience of discrimination and hatred that her clients experience. She is able to have more insight into Paul's struggle in their work together based on her ignorance and discomfort, and she decides to reach out to him. The two of them speak on the phone, and the therapist says she would like to apologize to Paul. She shares how she did not empathize with his experience and how that must have been upsetting for him. She would like to see if they could talk more about the process in person without charging him. Paul agrees to meet for one consultation session, and the therapist stays focused on Paul without being defensive. Paul is shocked to hear how open the therapist is to listening about his experience of the ruptures and the pain he felt during the sessions. He tears up when she asks if he experienced her nonverbal behavior as hurtful. He acknowledges that he did, and the therapist is able to explore his feelings of hurt and anger. After the session, Paul is grateful for their conversation but still does not want to restart the therapy.

In this example, we see how Paul ends therapy differently than in the initial termination. He feels more understood when the therapist owns her uncomfortableness with his sexual feelings based on her biases and ignorance. The difference in the ending is a direct result of the therapist becoming more insightful and reflective of countertransference and attitudes about sexuality/homosexuality/bisexuality. After supervision and therapy, the therapist is able to explore the painful impact that the therapy had on Paul. The therapist's empathy, self-awareness, openness, and curiosity facilitate a more intimate ending. The therapist helps the client rely on less avoidance during the termination and more honest engagement. The therapist, not withdrawing, welcomes Paul's anger, disappointment, and shame without forcing him to be silent about how he truly feels when being discriminated against. He is also able to say he does not want to work with the therapist at this time. Even though he still chose to end the treatment, the ending attended to Paul's feelings and was less negative than in the previous scenario.

As we can see from this example, therapist qualities can help or hinder the experience of ending therapy from the client's experience. The therapist's qualities, biases, and interventions can either foster emotional intimacy and change, or they can recreate painful dynamics that lead to premature dropout of treatment. A client's experience of ending therapy is always influenced by the complex interacting qualities of both the therapist and the client, but it is the therapist's job to do the best that they can to address these ruptures and issues so that clients can have the best possible experience in treatment, up to the last session.

IMPLICATIONS FOR RESEARCH AND TRAINING

Ending therapy can foster a client's gratitude toward a therapist, pride in achieving goals, hope for the future, and a positive experience with a caregiver. Unfortunately, this is not how all therapy ends. Many clients drop out of therapy before they have experienced the benefits of the treatment or resolved their presenting issues (Swift & Greenberg, 2012, 2015). Understanding how clients experience the therapy relationship and why they decide to end therapy is critical as we help clients navigate this important part of treatment. It is also important as we train the next generation of therapists to value termination and transfer.

Research Implications

Future research is needed to truly understand clients' experience of termination. We are only beginning to understand how important the end/ending of therapy can be. According to Renk and Dinger (2002), 35% of therapists did not give any reason for clients dropping out of therapy in their records. Murdock et al. (2010) found that therapists often provide biased assessments of termination, and they are often self-serving. Therapists may need to have more humility as they explore reasons why some of their clients ended therapy and how they feel when therapy ends. One solution is to collect information about termination from the client and supervisor. Qualitative and quantitative studies would help us understand how diverse clients experience the end of therapy. In addition, it is important for us to explore how prior therapy terminations influence new therapy relationships. How does prior premature termination influence the alliance with the new therapist? How does a negative therapy experience impact seeking out therapy when needed, attitudes about therapy effectiveness, and engagement in future treatment? Lastly, research is needed to understand what interventions and training initiatives facilitate the best terminations in different types of treatments for different presenting issues.

Implications for Training

Once we understand how terminations influence diverse clients with different presenting issues, we can train the next generation of clinicians to foster meaningful endings to treatment. Goode et al. (2017) suggested a collaborative approach to understanding and engaging in termination. These authors provided wonderful suggestions for therapists who want to improve their abilities to engage clients during this part of therapy. It may be helpful for therapists to understand what clients take with them years after therapy ends. Wucherpfennig et al. (2020) interviewed clients and found that clients often recalled valuing the therapeutic setting as an important healing factor. They described learning from the insight they gained, from the structure and clarity of goals in treatment, from the therapeutic relationship, from exposure therapy and tolerating the fears they came to therapy with, from identifying and changing maladaptive schemas, and from the therapists' direct and clear involvement. These are just a few things recalled, but they are important to consider when we ask clients why they stay in therapy, how they feel when they end therapy, and how we could have helped clients who drop out. When we honestly ask clients to share their experiences of termination, we also begin to understand the clients' experience of treatment effectiveness and their perceptions of our abilities to appreciate diversity, be open to ruptures, and facilitate repairs.

CONCLUSION

Termination of the therapy relationship is one of the most important events in therapy, and it is often the least studied and emphasized aspect of treatment when training therapists. We tend to focus on the early therapy alliance, case conceptualization, and treatment planning. Saying goodbye, following up with clients who drop out, or understanding the impact of therapist transfer has received much less attention. This chapter reviews the different types of therapy endings that occur. It also describes the many reasons clients may prematurely terminate the therapy relationship. In addition, the chapter begins to explore the client and therapist factors that influence termination. Client attachment style, cultural background, intersecting identities, and experience of the therapy relationship all influence decisions to end treatment and termination. Therapist comfort with loss, multicultural competency/humility, and ability to navigate ruptures also influence clients' decisions to end therapy and termination. Many factors influence treatment endings, and there are many different ways to say goodbye. It is time for us to focus more on this vulnerable moment and how it affects therapists and their clients.

REFERENCES

Ackerman, S. J., & Hilsenroth, M. J. (2001). A review of therapist characteristics and techniques negatively impacting the therapeutic alliance. *Psychotherapy: Theory, Research, & Practice, 38*(2), 171–185. https://doi.org/10.1037/0033-3204.38.2.171

Ackerman, S. J., & Hilsenroth, M. J. (2003). A review of therapist characteristics and techniques positively impacting the therapeutic alliance. *Clinical Psychology Review, 23*(1), 1–33. https://doi.org/10.1016/S0272-7358(02)00146-0

Alexander, F. G., & French, T. M. (1946). *Psychoanalytic therapy: Principles and applications.* Ronald Press.

Baldwin, S. A., Wampold, B. E., & Imel, Z. E. (2007). Untangling the alliance-outcome correlation: Exploring the relative importance of therapist and patient variability in the alliance. *Journal of Consulting and Clinical Psychology, 75*(6), 842–852. https://doi.org/10.1037/0022-006X.75.6.842

Barrett, M. S., Chua, W. J., Crits-Christoph, P., Gibbons, M. B., Casiano, D., & Thompson, D. (2008). Early withdrawal from mental health treatment: Implications for psychotherapy practice. *Psychotherapy: Theory, Research, & Practice, 45*(2), 247–267. https://doi.org/10.1037/0033-3204.45.2.247

Baum, N. (2005). Correlates of clients' emotional and behavioral responses to treatment termination. *Clinical Social Work Journal, 33*(3), 309–326. https://doi.org/10.1007/s10615-005-4946-5

Beck, J. S. (1995). *Cognitive therapy: Basics and beyond.* Guilford Press.

Ben David-Sela, T., Nof, A., & Zilcha-Mano, S. (2020). "We can work it out": Working through termination ruptures. *Psychotherapy: Theory, Research, & Practice, 57*(4), 491–496. https://doi.org/10.1037/pst0000297

Bordin, E. S. (1979). The generalizability of the psychoanalytic concept of the working alliance. *Psychotherapy: Theory, Research, & Practice, 16*(3), 252–260. https://doi.org/10.1037/h0085885

Bowlby, J. (1980). *Attachment and loss: Vol. III. Loss.* Basic Books.

Bowlby, J. (1988). *A secure base: Parent–child attachment and healthy human development.* Basic Books.

Boyer, S. P., & Hoffman, M. A. (1993). Counselor affective reactions to termination: Impact of counselor loss history and perceived client sensitivity to loss. *Journal of Counseling Psychology, 40*(3), 271–277. https://doi.org/10.1037/0022-0167.40.3.271

Bridges, M. R. (2006). Activating the corrective emotional experience. *Journal of Clinical Psychology, 62*(5), 551–568. https://doi.org/10.1002/jclp.20248

Clark, P., Cole, C., & Robertson, J. (2014). Creating a safety net: Transferring to a new therapist in a training setting. *Contemporary Family Therapy, 36*(1), 172–189. https://doi.org/10.1007/s10591-013-9282-2

Constantine, M. G. (2007). Racial microaggressions against African American clients in cross-racial counseling relationships. *Journal of Counseling Psychology, 54*(2), 142–153. https://doi.org/10.1037/0022-0167.54.2.142

Del Re, A. C., Flückiger, C., Horvath, A. O., Symonds, D., & Wampold, B. E. (2012). Therapist effects in the therapeutic alliance-outcome relationship: A restricted-maximum likelihood meta-analysis. *Clinical Psychology Review, 32*(7), 642–649. https://doi.org/10.1016/j.cpr.2012.07.002

Eubanks, C. F., Muran, J. C., & Safran, J. D. (2018). Alliance rupture repair: A meta-analysis. *Psychotherapy: Theory, Research, & Practice, 55*(4), 508–519. https://doi.org/10.1037/pst0000185

Flückiger, C., Del Re, A. C., Wampold, B. E., & Horvath, A. O. (2018). The alliance in adult psychotherapy: A meta-analytic synthesis. *Psychotherapy: Theory, Research, & Practice, 55*(4), 316–340. https://doi.org/10.1037/pst0000172

Fraley, R. C., & Bonanno, G. A. (2004). Attachment and loss: A test of three competing models on the association between attachment-related avoidance and adaptation to bereavement. *Personality and Social Psychology Bulletin, 30*(7), 878–890. https://doi.org/10.1177/0146167204264289

Fraley, R. C., & Shaver, P. R. (1997). Adult attachment and the suppression of unwanted thoughts. *Journal of Personality and Social Psychology, 73*(5), 1080–1091. https://doi.org/10.1037/0022-3514.73.5.1080

Fraley, R. C., & Shaver, P. R. (1999). Loss and bereavement: Attachment theory and recent controversies concerning "grief work" and the nature of detachment. In J. Cassidy & P. R. Shaver (Eds.), *Handbook of attachment: Theory, research, and clinical applications* (pp. 735–759). Guilford Press.

Fuertes, J. N., Costa, C. I., Mueller, L. N., & Hersh, M. (2005). Psychotherapy process and outcome from a racial-ethnic perspective. In R. T. Carter (Ed.), *Handbook of racial-cultural psychology and counseling, Vol. 1. Theory and research* (pp. 256–276). John Wiley & Sons.

Gelso, C. J., & Hayes, J. A. (1998). *The psychotherapy relationship: Theory, research, and practice.* John Wiley & Sons.

Goldfried, M. R. (2002). A cognitive-behavioral perspective on termination. *Journal of Psychotherapy Integration, 12*(3), 364–372. https://doi.org/10.1037/1053-0479.12.3.364

Goode, J., Park, J., Parkin, S., Tompkins, K. A., & Swift, J. K. (2017). A collaborative approach to psychotherapy termination. *Psychotherapy: Theory, Research, & Practice, 54*(1), 10–14. https://doi.org/10.1037/pst0000085

Greenberg, L. S. (2002). Termination of experiential therapy. *Journal of Psychotherapy Integration, 12*(3), 358–363. https://doi.org/10.1037/1053-0479.12.3.358

Harrison, R. L. (2020). Termination in 16-session accelerated experiential dynamic psychotherapy (AEDP): Together in how we say goodbye. *Psychotherapy: Theory, Research, & Practice, 57*(4), 531–547. https://doi.org/10.1037/pst0000343

Holmes, J. (1997). "Too early, too late": Endings in psychotherapy—An attachment perspective. *British Journal of Psychotherapy, 14*(2), 159–171. https://doi.org/10.1111/j.1752-0118.1997.tb00367.x

Holmes, J. (2009). *From attachment research to clinical practice: Getting it together.* Guilford Press.

Hook, J. N., Farrell, J. E., Davis, D. E., DeBlaere, C., Van Tongeren, D. R., & Utsey, S. O. (2016). Cultural humility and racial microaggressions in counseling. *Journal of Counseling Psychology, 63*(3), 269–277. https://doi.org/10.1037/cou0000114

Hummelen, B., Wilberg, T., & Karterud, S. (2007). Interviews of female patients with borderline personality disorder who dropped out of group psychotherapy. *International Journal of Group Psychotherapy, 57*(1), 67–92. https://doi.org/10.1521/ijgp.2007.57.1.67

Hunsley, J., Aubry, T. D., Vestervelt, C. M., & Vito, D. (1999). Comparing therapist and client perspectives on reasons for psychotherapy termination. *Psychotherapy: Theory, Research, & Practice, 36*(4), 380–388. https://doi.org/10.1037/h0087802

Joyce, A. S., Piper, W. E., Ogrodniczuk, J. S., & Klien, R. H. (2007). *Termination in psychotherapy: A psychodynamic model of processes and outcomes.* American Psychological Association. https://doi.org/10.1037/11545-000

Kazdin, A. E., Mazurick, J. L., & Siegel, T. C. (1994). Treatment outcome among children with externalizing disorder who terminate prematurely versus those who complete psychotherapy. *Journal of the American Academy of Child & Adolescent Psychiatry, 33*(4), 549–557. https://doi.org/10.1097/00004583-199405000-00013

Kazdin, A. E., & Wassell, G. (2000). Predictors of barriers to treatment and therapeutic change in outpatient therapy for antisocial children and their families. *Mental Health Services Research, 2*(1), 27–40. https://doi.org/10.1023/A:1010191807861

Keith, C. (1966). Multiple transfers of psychotherapy patients. A report of problems and management. *Archives of General Psychiatry, 14*(2), 185–189. https://doi.org/10.1001/archpsyc.1966.01730080073011

Knox, S., Adrians, N., Everson, E., Hess, S., Hill, C., & Crook-Lyon, R. (2011). Clients' perspectives on therapy termination. *Psychotherapy Research, 21*(2), 154–167. https://doi.org/10.1080/10503307.2010.534509

Lee, E., Tsang, A. K. T., Bogo, M., Johnstone, M., & Herschman, J. (2018). Enactments of racial microaggression in everyday therapeutic encounters. *Smith College Studies in Social Work, 88*(3), 211–236. https://doi.org/10.1080/00377317.2018.1476646

Marmarosh, C. L. (2017). Fostering engagement during termination: Applying attachment theory and research. *Psychotherapy: Theory, Research, & Practice, 54*(1), 4–9. https://doi.org/10.1037/pst0000087

Marmarosh, C. L., & Salamon, S. I. (2020). Repeated terminations: Transferring therapists in psychotherapy. *Psychotherapy: Theory, Research, & Practice, 57*(4), 497–507. Advance online publication. https://doi.org/10.1037/pst0000340

Marx, J. A., & Gelso, C. J. (1987). Termination of individual counseling in a university counseling center. *Journal of Counseling Psychology, 34*(1), 3–9. https://doi.org/10.1037/0022-0167.34.1.3

Mikulincer, M., & Shaver, P. R. (2016). *Attachment in adulthood: Structure, dynamics, and change* (2nd ed.). Guilford Press.

Murdock, N. L., Edwards, C., & Murdock, T. B. (2010). Therapists' attributions for client premature termination: Are they self-serving? *Psychotherapy: Theory, Research, & Practice, 47*(2), 221–234. https://doi.org/10.1037/a0019786

Norcross, J. C., Zimmerman, B. E., Greenberg, R. P., & Swift, J. K. (2017). Do all therapists do that when saying goodbye? A study of commonalities in termination behaviors. *Psychotherapy: Theory, Research, & Practice, 54*(1), 66–75. https://doi.org/10.1037/pst0000097

O'Keeffe, S., Martin, P., & Midgley, N. (2020). When adolescents stop psychological therapy: Rupture-repair in the therapeutic alliance and association with therapy ending. *Psychotherapy: Theory, Research, & Practice, 57*(4), 471–490. https://doi.org/10.1037/pst0000279

O'Keeffe, S., Martin, P., Target, M., & Midgley, N. (2019). "I just stopped going": A mixed methods investigation into types of therapy dropout in adolescents with depression. *Frontiers in Psychology, 10,* 75. https://doi.org/10.3389/fpsyg.2019.00075

Okosi, M. J. (2018). *The impact of racial microaggressions on therapeutic relationships with people of color* [Unpublished doctoral dissertation]. Rutgers University-Graduate School of Applied and Professional Psychology.

Owen, J., Imel, Z., Adelson, J., & Rodolfa, E. (2012). "No-show": Therapist racial/ethnic disparities in client unilateral termination. *Journal of Counseling Psychology, 59*(2), 314–320. https://doi.org/10.1037/a0027091

Owen, J., Tao, K. W., Imel, Z. E., Wampold, B. E., & Rodolfa, E. (2014). Addressing racial and ethnic microaggressions in therapy. *Professional Psychology, Research and Practice, 45*(4), 283–290. https://doi.org/10.1037/a0037420

Pekarik, G. (1992). Relationship of clients' reasons for dropping out of treatment to outcome and satisfaction. *Journal of Clinical Psychology, 48,* 91–98. https://doi.org/10.1002/1097-4679(199201)48:1<91::AID-JCLP2270480113>3.0.CO;2-W

Penn, L. (1990). When the therapist must leave: Forced termination of psychodynamic therapy. *Professional Psychology: Research and Practice, 21,* 379–384. https://doi.org/10.1037/0735-7028.21.5.379

Pistole, M. C. (1999). Caregiving in attachment relationships: A perspective for counselors. *Journal of Counseling and Development, 77*(4), 437–446. https://doi.org/10.1002/j.1556-6676.1999.tb02471.x

Porges, S. W. (2011). *The polyvagal theory: Neurophysiological foundations of emotions, attachment, communication, and self-regulation.* W. W. Norton & Co.

Porges, S. W. (2017). *The pocket guide to the polyvagal theory: The transformative power of feeling safe.* W. W. Norton & Co.

Quintana, S. M. (1993). Toward an expanded and updated conceptualization of termination: Implications for short-term, individual psychotherapy. *Professional Psychology, Research and Practice, 24*(4), 426–432. https://doi.org/10.1037/0735-7028.24.4.426

Renk, K., & Dinger, T. M. (2002). Reasons for therapy termination in a university psychology clinic. *Journal of Clinical Psychology, 58*(9), 1173–1181. https://doi.org/10.1002/jclp.10075

Safran, J. D., & Muran, J. C. (2000). *Negotiating the therapeutic alliance: A relational treatment guide.* Guilford Press.

Schen, C. R., Raymond, L., & Notman, M. (2013). Transfer of care of psychotherapy patients: Implications for psychiatry training. *Psychodynamic Psychiatry, 41*, 575–595. https://doi.org/10.1521/pdps.2013.41.4.575

Schore, A. N. (2000). Attachment and the regulation of the right brain. *Attachment & Human Development, 2*(1), 23–47. https://doi.org/10.1080/146167300361309

Schore, A. N. (2019). *Right brain psychotherapy.* W. W. Norton & Co.

Shahar, G., & Ziv-Beiman, S. (2020). Using termination as an intervention (UTAI): A view from an integrative, cognitive-existential psychodynamics perspective. *Psychotherapy: Theory, Research, & Practice, 57*(4), 515–520. https://doi.org/10.1037/pst0000337

Shulman, S., & Gold, J. (1999). Termination of short-term and long-term psychotherapy: Patients' and therapists' affective reactions and therapists' technical management (attachment style, therapy model). *Dissertation Abstracts International: B. The Sciences and Engineering, 60*, 2961.

Sue, D. W. (2010). *Microaggressions in everyday life: Race, gender, and sexual orientation.* John Wiley & Sons.

Sue, D. W., Capodilupo, C. M., Torino, G. C., Bucceri, J. M., Holder, A. M. B., Nadal, K. L., & Esquilin, M. (2007). Racial microaggressions in everyday life: Implications for clinical practice. *American Psychologist, 62*(4), 271–286. https://doi.org/10.1037/0003-066X.62.4.271

Swift, J. K., Callahan, J., & Levine, J. C. (2009). Using clinically significant change to identify premature termination. *Psychotherapy: Theory, Research, & Practice, 46*(3), 328–335. https://doi.org/10.1037/a0017003

Swift, J. K., & Greenberg, R. P. (2012). Premature discontinuation in adult psychotherapy: A meta-analysis. *Journal of Consulting and Clinical Psychology, 80*(4), 547–559. https://doi.org/10.1037/a0028226

Swift, J. K., & Greenberg, R. P. (2015). *Premature termination in psychotherapy: Strategies for engaging clients and improving outcomes.* American Psychological Association. https://doi.org/10.1037/14469-000

Tantam, D., & Klerman, G. (1979). Patient transfer from one clinician to another and dropping-out of out-patient treatment. *Social Psychiatry, 14*(3), 107–113. https://doi.org/10.1007/BF00582175

Tryon, G. S., & Kane, A. S. (1993). Relationship of working alliance to mutual and unilateral termination. *Journal of Counseling Psychology, 40*(1), 33–36. https://doi.org/10.1037/0022-0167.40.1.33

Vasquez, M. J. (2007). Cultural difference and the therapeutic alliance: An evidence-based analysis. *American Psychologist, 62*(8), 878–885. https://doi.org/10.1037/0003-066X.62.8.878

Vidair, H. B., Feyijinmi, G. O., & Feindler, E. L. (2017). Termination in cognitive-behavioral therapy with children, adolescents, and parents. *Psychotherapy: Theory, Research, & Practice, 54*(1), 15–21. https://doi.org/10.1037/pst0000086

Wachtel, P. (2002). Termination of therapy: An effort at integration. *Journal of Psychotherapy Integration, 12*(3), 373–383. https://doi.org/10.1037/1053-0479.12.3.373

Wallin, D. J. (2007). *Attachment in psychotherapy.* Guilford Press.

Wampold, B. E., & Imel, Z. E. (2015). *The great psychotherapy debate: Research evidence for what works in psychotherapy* (2nd ed.). Routledge. https://doi.org/10.4324/9780203582015

Wapner, J. H., Klein, J. G., Friedlander, M. L., & Andrasik, F. J. (1986). Transferring psychotherapy clients: State of the art. *Professional Psychology, Research and Practice*, *17*(6), 492–496. https://doi.org/10.1037/0735-7028.17.6.492

Westmacott, R., Hunsley, J., Best, M., Rumstein-McKean, O., & Schindler, D. (2010). Client and therapist views of contextual factors related to termination from psychotherapy: A comparison between unilateral and mutual terminators. *Psychotherapy Research*, *20*(4), 423–435. https://doi.org/10.1080/10503301003645796

Whaley, A. L., & Davis, K. E. (2007). Cultural competence and evidence-based practice in mental health services: A complementary perspective. *American Psychologist*, *62*(6), 563–574. https://doi.org/10.1037/0003-066X.62.6.563

Wucherpfennig, F., Boyle, K., Rubel, J. A., Weinmann-Lutz, B., & Lutz, W. (2020). What sticks? Patients' perspectives on treatment three years after psychotherapy: A mixed-methods approach. *Psychotherapy Research*, *30*(6), 739–752. https://doi.org/10.1080/10503307.2019.1671630

Xiao, H., Castonguay, L. G., Janis, R. A., Youn, S. J., Hayes, J. A., & Locke, B. D. (2017). Therapist effects on dropout from a college counseling center practice research network. *Journal of Counseling Psychology*, *64*(4), 424–431. https://doi.org/10.1037/cou0000208

Yalom, I. D. (2020). *Existential psychotherapy*. Basic Books.

Zilberstein, K. (2008). Au revoir: An attachment and loss perspective on termination. *Clinical Social Work Journal*, *36*(3), 301–311. https://doi.org/10.1007/s10615-008-0159-z

Zimmermann, D., Rubel, J., Page, A. C., & Lutz, W. (2017). Therapist effects on and predictors of non-consensual dropout in psychotherapy. *Clinical Psychology & Psychotherapy*, *24*(2), 312–321. https://doi.org/10.1002/cpp.2022

III

INTEGRATION AND DISCUSSION

13

Closing Thoughts About *The Other Side of Psychotherapy*

Jairo N. Fuertes

The chapters in this volume have provided excellent reviews of the literature and presented valuable ideas about clients' experiences and work in psychotherapy. In this chapter, I discuss what I believe to be the main themes that emerged from my study of the content. You should note that this discussion is a personal reflection on the material and that other professionals might highlight or interpret the same content differently. I leave it up to you to decide what themes and ideas seem most salient. In fact, I encourage you to do so. Given the quality of the work that our trustworthy authors have offered, I believe that you are in good hands in your journey to understand the "other side"; you might also come to understand our side better: the helper's work. My hope, and that of the chapter authors, is that you can become a better clinician, teacher, and researcher by developing your own understanding of what clients experience and process in psychotherapy.

This discussion reflects a few personal core beliefs about therapy. First, as I said in the Introduction, particularly in my analogy to the personal trainer and the physical gym, I believe that the client does a great deal of the work in treatment. Any given client can make the most talented and experienced clinician or, conversely, a rather novice and inexperienced helper look either good or bad; it is ultimately the client who makes therapy succeed or fail. Second, my view of treatment is also heavily tilted toward seeing the relationship in therapy as crucial to the process and outcome in treatment. And the client has a great deal to say about how the relationship develops and

https://doi.org/10.1037/0000303-014
The Other Side of Psychotherapy: Understanding Clients' Experiences and Contributions in Treatment, J. N. Fuertes (Editor)

operates in treatment. Third, my view of therapy is that most clients will make appreciable, demonstrable gains after about 3 to 6 months of treatment. Therefore, unless clients have an interest in taking a more thorough and deeper analysis of themselves, or if clients are particularly badly off, as in having personality disorder traits, problems with addictions, or a history of chronic mental illness or trauma, most clients who come to psychotherapy need not stay in therapy for long. I believe that the outcome literature largely supports these three personal beliefs (see Lambert, 2013; Wampold & Imel, 2015). With this in mind, the following discussion is organized around three broad themes that stood out for me: (a) the role of client agency in therapy, (b) client collaboration in adapting and tailoring therapy, and (c) the role that clients play in nurturing a collaborative and therapeutic relationship. I end the chapter by discussing some of the implications for research that were included in the chapters, and I offer a few of my own ideas for research.

THE ROLE OF CLIENT AGENCY IN THERAPY

Bohart and Tallman noted in Chapter 1 that the client is the common factor in treatment and probably why all therapies are almost equally effective. The client is, in fact, a creative collaborator and partner in the authors' "meeting of the minds" metamodel (MOM) view of therapy, which takes a more egalitarian view of the dyad than does the more traditional "interventionist" model. According to the MOM, clients work hard at identifying problems, generating possibilities, and imagining new scenarios and act according to the material they uncover in collaboration with their therapist. The client is active, not passive; the client brings creativity and self-expertise and can summon significant psychological resources to aid in the process of change. The client is ultimately the one who assimilates new perspectives and behaviors when the evidence points them to the value of changing and growing. The MOM takes a perspective that elevates the client as the most important member of the dyad and is cognizant and respectful of the autonomy and power of the individual. Clients decide what is meaningful and important to them, they formulate their own interpretations and understandings, and they are ultimately their own "interventionists." My take on what Bohart and Tallman proposed is that the therapist works as an expert companion and guide, who, through a series of interventions guided by the therapist's theory and techniques, facilitates and empowers the client to engage in what is often a similar psychological workout for all clients: to reflect more deeply, communicate more honestly, listen carefully, and begin to take small steps toward growth and change. The therapist sets up the workout, and the client learns and adopts it and modifies and intensifies it with the therapist's support and encouragement throughout the sessions.

Closely related to the MOM is the appreciation for client self-healing, as described by Greaves in Chapter 6. She made the remarkable assertion that clients in therapy spend less than 1% of their waking time a week with their therapist, which highlights the tremendous amount of time that the client spends out of therapy reflecting and working on their problems. Given the high level of change that occurs pre to post during the time the client is in therapy, it becomes clear how much work clients do on their own, between sessions and without their therapist. Greaves described two broad dimensions that emerged from her research, one that includes processes prompted by therapy but initiated by the client and a second dimension that includes processes that evolve in therapy and involve the client and therapist working in dialogic fashion. The autonomy and independence of the client in therapy is such that they experience problems, big or small, in highly idiosyncratic ways and attribute meaning to their problems in a highly personal, phenomenological manner. According to Greaves, therapists provide a variety of valuable services, including attentive listening and thoughtful analysis, empathy and challenges of thoughts and behaviors, and leverage of the therapy relationship in strategic ways to promote client change. But it is clients who ultimately work to fortify themselves and redefine and reinvent their lives, and only clients are in a position to do this for themselves.

Related to the central role of client agency and noted in the Introduction is that there is no monolithic "other side" perspective, no singular "client perspective," because clients experience therapy on the basis of their personality, circumstances, beliefs, and interactions with their therapist. In that sense, this book offers strategies for understanding the client, highlighting opportunities and optimal stances for collaborating and facilitating the valuable contributions of the client. As Greaves noted, clients will experience therapy and even individual sessions idiosyncratically, and to them, theirs is the only perspective that matters. Therapists do well when they listen to, invite, and attempt to understand clients' constructions about their problems and their ideas on how to proceed. Likewise, in discussing outcome, Constantino and his colleagues noted in Chapter 11 that clients' perceptions of healing, growth, change, and outcome are what is ultimately important. They also labeled clients' perceptions as idiosyncratic; that is, "objectively" a great deal of work may have taken place, and formal assessments may show substantial improvement, but "subjectively" clients will derive their own assessments and conclusions about how they feel, what they experienced and did in treatment, and the extent to which therapy was successful.

While we have all undoubtedly heard in our training about the importance of collaboration in therapy, the authors seem to take their conception of a client–therapist partnership much further. They seem to view collaboration by the client as not simply low reactance or high adherence and compliance but a true partnership where clients participate in every facet of treatment and where their feedback is regularly invited and integrated. In my view, it is certainly conceivable that there are instances in therapy—for example, due to the client's culture, personality, or preferences—when the client will desire a more "interventionist" or directive approach. However, the authors seem to suggest that even when therapist directiveness is desired (and careful consideration should be given to the "whom, what, when, and how" of directiveness), the client should still be encouraged to partner up to the fullest extent possible.

Greaves noted that clients, much like their therapists, help construct a relationship through respect, empathy, attention, and trustworthy behavior. However, they will perform "credibility" tests to see if the relationship with their therapist is solid and real. The concept of the real relationship from Gelso and Kline in Chapter 7 is relevant here. In this aspect of the relationship, genuineness expressed by both therapists and client, as well as the ability of each party to have perceptions that befit one another, are fundamental to the smooth process in treatment (the real relationship is described in more detail later). Furthermore, Greaves advanced the perspective of therapy that is like Bohart and Tallman's: a collaborative meeting of the minds experience, where both the client and the therapist contribute and make therapy work on behalf of the client. Greaves also noted that in a relationship that the client perceives as solid and real, the therapist does not have to be a wise sage or hero and can even get things wrong occasionally without negative consequences, as long as the therapist acknowledges the mistake and works through it with the client.

Oliveira and colleagues noted in Chapter 2 that clients not only find the content but they also provide the fuel for therapy: motivation. The authors identified a variety of needs as sources of motivation for the client and noted that clients' needs guide the collaborative formulation of goals for therapy. What is implied here is that motivation is ultimately a factor that the client must find to do the work, and without it, nothing will get done. However, the authors noted that motivation can increase as the relationship with their therapist grows so that it is not so much the level of motivation that clients bring to therapy but that a good level of motivation is sustained as therapy begins and the work intensifies. The authors also noted that because client ambivalence is frequently present, the therapist plays a significant role in helping the client work through their ambivalence and draw out some level of hope and motivation.

Anderson and Perlman noted in Chapter 4 that clients bring their own set of facilitative interpersonal skills (FIS) to therapy, which work in conjunction with therapists' FIS (and which have received considerable empirical attention in the literature). Clients' FIS were theorized by the authors to represent a strong and independent role in shaping the process and outcome of therapy. Without these client FIS skills and capacities, including warmth, creativity, hope, communication, and alliance-building capacities, psychotherapy is significantly limited. I found the implications of their writing compelling, one of which is that beyond a therapist's own FIS, clients' FIS give clients and therapists the set of tools to work with in advancing the work of therapy.

CLIENTS CONTRIBUTE TO THE ADAPTATION AND TAILORING OF THEIR THERAPY

Clients come to therapy with varying levels of motivation and desire for change. As Oliveira and his colleagues noted, clients are often deeply ambivalent about working on their problems, and a lack of motivation in a client can easily be one of the greatest challenges facing a therapist. Competent therapists understand the complexity of motivation in fueling change and tailor interventions to prepare clients for the arduous tasks of change. In Chapter 3, Norcross and colleagues also emphasized the value of assessing and empathically understanding the stage the client is in. Research on the stages has identified highly specific and effective interventions, as well as varying therapy relationship stances, that can be used to match the stage of change. The tailoring of interventions and relationship stances to the stage of client change provides a way to address problems with motivation, with the goal of moving the person toward planful action and the maintenance of outcomes. The transtheoretical model (Prochaska et al., 1995) that Norcross and his coauthors referenced also accounts for a client presenting at various stages of change in relation to several issues; for example, one client can present at a stage of precontemplation about giving up a toxic relationship while being at the contemplation stage about taking on a healthier diet and lifestyle and the stage of action with respect to career advancement. These scenarios add complexity to the treatment and often represent nonlinear trajectories in therapy (e.g., the client relapses or loses motivation in one or more areas). While the model is prescriptive, it is highly flexible and demands that the therapist understand the client and be flexible in tailoring interventions and adopting different roles given the stages of change the client presents. What I found compelling in this chapter is the idea that the client "decides" the stages of therapy, and the stages "decide" how the therapist approaches the client and which interventions to use.

Boswell and Scharff provided in Chapter 8 a strong rationale for including the client in assessment early on and continually throughout treatment. Client-focused assessment allows the client to speak about their assessment and their views of the problem(s). These authors made the remarkable assertion that therapists never treat "an average client"; clients' problems can be seductively interpreted from *t*-scores or means and standard deviations in manuals and textbooks. Therefore, the authors cautioned the therapist against classifying any one client with, for example, depression, with a "seen it a thousand times" mentality or other overgeneralizations. In client-focused assessment, practitioners give weight to the client's subjective experience, account for the client's beliefs and preferences, and discuss the client's and therapist's views about what is being assessed collaboratively. Including the client in discussing the nature of the problems improves the therapist's credibility and enhances the working alliance by increasing the client's confidence and engagement in therapy. Partnering with the client in regular assessments of the work also improves the therapist's understanding of individual differences and allows the therapist to better tailor interventions and respond to the client's unique needs. According to the authors, an inclusive assessment posture increases client motivation and participation, calibrates expectancies for treatment, and provides crucial information about the stages of change for the client.

In Chapter 9, Levitt and her colleagues discussed clients' experiences of therapists' helping skills and how attending to clients' perceptions can enhance therapist tailoring of interventions and their overall responsiveness. The authors also emphasized the importance of adjusting modes of relating and intervening to the needs of the client, and like other authors in this book, they also see the relationship as a key component that enhances understanding and responsiveness. Levitt and her collaborators remind us that skills in empathy, probing, immediacy, and metacommunication can promote client agency, expression, and exploration; through the relationship that develops, clients develop more charitable views of themselves, the therapist, and others. Dr. Levitt and colleagues seem to place great value in therapist genuineness, particularly in acknowledging and leveling cultural and professional power and privilege with the client. This reminds me of what Egan (2010) called the need to create a "fair society" in therapy, where differences are acknowledged, shared, explored, and integrated into the work. Following Egan's line of thought, which Levitt et al. also discuss, clients bring identities, not just problems, to therapy; these aspects of their person matter and should be recognized and integrated into sessions. Levitt and her collaborators noted that by attending to factors central to an individual's identity, such as race, ethnicity, gender, social class, and sexual orientation, therapists gain a more complete picture of their clients, and clients, in turn, can gain a clearer appreciation of themselves.

Constantino and his coauthors noted in Chapter 11 that clients with the same diagnosis attribute their problems to different events and etiologies. Clients also have personalized expectations and views of what constitutes successful therapy. There does not seem to be a singular, typical, or "average" trajectory of change in outcome, at least when clients' freely offered perspectives of change are collected and examined. Constantino et al. pointed out that in studies of client recall of effective therapy, clients noted themes of a safe, supportive, collaborative therapy relationship and working together with their therapists, including on treatment decisions. Clients also recalled effective treatment involving therapists who invited facilitative conversation about the treatment and allowed clients to express different opinions, views, and even disagreements. These views were discussed, processed, and resolved to some extent. What strikes me as remarkable is that clients do not readily recall specific therapist techniques or interventions, but instead, they recall the quality of the relationship and how they felt with their therapist, and they have broader memories of working together and collaboratively with them.

It is also fascinating to read that it is not just therapists who influence their clients. Clients have an influence on therapists' view of therapy, on their estimates of how well the client is progressing, and even on which interventions to use or avoid. Several authors, including Goodyear and Sera in Chapter 10, as well as Gelso and Kline (Chapter 7) and Anderson and Perlman (Chapter 4), noted that clients can influence how therapists feel about themselves, their beliefs, and their relationships and even the level of distress and trauma they experience by working psychologically intimately with their clients. In particular, Goodyear and Sera noted that clients are not passive or inert participants; they influence the therapy. Competent therapists respond to their clients' constant verbal and nonverbal behavior ("one cannot not communicate") and the feedback they provide. The authors noted that therapists' responses or reactions to clients' influence can be intentional or unintentional, and therapists can be affected momentarily or in a more enduring manner by clients' circumstances, values, and beliefs. In fact, the authors noted that most therapists admit in surveys of the profession to the influence they have experienced from their clients. Goodyear and Sera shared the Japanese proverb 持ちつ持たれつ [*mochitsu-motaretsu*], which says there is interdependency and mutuality between individuals in all relationships. To some readers, this point may seem obvious. But it is worth reiterating that in therapy, it is no different; each person affects the other, and together they continually shape and construct their relationship. The authors also emphasized the value of partnering with the client by receiving regular feedback using formal processes such as routine outcome monitoring, remaining attuned to how the client feels and how the therapist feels in return, and soliciting feedback from the client about expectations, preferences, progress, and ideas about how to proceed.

CLIENTS AND THERAPISTS COCONSTRUCT AND NURTURE THE THERAPY RELATIONSHIP

In Chapter 5, Mallinckrodt described psychotherapy as involving an attachment experience and what transpires between the client and the therapist as a corrective emotional experience (CEE), wherein attachment to the therapist becomes more stable and secure. He noted that client attachment to the therapist is positively associated with in-depth exploration and treatment outcomes. In its simplest form, his model suggests that clients can "hyper-activate" based on attachment insecurity and experiencing therapists as too distant; the process of therapy leads them from gratification to frustration as therapists strategically enhance therapeutic distance. Or clients can "deactivate" on the basis of attachment insecurity and experiencing therapists as too close and move from relief to anxiety as therapists intentionally decrease the therapeutic distance. According to Mallinckrodt, for hyperactivating or deactivating clients, the CEE is either a growing sense of comfort with autonomy or an increased comfort with closeness and intimacy. In both instances of either hyperactivation or deactivation, clients gain an "earned security" by establishing a more secure attachment to the therapist that can then be generalized to relationships outside of treatment. Notably, Mallinckrodt pointed out that while achieving a healthy, secure attachment style is ideal, it is not entirely necessary as an outcome for therapy to be successful and the client to feel improved. He noted that clients can develop more adaptive cognitions, behaviors, and planful interactions to work around and compensate for deeply ingrained attachment insecurities.

Gelso and Kline pointed out that clients contribute to the therapy relationship. This may seem obvious because a relationship, by definition, requires at least two people to be involved in some way. But in our therapist-centric, interventionist way of thinking about therapy, we often focus on what we do to establish and maintain the relationship and not much on what clients contribute. The authors discussed the tripartite model of the relationship, which includes what is termed the real relationship, the working alliance, and the transference–countertransference configuration. The aspect of the relationship that stood out for me is the real relationship. It is referenced indirectly in several chapters, including Greaves's model of self-healing, which is predicated on clients experiencing a sound and "real" relationship with their therapists, as well as Mallinckrodt's contention that attachment is foundational to all relationships and that insecurities fuel transferences, which represent the antithesis of the real relationship.

In Mallinckrodt's model, what is left after more secure attachments are established in treatment is a more real and genuine relationship, exactly what defines the real relationship. The real relationship is called "the foundation" by Gelso and Kline; it is the person-to-person experience that clients and therapists have of each other as people. According to the authors, the real relationship is present from the first moments of therapy, perhaps even before the first meeting takes place (e.g., over the phone or even email in setting up the first appointment, the future client may like or resonate with the accurately perceived tone and demeanor of the therapist). Gelso and Kline noted that the client contributes to the real relationship by sharing as genuinely as possible, making efforts to see the therapist as the therapist is, and contributing to the warmth, genuineness, and nondefensiveness that is at the heart of the real relationship.

Gelso and Kline also discussed the other two strands of the relationship, the working alliance and the transference–countertransference configuration. These last two components are crucial to the success of treatment, but the outcome research to date shows that the real relationship is the most predictive of a good outcome. In the working alliance, which is characterized by agreement on the goals and tasks of therapy and the development of an emotional bond, clients are central in setting goals and identifying ways of meeting them (i.e., the tasks). They find and sustain the motivation to initiate changes, and they have to summon the wherewithal to trust and bond with their therapist in an alliance. Their ability to work through insecurities and put aside past injuries from relationships (and this involves a real relationship and, to some extent, working through transference) and their willingness to give the therapist the benefit of the doubt are essential in forming and sustaining the alliance. The authors noted that trust is also key for clients to work through the low points of therapy, that middle phase identified by research where the alliance wanes as the demands and rigors of the work put stress on the relationship. Client trust, capacity for forgiveness, and an already established working alliance also seem essential in being able to work through ruptures.

The third aspect of the relationship is the transference–countertransference configuration. Gelso and Kline described transference as "the window into the client's conflicts" that often includes unconscious conflict, trauma, and a variety of emotional "unfinished business" from the distant or recent past. Client factors also associated with transference include exaggerated internal schemas that generate fear or the need to demean the self or others. And it is perhaps in the throes of transference when the patient must remain strong and work hardest with the therapist to work through intense emotional material that has been activated and/or dredged up from the past. In terms of therapist transference and/or countertransference, the authors pointed out that the client can trigger, fuel, or exacerbate therapists' distortions and unconscious reactions in therapy. In the hands of a competent therapist and the context of an otherwise good working relationship, working collaboratively by referencing therapist transference–countertransference can be valuable to the relationship and the client, so long as it is done in a clinically indicated manner with the client's interests in mind. Thinking about the hard work of therapy and the intense emotions generated intrapsychically and interpersonally for the client, I can appreciate even more the strength, hope, and capacities for trust and for connecting that clients bring to and refine in treatment.

As in the gym analogy I presented in the Introduction, a lifetime membership to a gym or psychotherapy is rare. Therapy ends due to a variety of issues, often within months, unless the client desires and pursues a longer and more thorough analysis. However, a lifelong commitment to personal self-care and psychological fitness is often obtained from psychotherapy. In physical fitness, the gym and personal trainer may no longer be needed as the person learns to work out and take care of themselves physically on their own. The same is true in psychotherapy: The client learns to work out psychologically and stay emotionally fit on their own. In Chapter 12, Marmarosh tied the quality and experience of termination to the quality of the experiences in therapy, particularly the relationship with the therapist. She noted that therapy is remarkably successful and that most terminations are also successful (i.e., termination is mutually agreed on and clinically indicated, and the client is ready for the end of treatment). But there are instances when therapy is not as successful, and the process and course of less successful therapy are associated with client dropout. While there is a dearth of research on dropout, the factors that seem implicated with unsuccessful therapy and unwanted termination include the client (e.g., psychopathology, severity of problems, attachment insecurity), therapist (e.g., insensitivity, own attachment problems, inability to repair ruptures with the client), or relationship (e.g., weak or unattended to ruptures in the working alliance, transference or countertransference issues that are not identified or resolved). Marmarosh noted that not all premature terminations are the same, although the research is also limited in this area. She noted that in multicultural therapy, clients who experience insensitivity, bias, lack of cultural knowledge, and microaggressions from their therapists are more likely to drop out of therapy.

IMPLICATIONS FOR RESEARCH

All authors pointed out that research that takes the client's perspective is sorely lacking, and all made excellent recommendations for future research. They also made recommendations for clinical practice and training in each of their respective chapters. To address many of the questions that remain unanswered, the authors pointed to the need for studies that employ qualitative methodologies and allow clients to offer and express their perspectives about psychotherapy freely. What seems to emerge collectively from their recommendations for research is the need for a new collection of stories in which clients discuss their views of the entire process and outcome of psychotherapy. In essence, there is a need to lift the veil from the "other side" of psychotherapy. Next, I note some of their recommendations and offer a few of my own ideas.

Bohart and Tallman noted that research is needed to understand how clients summon their creative capacities and self-knowledge in therapy and how therapists are able to integrate these client activities and contributions to advance treatment. Greaves described how clients engage in self-healing, but clearly, more research is needed to advance our understanding of how clients work, practice, and make progress, particularly between sessions. She pointed out how little time clients actually spend with their therapists and how much progress toward healing clients achieve between visits. While there is ongoing research examining client gains during and after therapy (Lambert, 2013), clearly, more work is needed in this area. Specifically, there seem to be opportunities for research grounded on narratological and phenomenological approaches (see Betz & Fassinger, 2012) with an explicit focus on revealing clients' healing processes and activities in treatment. This research could also examine instances when therapy is not successful and how or why client healing was somehow thwarted during and between psychotherapy sessions.

Levitt and her colleagues recognized the need for more qualitative meta-analyses to highlight how clients work and what they experience from their side of psychotherapy. These analyses could provide further insight into the subjective experience of the client—for example, by capturing context-driven experiences that are shaped by content, processes, or interpersonal events and may explain variations in client agency, the process by which clients come to value their own subjective experiences, and how they come to summon their self-healing capacities. Boswell and Scharff recommended the regular use of monitoring practices in treatment. They noted that while the emphasis has been on routine outcome-monitoring feedback systems, there is clearly a need and opportunity for implementing "idiographic" outcome monitoring within sessions, using a collaborative approach that involves the client. Research is needed on how such idiographic assessment can take place and be used in treatment and how and when client participation can be solicited. Collaborative monitoring can gauge the level of progress in the therapy or the need for modifications in intervention, and the authors noted that clients generally welcome participation in progress monitoring because it communicates therapist attentiveness and a commitment to help.

Constantino and colleagues noted the need for client-constructed measures of outcomes and mechanisms instead of therapist- or researcher-constructed ones, which is largely what we have now. By encouraging freely offered perspectives on what clients find helpful and involving clients as coleaders in examining outcomes and mechanisms, we can enhance how we measure process, progress, and outcome. These authors also pointed out that there is an opportunity for involving clients in adapting current researcher- or therapist-derived measures, possibly making them more inclusive of relevant content, more sensitive and accurate, and more consumer oriented. Relatedly, Constantino and his coauthors suggested that researchers use clients' perspectives and feedback to redefine existing therapist constructs in psychotherapy, such as the relationship, satisfaction, adherence, progress, and outcome. These authors also reminded us of the value of using interpersonal process research (IPR; Elliott & Shapiro, 1988). This method would allow researchers to understand better clients' experiences and perspectives during the process of therapy while these experiences are "still fresh" in their minds. IPR could provide us (and clients) with insight into their internal frame of reference while they are still actively engaged in therapy. These authors also referenced Levitt et al. (2016), who recommended including in qualitative research more underrepresented and marginalized populations, with a focus on understanding how the intersection of power, privilege, and the spectrum of difference influences clients' experiences of what works, when, and how. Constantino and his collaborators also suggested the inclusion of diverse and historically oppressed groups in research to advance and address the need for social justice in psychotherapy, as well as to broaden and enrich concepts that are respectful and inclusive of diversity and culture.

Gelso and Kline also suggested that research be conducted taking the client's perspective, including the use of discovery-oriented approaches where clients can share their views and experiences of the relationship in their own words and "where conclusions are drawn inductively based on clients' viewpoints rather than predetermined researcher-framed hypotheses and measures." There is a need for research to examine all three facets of the relationship at the same time, which would tell us (and clients) how these three strands operate and interrelate, as viewed from the lens of the client. With respect to attachment, Mallinckrodt pointed out the need for qualitative research that examines clients' first-person experiences and work in earning their secure attachment to therapists and how these gains in security to the therapist translate into advances in attachment with others. Qualitative research could also explore how clients work through and obtain their growing capacities for intimacy or independence, depending on the severity of deactivation and hyperactivation that clients bring to treatment.

CONCLUSION

The "other side" is a part of the whole in psychotherapy, and to understand therapy holistically, we must understand both sides: the therapist's and the client's. I hope this book has stimulated your thinking about what clients experience and contribute to psychotherapy. While the emphasis has been on clients, they are obviously not operating solo, without us or our help. Therapists bring a great deal of knowledge and training, and clients bring the all-important "local knowledge" to the sessions: their knowledge of themselves, their families, and their personal histories; a wealth of experiences; and skills and capacities that can be harnessed and/or refined to the benefit of the work. While we can speak of clients as self-healing and self-experts—and we do so because clients ultimately know themselves best and decide the extent to which they will change and heal—their work does not occur in a vacuum. Client growth occurs in the context of a warm, supportive, and at times, challenging relationship with their therapist.

Stanley Hunt, one of my practicum supervisors at the University of Maryland, once said, "Jairo, psychotherapy can be a bit of a mean business; we have a hand in setting up the battles, and the client ends up doing all the fighting." The fact that I remember this quote 25 years later shows that it made a good point—and maybe I also remember it because it had a bit of humor to it. Over the years, his comment has stayed with me, and I have come to appreciate it even more; whenever I remember it, it has spurred me to try to do more for my clients. We do have a hand in setting up the client in a battle— for example, by encouraging them to examine existing conflicts, take on persistent negative thoughts, change deeply ingrained templates that guide their reactions and behaviors, and take on the challenge of change and personal growth. This book has reaffirmed that the battle has to be agreed to by the client, who has a significant say in every facet of therapy, and while the client has to do much of the work in therapy (i.e., the workout as alluded to in the analogy to the physical gym), the more established literature on therapists' work shows that our help makes a difference in helping the client win the battle and that we do so by bringing our better selves to the sessions, including our knowledge, skills, energy, and commitment.

REFERENCES

Betz, N. E., & Fassinger, R. E. (2012). Methodologies in counseling psychology. In E. M. Altmaier & J. C. Hansen, *The Oxford handbook of counseling psychology* (pp. 237–269). Oxford University Press. https://doi.org/10.1093/oxfordhb/9780195342314.001.0001

Egan, G. (2010). *The skilled helper: A problem management and opportunity development approach to helping* (9th ed.). Brooks/Cole Cengage Learning.

Elliott, R., & Shapiro, D. A. (1988). Brief Structured Recall: A more efficient method for studying significant therapy events. *The British Journal of Medical Psychology, 61*(2), 141–153. https://doi.org/10.1111/j.2044-8341.1988.tb02773.x

Lambert, M. J. (2013). The efficacy and effectiveness of psychotherapy. In M. J. Lambert (Ed.), *Bergin and Garfield's handbook of psychotherapy and behavior change* (6th ed., pp. 169–218). Wiley.

Levitt, H. M., Pomerville, A., & Surace, F. I. (2016). A qualitative meta-analysis examining clients' experiences of psychotherapy: A new agenda. *Psychological Bulletin, 142*(8), 801–830. https://doi.org/10.1037/bul0000057

Prochaska, J. O., Norcross, J. C., & DiClemente, C. C. (1995). *Changing for good.* HarperCollins.

Wampold, B. E., & Imel, Z. E. (2015). *The great psychotherapy debate: The evidence for what makes psychotherapy work* (2nd ed.). Routledge. https://doi.org/10.4324/9780203582015

INDEX

ABOUT THE EDITOR

Jairo N. Fuertes, PhD, ABPP, LMHC, is a professor of psychology in the Gordon F. Derner School of Psychology at Adelphi University and a clinical assistant professor of medicine in the Donald and Barbara Zucker School of Medicine at Hofstra/Northwell. He is senior associate editor of *Behavioral Medicine* and served on editorial boards for other top-tier journals, including *Psychotherapy* and *Psychotherapy Research*. Dr. Fuertes is a fellow of the American Psychological Association (APA; Divisions 12 [Society of Clinical Psychology] and 29 [Psychotherapy]) and has served as chair of the Education and Training Committee and as diversity domain representative in APA's Division 29. He is a licensed psychologist and mental health counselor in New York State and is board certified in both clinical and counseling psychology by the American Board of Professional Psychology. For over 20 years, he has been a staff psychologist and clinical supervisor at the Counseling Center at Baruch College, The City University of New York, and he maintains a bilingual private practice in Garden City, New York.

Dr. Fuertes is an immigrant from Colombia, South America. He arrived in the United States at the age of 10 and graduated from the public school system in Montgomery County, Maryland. He is also a "Triple Terp," having obtained his bachelor's, master's, and doctoral degrees from the University of Maryland at College Park. He is a professional percussionist and has recorded several albums over his musical career. He lives with his wife, Hnin, and their two daughters in Garden City.